Christina Polvak 2005

A Wind in Africa

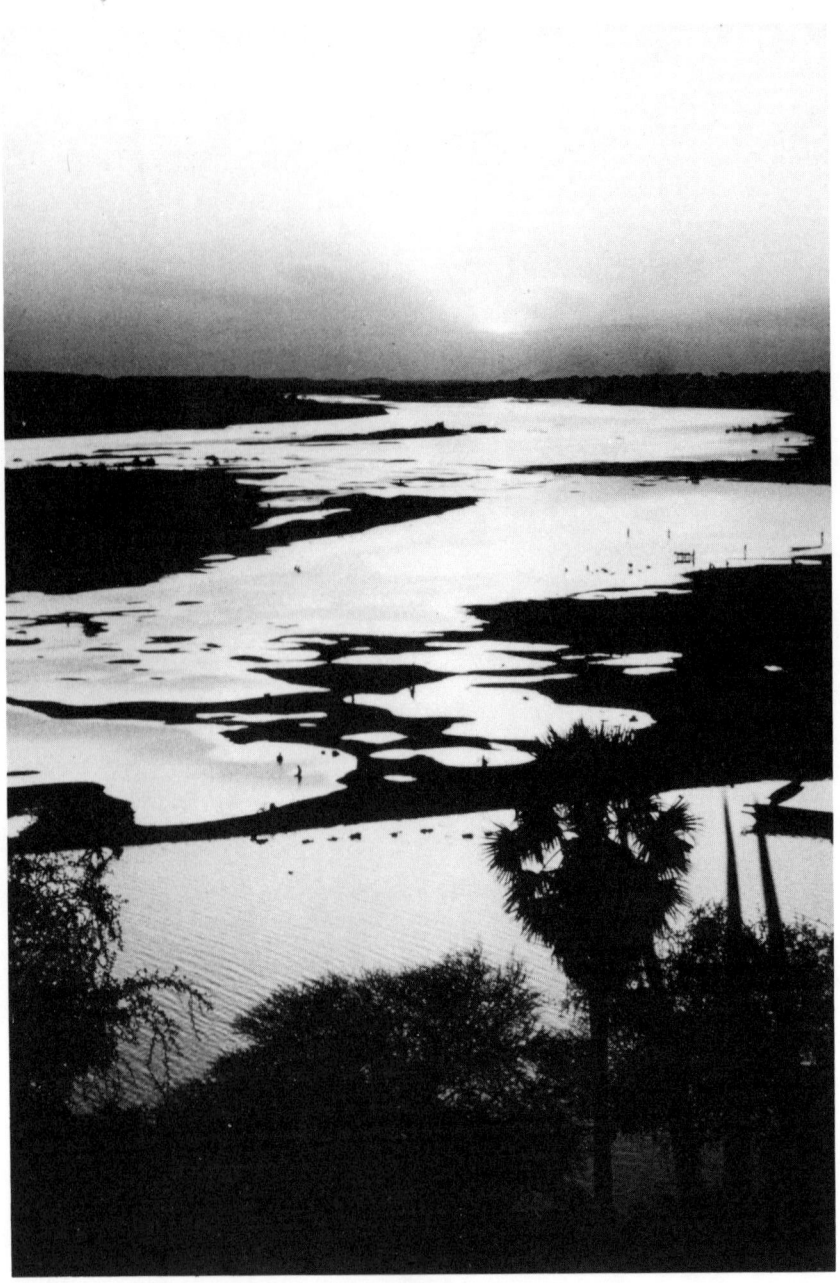
Sundown over the Niger River.

A WIND IN AFRICA
A Story Of Modern Medicine in Mali

by

PASCAL JAMES IMPERATO, B.S., M.D., M.P.H. & T.M.

With Photographs By The Author

First Deputy Health Commissioner, City of New York, Department of Health; Assistant Clinical Professor, Departments of Medicine and Public Health, Cornell University Medical College; Assistant Attending Physician, The New York Hospital; Lecturer, Department of Community Medicine, Mount Sinai School of Medicine, City University of New York; Consultant, United States Agency For International Development, Department of State; Diplomate of The American Board of Preventive Medicine; Fellow of The American College of Physicians; Fellow of The Explorers Club of New York.

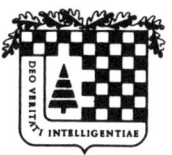

WARREN H. GREEN, INC.
St. Louis, Missouri, U.S.A.

Published by

WARREN H. GREEN, INC.
10 South Brentwood Boulevard
Saint Louis, Missouri, U.S.A.

All rights reserved

© 1975 by WARREN H. GREEN, INC.
Library of Congress Catalog Card Number 73-24001
ISBN No. 087527-139-1

Printed in the United States of America

DEDICATION

This book is dedicated
with great affection to

ED and LEE CLARK

Who have given so much
of themselves to the
peoples of Africa

MEMORIES OF THE ENDEMIC DISEASE SERVICE

My very dear friend,
Your letter permitted me,
In my solitude,
Contrary to my habit,
To experience a pleasure
Always good to seize.

Also for your missive,
My tired pen,
Replies to you by these verses,
From the small universe
Where now I am.

I would like that this might prove,
That my heart is always,
As on all beautiful days,
On African soil.

It is not by stale excuses,
That my regrets are expressed,
Of the time where our legs,
Carried us through the bush,
To put us on the trail
Of the poor sleeping sickness victims,
That I say incredible,
If one might still be alive.

Though satisfied,
My soul has some good fortune,
Like the harvester,
Who because of his courage,
Has saved from the storm,
The good grain just ripe,
Of which all have need.

From the depths of my retirement,
Yes certainly I miss,
My African friends,
Even the most difficult,
Tell them that in the Endemic Disease Service,
Our souls are united,
By a glorious past,
And that it is out of place,
Not to wish to believe it.

And from the banks of the Loire,
I give you my wishes,
My most affectionate wishes,
And also to the family,
So brave and noble,
Of the world of the Endemic Disease Service.

Jean Lastouillas

MEMOIRES DES GRANDES ENDEMIES

Mon bien très cher ami,
Ta lettre m'a permis,
Dans notre solitude,
Contre mon habitude,
D'éprouver un plaisir
Toujours bon à saisir.

Aussi pour ta missive,
Ma plume un peu poussive,
Te répond par ces vers,
Du petit univers
Où maintenant me trouve.

Je voudrais que ça prouve,
Que mon coeur est toujours,
Tout comme aux plus beaux jours,
Sur la terre Africaine.

Ce n'est pas par rangaine
Qu'exprimant mes regrets,
Du temps où nos jarrets,
Nous portaient dans la brousse,
Pour marcher sur la trousse
Des pauvres sommeilleux,
Que je dis fabuleux,,
Qu'on soit encore en vie.

Cependant assouvie,
Mon âme a du bonheur,
Comme le moissonneur,
Qui grâce à son courage,
A sauve de l'orage,
Le bon grain mûr à point,
Dont tous avons besoin.

Du fond de ma retraite,
Oui bien sûr je regrette,
Les amis Africains,
Même les plus taquins,
Dis leur qu'aux Endemies,
Nos âmes sont unies,
Par un glorieux passé,
Et qu'il est déplacé,
De pas vouloir le croire.

Et des bords de la Loire,
Je t'adresse mes voeux
Les plus affectueux,
Ainsi qu'à la famille,
Si brave et si gentille,
Du monde trypano.

Tours, France

Jean Lastouillas

BY PASCAL JAMES IMPERATO

A Wind in Africa
(1975)

The Treatment and Control of Infectious Diseases in Man
(1974)

The Cultural Heritage of Africa
(1974)

Last Adventure (editor)
(1966)

Doctor in the Land of the Lion
(1964)

Foreword

The adventure that unfolds in these pages is not only complex and exciting, but it is also highly significant. To my mind at least it is an ideal example, as heartwarming as it is splendid, of what the American posture abroad can be and should be. Calling upon our better qualities, it was not only carried through to success, but achieved that success with a becoming modesty — a virtue too rarely present these days in the ventures of great nations. Here the humanitarian motive was uppermost.

The purpose of the medical mission to Mali was, one, to vaccinate the entire population — 4,500,000 men, women, and children — against smallpox and yellow fever and to vaccinate all children six months to six years old against measles; and, two, to deliver mobile health services, again, to the entire population. A sizable order in any circumstances, but here success depended upon the solution of problems — diplomatic, social, technical, practical — of sufficient intricacy to challenge the Paul Bunyan spirit in anyone — the sort of challenge, in other words, to which the American traditionally responds, and in this instance, at any rate, certainly did.

There was, first of all, the country itself, very newly carved out of old French West Africa, stretching from Sahara sands in the north to the Niger River and the forests of the coast in the south — a confederation of 42 districts or *cercles* loosely tied together by a tired bureaucracy established by the French. The official language was — and still is — French. And in other cultural ways the French influence was still strong, though by the early sixties the Red Chinese presence was proving magnetic.

Climate and terrain offered their own challenges — the climate hot and dry or hot and humid, really comfortable to denizens of the temperate zones only during the cool season, December, say, to March. As to the terrain, it was desert and mountain, grassland and swamp, and especially river. Indeed, such a factor is the Niger River in the ecology of the country that it can be truly said that the vast area affected by it has two terrains, shifting seasonally with the rise and fall of the waters.

The diversity of the land is matched easily by the diversity of the people. Christians, Mohammedans, deists, fetishists as to religion, they own a variety of social organizations — often family- or tribe-oriented that run the gamut from Stone Age to the pre-Industrial Revolution agrarian mode. Venturing into some villages, jet gun in hand, was not unlike Margaret Mead's uneasy sojourn with the Mundugumor of New Guinea in the early Thirties. Yet the villages were *there,* posing cultural problems, yes, but at least physically stable. The large numbers of nomads were something else, for these trekking herders of sheep and cattle must be caught up with, evangelized, and immunized, all on the wing, so to speak.

And to these factors must be added, finally, that at the outset the bureaucracy, quite aside from its affliction by advanced arteriosclerosis, was indifferent to the mission when not downright hostile; and that all technicians, medical or mechanical, had to be recruited within the country and trained from the ground up. There were 268 health workers among them, including vaccinators, medical auxiliaries, and nurses, and some eighteen drivers and mechanics. All of their equipment, of course, had to be supplied by the United States.

For all of this, the mission was indeed an outstanding success. In the course of five years, the Smallpox Eradication-Measles Control program tallied up 4,262,000 smallpox and 1,080,000 measles vaccinations, administered in over 8,000 villages and nomad camps. In addition, mobile health services of both a curative and a preventive nature were brought to 3,000,000 people, who were treated for a variety of diseases. As adjuncts to these major enterprises, immunization campaigns were mounted against cerebrospinal meningitis in 1968; against an epidemic of yellow fever in 1969; and against cholera in 1970 and 1971, when a million vaccinations against this last disease were administered.

The total cost of this comprehensive program to the American taxpayer was a mere one and a half million dollars — including the cost of vaccines, 24 trucks, automatic jet injector equipment (65 jet guns), camping equipment, and medical supplies. Oh that we might always achieve abroad so much for so little! For the dividends were indeed great. Not only were there rewards in the contribution made to the health of the world, but there were political benefits as well. As a corollary to the main humanitarian objective, there was also a victory in the battle of East and West. Red Chinese influence in Mali was considerably less by the conclusion of the program.

With one exception, these objectives were achieved within budget. The exception was *time,* and the young doctor in charge of the mission saw his original tour extended — others, with some justification, might call it "his sentence" — some two to three years. This he accepted cheerfully; and I must make some point of it. For though this is the young doctor's, Dr. Pat Imperato's, book and, therefore, essentially an autobiographical narrative, the personal pronoun *I* is rarely encountered.

I know of few such narratives in which self so seldom intrudes. The unwary might easily think that the events recorded here happened of themselves, without human direction or motivation.

Yet in so many ways the man *was* the mission; and in choosing Dr. Imperato for it the United States Public Health Service was superbly perspicacious. To be sure, he was highly qualified in tropical medicine; to be sure, he was fluent in French. He had experience of Africa, moreover, albeit East Africa, specifically Tanzania and Kenya, and a sympathy for it. And, having this experience, he volunteered for what was certain to be an arduous experience. All these attributes counted heavily, of course; yet there was in Pat Imperato one transcendent quality without which his other qualifications might have proved meaningless, at the same time that it is one that is easily overlooked, and this is his involvement in mankind. Gently and unostentatiously, Pat Imperato is dedicated to humanity and its welfare. He believes literally in the dignity of man and in his essential worth. He is, therefore, patient, he is tolerant, he respects the other man's point of view, he is kind, and he is forbearing — all buttressed by a quiet strength and resolve. Within these pages, though he will never point them out, you will find occasion after occasion where this dedication was paramount.

For his work in Mali, Dr. Imperato was awarded the Meritorious Honor Award and Medal of the United States Agency for International Development in 1970 and the Meritorious Honor Award and Medal of the United States Department of State in 1971.

Well earned, these awards. If anywhere in the world traces of what was once aptly called the Ugly American are still to be found — and pray God that they are not — not a vestige of him was to be seen in our medical experience in Mali, 1966-71.

JOHN C. WILLEY

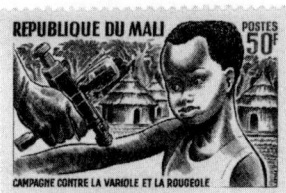

Commemorative stamp from Mali concerning the vaccination campaign.

Preface and Acknowledgements

This book is about Mali as it seemed to me when I was there. It was compiled in a gradual manner over a period of seven years from my memory of experiences and from the daily diary which I kept for the six years, from 1966 until the end of 1971. This final form of the book was written in 1972 and 1973.

I arrived in Mali in December, 1966 and lived and worked there in a continuous fashion until November, 1971. As this is written in 1973, I have returned to Mali for two months in order to continue my medical and anthropological research projects. My stay in Mali was by no means insular since my responsibilities required my traveling to and working in other African countries from time to time, including Senegal, Gambia, Mauritania, Guinea, Sierra Leone, Liberia, Ivory Coast, Upper Volta, Ghana, Togo, Dahomey, Niger and Nigeria. This broadened my African experience considerably and provided me with a basis for viewing Mali with greater insight. During the years I was in Mali, the country underwent a drastic change in its political philosophy which affected the quality of life of its people. As a result of the military coup d'etat of 1968, Mali abandoned its strong Marxist orientation and adopted a more moderate form of socialism. How drastic this change has been is exemplified by the incredulity with which most recently arrived foreigners listen to descriptions of what life was like before. The pre-1968 political life of independent Mali has now become historical and I have made special efforts to describe both accurately and objectively what it was like in the country for both Malians and foreigners at that time.

Although I was sent to Mali to direct a smallpox eradication and measles control program for the United States Agency for International Development, I ultimately became responsible for directing a mobile health program which delivered a variety of diagnostic, curative and preventive medical services to the entire population of Mali, including immunizations against smallpox, measles, yellow fever, cholera and meningitis. This smallpox eradication and measles control program was not unique to Mali, but was funded by the U.S. government for twenty countries in West and Central Africa. The regional nature of the program and the presence in other countries of my colleagues from the Center for Disease Control of the United States Public Health Service brought me into close contact with the health problems of the entire area.

In Mali, the program's activities were carried out by mobile teams of infirmiers and vaccinators working in a carefully structured organization which eventually reached most of the country's population. All of our activities were organized within the framework of Mali's national mobile medical service, the Service des Grandes Endemies. The professional cadre of this service was composed primarily of experienced infirmiers who over the years had visited virtually every village in the country. When all of the infirmiers of the Service des Grandes Endemies were gathered beneath one roof, there was hardly a village in Mali which one could mention which was not familiar to someone present. My working closely with this group of Malians, who themselves had a profound knowledge of their own country and its peoples, greatly enlarged the richness of my own experience. My acceptance in villages and nomad camps was not only enhanced by my service-rendering role as a physician, but also because of my association with infirmiers who were known and respected. This combined with the nature of my work gave me access to parts of the country little known to foreigners. I worked in each of the country's forty-two cercles and two hundred and twenty-eight arrondissements and traveled by truck, plane, canoe, boat, on horses, camels, donkeys and on foot. It is difficult to estimate the total distance I covered in Mali, except by truck which totaled about 150,000 miles. The consequences on my health of this extensive and difficult travel were considerable because of the harsh climate and difficult terrain. I was medically evacuated from Mali three times during the five years, twice to the U.S. Air Force Hospital at Wiesbaden in Germany and once to New York, but fortunately I was able to return each time and resume my work.

It would be difficult to condense the many and unique experiences I had in Mali into a book of this size and consequently I have limited myself to the important high points. In this regard I owe a great debt of gratitude to Mr. John C. Willey, a loyal friend, who over the years this book was being prepared advised me on its preparation, corrected many drafts and guided me through the preparation of the final form.

I am very thankful to him not only for his wholehearted support and help in the writing of this book, but also for the encouragement, support, understanding and friendship which he and his late wife, Fern, gave me during the years I was in Africa.

The successful accomplishment of my mission was due in large measure to the support of many people to whom I wish to express my thanks. I would like to thank my colleagues at the Center for Disease Control for all their help, especially Mr. Donald Eddins, Mr. William Desprez, Dr. William Foege, Mr. Billy Griggs. Dr. D. A. Henderson, Dr. Ralph Henderson, Mr. James Hicks, Dr. George I. Lythcott and Dr. J. Donald Millar. Dr. Henry Gelfand was an inestimable source of help and gave generously of his advice. He was a patient house guest who tolerated Bamako's sudden cessations of electrical power and water supply with great equanimity. He even managed to look pleasant when eating stale bread for breakfast during one of Bamako's flour shortages. I am grateful to the members of the staff of the Smallpox Eradication Program of the Center for Disease Control for all their help, especially Miss Jane Cooley, Mrs. Evelyn Harrison, Mrs. Fay Hendricks, Mrs. Mary Ann Lyle and Mrs. Shirley Kaufman.

I want to thank Bob and Mona Helmholz for their help and gracious hospitality during my many visits to Senegal and Tony and Elaine Masso for their warm hospitality to me in Niger. Dr. and Mrs. Thomas Drake and Mr. and Mrs. Edward Musante helped me during my visits to Senegal and Mauritania and Dr. and Mrs. Donald Moore assisted me on my early visits to Niger. I am much indebted to Mr. and Mrs. Nathaniel Rothstein for their warm friendship and always open home in Lagos, to Dr. Margaret Grigsby for her help in Ibadan and to Dr. and Mrs. Hans Mayer for their hospitality and help in Liberia and the Ivory Coast. Mr. Jean Roy was a gracious host to me in Dahomey and Mr. and Mrs. Thomas Leonard were of great help to me in Upper Volta. I would like to thank Mr. and Mrs. Dennis Olsen for their hospitality to me in Monrovia.

I want to express my special gratitude to Dr. Benitieni Fofana, Minister of Public Health and Social Affairs of Mali for his wholehearted support, interest and friendship. I am thankful to Dr. Daouda Keita, Director General of Public Health and to Dr. Ousmane Sow, Director of the Division of Socio-Preventive Medicine for their close collaboration. Dr. Paul Jean-Joseph, Director of the Protection Maternal et Infantil worked together with us in planning, organizing and implementing the measles control program in Bamako and the rural areas of Mali and for his dedicated efforts I am most grateful. The late Dr. Somine Dolo, Minister of Public Health and Social Affairs, gave me his full support at the inception of the program. I want to thank Dr. Garba Keita, Dr. Sidi Boucanem, Mons. Ingre Dolo and Messrs. Damas, Sylla, Tounkara, Doucoure and Diallo of the Ministry of Public Health and Social Affairs for all their help. To Mons. Lamine Sidibe of the Section Statistique of the health ministry I owe a debt of gratitude for compiling the program's statistical data. The advice and assistance of Dr. Jean J. Leveuf, technical advisor to the health ministry, were of great help to me in program planning. I am grateful to the late Dr. Jiri Nedvideck of the World Health Organization for the benefit of his experiences in smallpox eradication in Mali and for his insights. He was a pleasant traveling companion and enlivened many of my early bush trips in Mali with his conversation and observations. His premature death was a great loss to all of us who knew him.

I would like to acknowledge the help of the following persons in conducting immunization programs in Bamako: Dr. Seydou Diakite, Director of School Health, Dr. Malet Keita and Dr. Yalla Sidibe, former Directors of the Service d'Hygiene, Mons. Yacouba Rouamba, Director of the Division of Health Education, the late Dr. Arouna Toure, medecin chief of the cercle of Bamako, Dr. Diop and Dr. Amidou Ba, former Regional Directors of Public Health of Bamako and Dr. Suleyman Sow, former chief medical officer of the Malian army. I would like to thank the central office staff of the Division of Socio-Preventive Medicine for their help in planning and executing all of the mobile health campaigns. I want to especially thank Mons. Sira Bamba Cissoko, Mons. Kola and Mons. Asymou Toure for their help.

To Mons. Jean Paul Lastouillas a special debt of gratitude is owed for his cooperation and help over the years in virtually every aspect of the program. I want to express my thanks to both him and his wife for their warm friendship and understanding.

The staff of the Service d'Hygiene in Bamako assisted us in all of our campaigns and I am grateful to them for their help. Mons. Ibrahim Diallo, Assistant Director of the Service d'Hygiene and his gracious wife gave fully of their support and understanding and I am thankful to them. Their four children found a second home in our offices at the Service d'Hygiene and eased the gravity of many a crisis with their laughter and search for candy in the desk drawers. The infirmiers and medical assistants of the Bamako sector of the Service des Grandes Endemies made a significant contribution to the program's success. I want to especially thank Dr. Baba Oumar Toure, Mons. Mamadou Goundiam and Mons. Mety Keita.

Mons. Dramane Samake, Mons. Poundiougou Pangalet, Mons. Seydou Dembele and Mons. Teninkou Togola supervised many of the teams in the field and I wish to acknowledge their fine contribution to our success. Mons Djigui Diakite was an able vaccinator and excellent interpreter who traveled with me over much of central Mali and greatly assisted me not only in directing the medical programs, but also in conducting my medical and anthropological studies. Mons. Modibo N'Faly Keita came to us as a driver and over the years was transformed into an excellent mechanic, interpreter and medical assistant. He drove me over much of Mali in a Dodge truck from Kayes to Gao without a serious mishap. I also want to thank Messrs, Kassim Sangare and Djadouga Fane who drove me over some of the most difficult terrain in Mali.

To all of the regional governors, cercle commandants and arrondissement chiefs, I owe a vote of thanks for their cooperation. I am especially thankful to all of the medecin chefs of Mali's forty-two cercles and to the medecin chefs of the eleven sectors of the Grandes Endemies service who actively participated over the years in the program. I want to thank the regional directors of public health, Dr. Mohamed Soumare (Kayes), Dr. Kante (Segou), Dr. Marcel Gabriel (Sikasso), Dr. Seydou Diallo (Mopti), Dr. Malhamane Diarra (Gao) and Dr. Nianankoro Fomba (Gao). I am particularly grateful to Dr. Mohamed Soumare and his wife for their kindnesses to me and to Dr. Malhamane Diarra and his wife who extended the hospitality of their home to me on many occasions.

Special thanks go to the following medecin chefs and infirmiers for their invaluable help: Dr. Bakary Coulibaly (Nioro), Mons. Bekaye Samake (Yelimane), Mons. Bamba Cissoko (Kenieba), Dr. Djigui Diabite (Kita), Mons. Cheickna Maiga (Bafoulabe), Dr. Kilisi (Dioila), Dr. Briere de l'Isle (Koutiala), Mons. Brehima Dategue Kone (Yorosso), Mons. Amadou Karambe (Yorosso), Mons. Bakary Kante (Koutiala), Mons. Badara Aliou Sako (Koutiala), Mons. Tiecoura Konate (Yorosso), Mons. Amboubou Poundiougou (Koutiala), Dr. Ousmane Sow (Segou), Dr. Safoune (Macina and San), Dr. Thiero (Segou), Dr. Dibo (San) and Dr. Lamine Keita (Timbuctoo). Mons. Jean Pierre Ouedraogo, head of the Grandes Endemies station in San assisted us in investigating smallpox epidemics in the arrondissements of Baramandougou, Koula and Kimparana and in conducting the vaccination campaigns in the cercles of San and Tominian. I thank Noumon Sissoko, Mentaga Diabate and Dramane Niambele, infirmiers of the Grandes Endemies, San, for their help.

For the success achieved in the Dogon country, in the cercles of Bandiagara, Koro, Bankass and Douentza, I wish to express my gratitude to Mons. Mabo Kassambara, medecin chef of Secteur Numero Neuf of the Grandes Endemies. Mabo gave his work an extraordinary dedication and our program his full support. He was a gracious host and a pleasant traveling companion whether bouncing in the trucks along the rough tracks or climbing up the cliffs. I am indebted to the infirmiers of the Grandes Endemies in Bandiagara, to Mons. Koniba Bamba, Mons. Soliman Angaiba, Mons. Domo Ouloguem, Mons. Zakari Dolo, Mons. Binem Dolo and Mons. Sene Tabile for their fine work among the Dogon and Peul of the Bandiagara Cliffs. A special word of thanks is due Mons. Ogobara Dolo of Sanga for his help in planning the campaign on that area of the cliff. I am grateful to the medical assistants in Koro and Bankass who assisted me in conducting smallpox epidemic investigations in extremely difficult terrain.

The long and difficult campaign in the inland delta of the Niger was an extraordinary success due to the efforts of many people. To all those who worked in this campaign I extend my sincerest thanks. I would like to thank Dr. Guide, medecin chef of Mopti, Mons. Domo Telli, head of the Grandes Endemies, Mopti, Mons. Mamadou Sangare, infirmier of the Grandes Endemies who accompanied me on several trips into the inland delta. The assistance of Mons. Belco Tambaoura of the Assistance Medicale, Mopti was greatly appreciated. Mons. Mama Tangara of the Service des Eaux et Forets and Mons. Djenepo, President of the Mopti Fishing Cooperative gave us their invaluable help in organizing the immunization campaign for the Bozo fishermen on the Niger between Diafarabe and Lake Debo. For their putting their canoes and boats with outboard motors at our disposition, I am extremely grateful. Thanks go to the interpreters and assistants who accompanied me through the inland delta. I am particularly thankful to Mons. Khalil Dicko of the Grandes Endemies, Kona, who accompanied me on many occasions to the eastern shores of Lake Debo and to Gagni Diallo who assisted me in Dialloube, Fatoma and Korientze. Through them filtered most of my medical and anthropological studies on the Peul. I thank Nouhou Diallo who guided me through the flood plains of the arrondissements of Youvarou, Guidio-Sare, Sarafere and N'Gouma and I am very grateful to the unknown and remarkable woman guide who took me safely over the flood plains from Bambara-Maounde on Lake Do to Korientze. Mons. Moussa Maiga was a helpful guide in the cercles of Ansongo, Bourem and Gourma-Rharous and Abdoudramane Maiga assisted me in Douentza.

The Rev. and Mrs. Francis McKinney of the Protestant Mission, Sanga, and Rev. and Mrs. John McKinney were extremely helpful to me in the Dogon country, especially when I was ill. I am grateful to them for all of their help. In Sikasso, Rev. and Mrs. Earl Gripp always opened their doors to my staff and I at their mission station at Tyefala. I am thankful to them and to Miss Carol Proebe, R.N. of Tyefala. In Bamako, Rev. and Mrs. Edward Tschetter of the Protestant Mission extended their help and warm hospitality for which I am very grateful. Rev. and Mrs. Frank Marshall were always helpful on my visits to Timbuctoo. Père Huet of the Catholic Mission, Kimparana, was of help in investigating epidemics of smallpox in the Miniankala. Père Marcoux assisted me in controlling measles epidemics in Faladie and Père Spahn acted as a helpful guide for the program when the teams crossed the desert from Hombori to Gao. I want to especially thank Père Franz Van der Weijst of the Bougouni Catholic Mission for his many years of warm friendship and support.

Gratitude goes to my household staff for having made my home in Bamako pleasant. The loyalty, courtesy and generosity of Ahmadou Sanogo, my house servant and his family cannot be measured. To him and his wife Amineta and their family in Boussin, Segou, I express my sincerest thanks. I want to thank Mons. Brahima Mallet and Mons. Camara for their dedicated service.

I am extremely grateful to Mr. Jay Friedman and Mr. Mark D. LaPointe for their invaluable contribution to the success of the program. As the program's operations officers, they performed many functions ranging from the investigation of epidemics of measles, smallpox, yellow fever and meningitis to managing all of the equipment and supplies which came by sea and air from the U.S.A. I want to particularly thank Jay for his important contribution to the campaign in the inland delta of the Niger and Mark for having administered the campaigns in Kayes and Sikasso. Diane LaPointe was a gracious hostess and warm friend whose understanding was valued and appreciated.

The help and cooperation of the personnel of the United States Embassy in Bamako were invaluable and I want to thank all of the fine people who served at the post between 1966 and 1973. My special thanks go to Ambassador and Mrs. C. Robert Moore for all their efforts on our behalf at the beginning of the program and for their advice, interest and encouragement. The support of Ambassador and Mrs. Robert O. Blake during the phasing out of the program was sincerely appreciated as was Ambassador Blake's dynamic interest in Mali's health problems.

To Ambassador and Mrs. G. Edward Clark, I am deeply grateful for their wholehearted support, constant encouragement and sincere concern for the health and well being of the people of Mali. Their sincere friendship is greatly cherished.

The deputy chiefs of mission and their wives and families assisted us in many ways. Mr. and Mrs. Oliver Crosby were of great help to us at the beginning of the program. Mr. and Mrs. Joseph Christiano took a keen interest in all of the program's activities and gave us their sincere support. Mr. and Mrs. Jay Katzen were extremely helpful to us during their stay in Mali and extended many kindnesses to me. I am grateful to Jay for the invaluable assistance he gave me in arranging my 1973 trip, and to him and his wife for extending the warmth of their home to me.

I sincerely appreciate the help given to us by the embassy administrative officers, Messrs. Bryant Collins, Thomas Baron, Philip King, Michael Curtis, Gerald Keathley and Douglas Stevens. Thanks are also given to the following embassy officers: Messrs. Robert Brown, Benjamin Hardy, Andre LoGallo, John Zerolis, John Yates, James Smith and Pat Patty.

Bob Baker of USIS gave his dedicated services to the program in so many ways. To Patty Baker, I am especially thankful for putting my home in Bamako in order and for insuring my state of good nutrition. When Bob and Patty left Bamako it was with much emotion, taking with them special memories of their stay in Mali.

Mr. Harold Engel, Public Affairs Officer, gave the program considerable assistance and arranged for the production of the program film, *The Fight Against Endemic Disease In Mali*. His wife, Louise, provided us with secretarial assistance. His successor, Lewis Pate, was due to arrive in Bamako the day of the coup d'etat and as a result spent a week in Abidjan when the plane was forced to overfly Bamako. Lew and his wife Sonja became my close friends in Bamako and I am indebted to them for many kindnesses. I want to thank Lew's successor, John Garner and his wife, Georgette, for their kindnesses to me and Frank Strovas, Lewis Luchs and Roger Russell of USIS.

During the early years of the program, we were given much help by the staff of the USAID mission to Mali and I want to particularly thank Mr. Peter Daniells, Mr. Stanley Clark, and Mr. Rudolph Ellert-Beck. Rudy Ellert-Beck facilitated the beginning of the program through his direct assistance to us and by giving us the benefit of his experience with the previous Malian measles vaccination program.

My very special thanks go to Miss Maxine Bradrick, R.N., who, as the U.S. Embassy nurse in Bamako from 1967 to 1975, took good care of the doctor when he was ill. Maxine helped us in so many ways that it is difficult to enumerate them, but I want to particularly thank her for her many kindnesses to my Malian staff and for her help in the immunization programs in Bamako and Timbuctoo. Maxine became an institution in Bamako because of her dedicated service to both Americans and Malians alike.

Mrs. Sadie Rogers, R.N. and Mrs. Susan Forrester, R.N. helped us in many ways and I thank them. To Miss Joyce Murray I owe a debt of gratitude for her help with the office work and with the management of many of the program's activities. Madame Assa Keita Traore was our secretary for three years and I want to thank her for her fine work. Mons. Louis Derebergue assisted us in many ways with travel arrangements and other administrative matters. Madame Parthenay and the late Madame Bujard translated many of my scientific papers and program documents into French and assisted us with much of the office work. I wish to thank all of the Malians in the U.S. Embassy in Bamako, especially Mons. Berthe, Messrs. Sadio Cissoko, Malik, Dau, David, Ly, Christian, George, Sako, Tidjani, Madame Hacko, and Madame Coulibaly for all of their help.

I want to thank my family for their wholehearted support and encouragement over the years. My late mother, Madalynne M. Imperato, and my late uncle, Dr. P. J. Imperato, gave me their complete understanding and were a constant source of encouragement and inspiration. I am grateful for the warm encouragement given me by Mrs. Marion Baxter and Dr. C. William Lacaillade.

My sincere thanks go to all of those Malians in hundreds of villages and nomad camps from Kayes to Kidal, men, women and children, farmers, fishermen, herdsmen, traders and civil servants who opened their homes to me and allowed me to enter their lives.

Special thanks are extended to Mrs. Lylian M. Imperato and Mrs. Sally Koch for their help in preparing the manuscript.

PASCAL JAMES IMPERATO

"Ko domba be ko dombali hakili wa."
—*Bambara Proverb*

Contents

	Foreword	ix
	Preface and Acknowledgements	xiii
I.	The Village on the Dune	1
II.	Looking Up the Facts	14
III.	The Crocodile City	31
IV.	Hard Times	53
V.	A Miracle Is Born	73
VI.	On the Trail of the Nomads	86
VII.	The Thoughts of Mao	113
VIII.	A Beginning	138
IX.	The Festival of Return	161
X.	The Wind Illness	170
XI.	Land of the Cliff Dwellers	183
XII.	The Venice of Mali	204
XIII.	Illness	217
XIV.	A Life at Home	226
XV.	The Song of the Minstrel	244
XVI.	A Sorcerer's Revenge	257
XVII.	The White Goddess	265
XVIII.	A Difficult Vaccination Campaign	275
XIX.	Cholera	295
XX.	Timbuctoo	306
XXI.	Into the Niger Bend	323
XXII.	Farewell	341
	Bibliography on Mali by the Author	354
	Index	357

A Wind in Africa

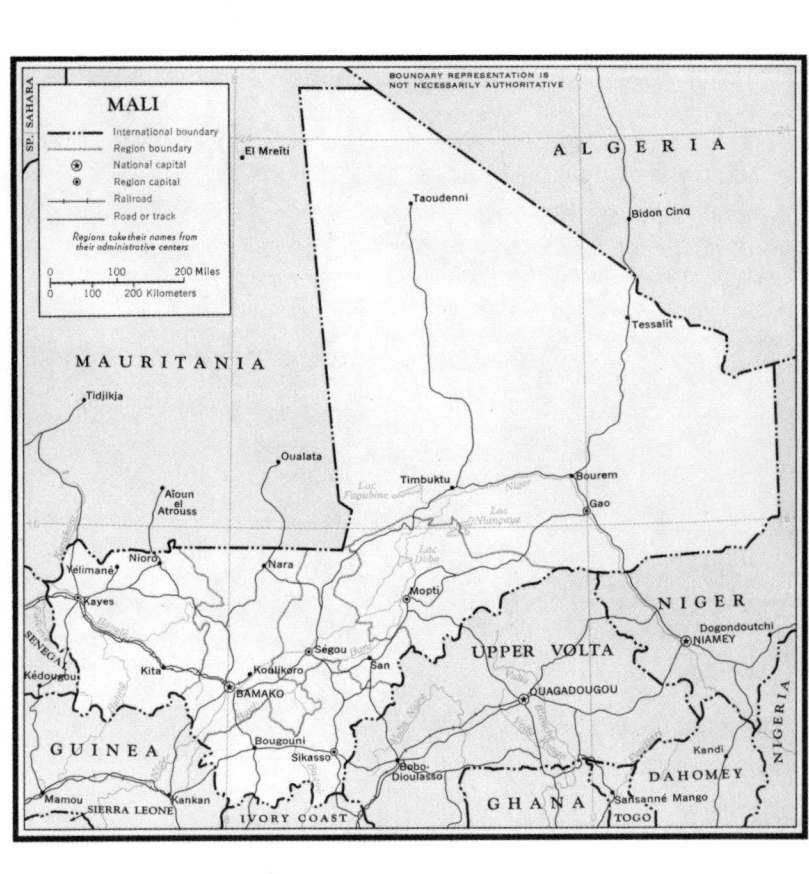

Chapter I
The Village on the Dune

In 1967, a serious epidemic of smallpox broke out in the far eastern part of Mali. It appeared on the sand dunes where the Niger hurries its usual slow pace before tumbling over the narrow cataracts at Labezanga. The river here flows southeasterly out of Mali into the Niger Republic. It is a world of silence and stillness where not even the river makes any noise as it cuts its way through soft sand dunes and disappears into a midday horizon of quivering heat waves and dancing mirages. The Sahara is next door; harsh, patient and unfeeling. When you look at it you see a frightening lonliness. But there is also a whisper in the air, daring you to a challenge, tempting you to come and discover its secrets for yourself. And it is this which pulls you into the heart of the desert.

The Tuareg nomads who took up the challenge are still there and have made the Sahara their home. The less daring Songhoi people stayed next to the river and built their villages on islands which gave them the security and stability they desired. These villages were impregnable fortresses with the Niger surrounding them like some great moat.

Whenever the Tuareg bands descended out of the desert the Songhoi retreated to their islands from where they watched the river defeat their enemies and their hoards of camels. This way of life changed when the French arrived at the turn of the century and imposed colonial law and order over the middle Niger. Since those days, the Songhoi have moved out of their island villages and spilled out over the green banks on either side of the river. They have never wanted anything of the Tuaregs' impractical spirit of adventure and unreflecting boldness and so even today the Sahara is not their home. Although they are now subsistence farmers and fishermen, their great empire once stretched up the river for a thousand miles. But the days of empire are gone, replaced by a world of grass beehive shaped huts, cow dung fires, a subsistence way of life and Islam.

The country doesn't improve as you go south until you get well beyond Niamey, the capital of the Niger Republic. The river never tires of its barren world of sand, gravel and thorn trees. It resumes its slow pace, a flow which is almost imperceptible and if you are on it you have the uneasy feeling of being cut off from everything present. Only your own past is with you, flashing by in your mind like a disorganized dream. There are no ruins nor relics to be seen, no traces of man's previous existence to stir up memories of the past. In most places there is no present day flurry of activity, let alone a past. It is a lonely world of dunes and laterite hills in which nature doesn't change but simply turns over on itself in an endless unchanging cycle. There are herds of giraffe on the river's left bank and early in the morning they move down the dunes to the river to drink. They come slowly and deliberately, beautiful in their docility and alertness, as silent as everything else in this great wilderness. You see hippos and crocodiles lying side by side on the sandy beaches and flocks of herons and lonely storks looking bored in the monotony of the stagnant marshes. The few canoes on the river move slowly, past scattered villages which sit high up on the soft backs of the dunes. Only the gentle breeze blowing up and down the shallow valley breaks the silence as it whistles through the thorn trees and flutters people's garments.

One day a Malian boy named Mamadou Dabala sailed down this river with his mother in a canoe and went into the Niger Republic to visit relatives in the town of Tillaberi. He had never taken a long trip before and the six days spent on the river were full of excitement and fun. Passengers were always getting off and new ones coming on and at each stop there were different things to see and an endless number of stories to be heard. Although this was quite an experience for Mamadou he felt homesick and often thought about his little sister and his friends. By the time the canoe had reached Tillaberi he was longing to return home.

Tillaberi is a big place compared to Mamadou's village back on the dunes in Mali. In a relative sense it is a very important trading center because it stands both on the river and on the road to North Africa where the truck and camel caravans meet the canoes which sail the Niger. It is a crossroads for men and goods coming down out of the Sahara and up from the savanna and forest. The market in this town is a lively conglomeration of straw stalls standing in the cool shade just a few feet from the river. Here black skinned Africans and fair complexioned desert nomads sit side by side, buying and selling spices and dates from North Africa, French flashlight batteries, leather goods and cloth, millet, rice, peanuts, pottery, basketware of every imaginable size and shape, salt from Bilma and Taoudeni, charms and jewelry and attractive swords made locally from old automobile springs. Whenever the weekly fair takes place there is the great excitement associated with varied peoples arriving and leaving with their wares. The Peul herdsmen come down from the faraway valley of the Azaouak with their cattle and calabashes of milk and the Tuareg from the inner Sahara with their camel caravans loaded with dates and salt. The Tuareg are a very confident looking people tinged with a visible trait of conceit. The men's eyes are impressive, standing out as small penetrating beads through a slit in the yards of indigo colored cloth which veil their faces and cover their heads. This dress gives them the air of bluff, of unpredictability, strength and cunning, which is as they want it, since it frightens off any would-be challenger. They are the undisputed masters of the camel caravans in this part of Africa. But for Tillaberi and the other towns and villages which lie along the Niger, the real caravans no longer arrive with them from the north. Rather, they came up from the south out of Niamey, convoys of five-ton Renault trucks, full of buyers, traders and merchandise from as far away as Ghana, Dahomey and the Ivory Coast.

An eight-year-old boy finds unlimited enjoyment in an African market. Mamadou went through the stalls where he met and saw people who came from places he had never heard of before. He stuck his fingers into the aromatic dishes the women sold, kous kous, millet cakes, rice and sauces and drank milk from the common drinking calabashes the Peul women carried. When the market wasn't in session he filled his hours of boredom wandering through the town. He often went into the white cement block buildings built many decades ago by the French colonials. He asked his mother why people had built such houses which were hot inside unlike the cool straw buildings they had at home. She said they had been built by the white people who liked buildings such as these which were hot inside with big windows broken into their walls. He found it strange that the white people had never built fires inside these buildings to keep the mosquitoes away.

There was nothing unusual about Mamadou getting sick. Boys his age were always coming down with fevers which came and went in a few day's time. But this time the fever and headache didn't leave and his mother became very anxious. She sent word up to their village with the leader of a caravan saying that the boy was ill and then went to the market to buy some herbs and charms from the Hausa medicine men from Nigeria. She also called a *marabout,* a Koranic teacher, an old man well versed in all kinds of illness, who imparted a sense of security when he entered the concession. "The fever will pass," he said and it was believed because this man knew what the destiny of life was all about. But the fever didn't disappear and by the time the boy's father had arrived in Tillaberi he was worse. There were no hesitating doubts about what had to be done. The father realized at once that the boy might die. But he also believed that if he could get him back to their village then all of the known and trusted forces could be mustered to cure him. The need to get home quickly was a pressing one charged with tremendous emotion. The father only remained in Tillaberi for a few hours and then bundled his son up in blankets and set off in his canoe. It was a frantic dash to get back home to Lellehoi and every inch of the landscape which lay between them and home was like a hostile impediment. Anyone who has ever rushed a sick child to the hospital knows what this feeling is like. There is only one thought in mind and that is to get the child to where he can be helped. Whether the child is in danger is immaterial to the emotional reaction of the parents. In their eyes he is and the only chance of hope lies ahead at the hospital. There were no hospitals in Lellehoi, only marabouts and healers. But they stood for the same thing because they were trusted and in everyone's eyes could heal Mamadou if he could be put into their hands.

    The canoe moved slowly against the current, thrust ahead by Mamadou's father who stood in the back pushing his long bamboo pole deep into the sandy bottom of the river bed. The boy's skin was covered with hundreds of pock marks, large ugly blisters which distorted his features beyond recognition. He lay on a heap of blankets in the middle of the canoe, trying to find a position in which to be comfortable. The gentle river breeze tortured him when it came into contact with the swollen blisters. Even the slightest well meant touch of his mother's hand made him cry out from pain. The blisters covered the inside of his mouth and throat, making it difficult for him to eat or drink anything. There was a sense of utter frustration in that canoe because they had never seen a sickness like this before and didn't know what to do for their only son. They were only positive of what the marabout in Tillaberi had told them. The boy had been cursed by an evil genie who had sent this illness out with the wind.

They pulled their canoe ashore whenever the sun dipped towards the right bank of the river. They always spent their nights on lonely stretches of the river bank, well away from the villages. They feared going into the villages with the boy because he had been cursed by an evil genie. People would turn them away, fearing the curse might fall on them and their children.

By the time the canoe had gotten to the rapids at Labenzanga, Mamadou no longer spoke. He didn't ask about his sister nor demand when they would be home. His breathing was heavy, his mouth parched and dry and his skin oozing liquid from hundreds of swollen blisters. He didn't scream anymore whenever they carried him because now he was in a coma. The last night before they reached Lellehoi they met a man who was fishing from his canoe in the middle of the river. When he saw Mamadou lying in the middle of his parent's canoe he was deeply moved and asked them to pass the night next to his hut in the village of Hounkoum. Later that night when Mamadou lay next to the cooking fire, the man took another look underneath the blanket. He shook his head. He had never seen anything like this disease before in his life. His own three children peeped out of their grass hut and glanced at Mamadou for a long time, but they weren't frightened by what they saw. Instead they laughed among themselves and said that he looked like a crocodile. They wanted to touch his skin to see if it really felt like a crocodile's and so later on that night when everyone was asleep they crawled out of their hut and approached the small motionless form on the mat next to the fire. The oldest of them rubbed his hand across Mamadou's leg. The pus spread all over his hand and he tried to wipe it off on his robe.

The next day the family arrived home and the boy was taken to his hut. The marabouts came and looked at him, but admitted that they had never seen an illness like this before. They promised to do their best, but guaranteed nothing. The genie had been at work for a long time and so even the best of their charms was at a great disadvantage. When word got out in Lellehoi that Mamadou Dabala was back from Tillaberi with a strange illness, people came by the score to look and see for themselves. Three days after he arrived home, Mamadou died, at a time when his parents had already despaired of his ever being saved. They buried him on the far side of the dune and put heavy stones over the grave to protect the body from the hyenas and jackals.

Although no one knew it at the time, the smallpox virus had been seeded into two villages along that stretch of the Niger. Most of the people in this area had never been vaccinated before in their lives. It was only a question of time before the disease would break out in epidemic proportions. Because so many people had been exposed, it was a certainty that it would strike with force and swiftness and take everyone completely by surprise.

Two weeks after Mamadou died a group of young men came to Lellehoi in a canoe from the village of Houkoum. They brought disquieting news for the chief of the village. The man and the three children who had seen Mamadou in Hounkoum now had the same disease caused by the evil genie. When word of this got out in Lellehoi pandemonium broke loose. People rushed to the marabouts for charms and talismans and offered goat blood sacrifices to the good genies who lived at the bottom of the Niger. They hoped and they waited. Several days went by and nothing happened and so everyone thought the danger was over. The good genies had put an end to the curse. But one morning Mamadou's sister and the three children who lived in the hut nearby developed fevers and headaches. Within several days their

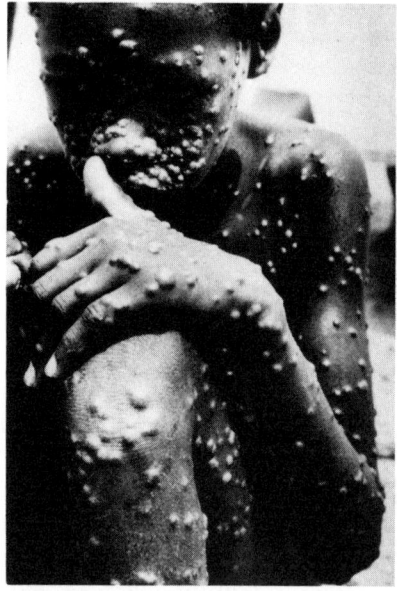

FIGURE 1. The early eruptive stage of smallpox in a young boy in the cercle of Ansongo.

skins were covered with the same horrible rash that had killed Mamadou. Then more people fell ill, until they numbered over a hundred. The elders assembled together to discuss what they should do to stop the curse. They decided to sacrifice a cow to the good genies who lived atop the nearby mountains. But in spite of the sacrifice the epidemic continued, people died, others were left blind and many others scarred. It didn't occur to anyone to inform the government commandant at Ansongo because this was a supernatural matter over which only the marabouts and elders had jurisdiction. The people of Lellehoi and Hounkoum lived with their group disaster for several weeks before anyone in the outside world knew anything about it.

One of the elders of Lellehoi, Abdoulaye Maiga, had been away in the town of Gao when the epidemic broke out. When he had finished selling his sheep and goats in the market there he started on his way back home. Even before he had crossed the river, word had reached him that there was a terrible plague in Lellehoi. He only had to look at it once to know what it was. It was smallpox, the same disease he had seen in Dakar when he was a soldier in the French army during the war. He also knew that there was only one way to stop an epidemic of this kind, but convincing the chief and the other elders was not easy. After two days of incessant palavering, the chief finally agreed to go to Ansongo and tell the commandant that there was an epidemic of smallpox in Lellehoi. The trip by camel and canoe took a day and then, when they arrived, the commandant was busy attending a political meeting and couldn't see them until the following day. When the commandant finally got to Lellehoi, he was appalled by what he saw. Smallpox was everywhere, in virtually every family, in every part of the village. He then discovered that it wasn't confined only to Lellehoi and Hounkoum, but that it had spread to other villages along the river.

Abdoulaye Maiga was a very resourceful man by nature and his wartime experiences had taught him to fall back on his own capacities in a difficult situation. The commandant had promised the chief and the elders that he would send a telegram to Bamako, the capital of Mali, and ask for vaccine to stop the epidemic. But the commandant had promised so many things so many times before and was never able to deliver on his promises. They had no reason to believe that it would be any different now. Abdoulaye knew that the Tuaregs protected themselves from smallpox by variolating. So, he rode out into the desert with several other men and three days later returned with four Tuareg blacksmiths who knew how to perform the operation. What the

Tuareg blacksmiths did in Lellehoi had been done many times over the centuries in many parts of the world. They took thorns from the acacia trees and stuck them into the blisters of people sick with smallpox. They turned the thorns around several times and then scratched the thick liquid into the skins of those who hadn't had the disease yet. Most medical authorities in the world would condemn Abdoulaye and the Tuaregs for what they did in Lellehoi, but when I arrived there several days later to launch a mass vaccination campaign in order to stop the epidemic, the question of condemnation was not so clear-cut. Their intentions had been good and what they had done was sanctioned in their society. They knew through experience that once they had variolated a person he developed a reaction on his skin not unlike that seen with a normal vaccination. When the operation was well done the local reaction disappeared, leaving only a small scar and the person never contracted smallpox. Occasionally, some of those variolated developed a serious form of smallpox and often they developed a mild type of illness. Abdoulaye and the Tuaregs believed that the procedure gave people a better chance of surviving the epidemic than if nothing were done at all.

Variolation has been practiced in the world for close to three thousand years. Medical authorities and historians say that it passed from the Hindus to the Chinese and then across Asia to Turkey. In 1717, it was observed in Constantinople by the wife of the British Ambassador, Lady Mary Wortley Montague. Lady Mary had a flair for the exotic and she hadn't been in Turkey more than a few weeks when she wrote up her observations and made known her resolve to introduce the practice into England. Recent historical evidence indicates that while Lady Mary championed the cause of variolation in England, others played a more important role in popularizing the practice. Eventually, even members of the royal family were variolated. The idea made its way over to the United States where Cotton Mather became one of its chief proponents. The possible risk of getting smallpox from variolation has virtually guaranteed that the practice will be eternally surrounded by controversy. And, over the years, this is what has happened. While one couldn't condemn the Tuaregs, one could show them that vaccination was better than variolation.

When I arrived in Lellehoi, it was the begining of the rainy season. I stood on top of the dunes and looked out for miles in every direction across the broad flat tops of the thorn trees. There were no heat waves nor scintillating mirages to mar the view. From Lellehoi, I saw the

Niger coming down out of the blue horizon and flowing past Ansongo between the rocky pillars which the explorer Heinrich Barth described a century ago as the iron gates of Akarambay. There is great majesty to the river at this time of year. The sky is serene, reflected in the river's surface, a powder blue accented with limpid puffs of white cloud. Everything is green and blue, the sand and gravel submerged beneath a cover of wet grass. There is tremendous clarity in the air and the scent of grass and flowering herbs spices the mornings before the last star disappears from sight. Mountains you never thought existed come into view and what you once thought to be nothing more than a dull continuum of flat monotony shows itself to be a delightful rhythm of green valleys and sloping hills. You feel tremendously alive in the mornings up there on the edge of the desert. Your lungs take in volumes of cold air and you shiver beneath your blankets as you might on a cold winter morning in New York. It is all a rainy season luxury and you enjoy it to its fullest while it lasts.

The grass in the pre-dawn hours is all wet down with beads of dew before the sun begins to throw its light horizontally over the mountains. It is the hour for the bees and pigeons. They fill the air with a hum and a repetative tolling which is pleasing to the ear as you open your eyes for the first time and gaze up at the great vault beyond your mosquito net. You look out at this world of natural radiance and find it hard to believe that in a few month's time a slight tilt of the earth will cause the grass to burn up, send the birds and pigeons away, blot out the blueness of the sky and fill the whole with suffocating heat and dust. It was difficult for me to come to terms with the harsh reality that this serenity cradled in its bosom a terrible human tragedy.

I crossed the river on a barge and then drove through the soft sand over a cattle track. It was late in the afternoon and the herds of cattle, sheep and goats moved with a slow shuffling gait up the side of the dune. The village came on us all at once, spreading out over the broad flat surface of the dune as a repetative design of gray oval forms. Off on the distant trails were camel caravans, gliding their way across the grass-covered sand and small groups of women bouncing their way home on the backs of overloaded donkeys. When the people heard the noise of the motor, they came out of their huts and surrounded the truck. When I looked at them, I would never have been able to sense that any great disaster had taken place had I not been in Africa for a long time. In a comparative sense, they were quiet and had an air of hidden knowledge about them. Under any other circumstances, there would have been a noisy and lively outburst of activity, an outpouring of vitality and enjoyment at the arrival of a stranger in the village. But here there was nothing but patient silence.

The chief and the elders moved out of the crowd as a dignified body in flowing robes, turbans and mufflers. They were very black but their fine aquiline features struck you as a faint far whisper of the Moroccan presence on this river in the sixteenth century. We finally sat down cross-legged on several straw mats which some small boys stretched out on the sand beneath an enormous thorn tree. When the elders spoke, there were more than just words falling from their lips. Their patience, fatalism and resolve came through as measured breaks in their description of the ordeal they were living through. These men had learned to live with an unknown terror and with heartbreak. And, although they were benumbed by what had happened, they had dealt with it on their own terms and to their way of thinking had come through it all as the final victors. They were patient with me as I began

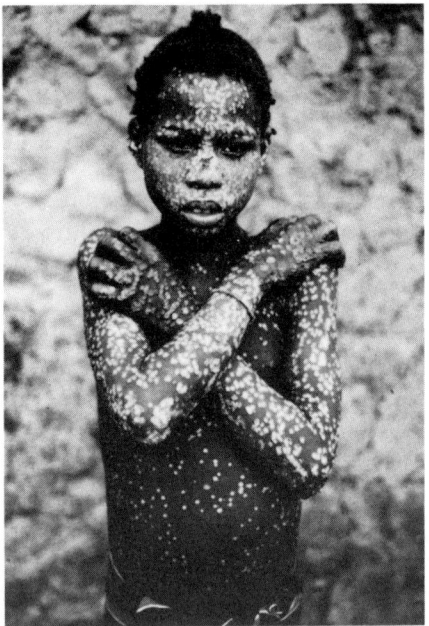

FIGURE 2. A young Malian girl in the recovery stage of smallpox. The severe depigmentation follows the desquamation of scabs. Repigmentation occurs over a period of several months.

the long and drawn-out inquiry which was to go on into the late hours of the night. It is always a marvelous thing in Africa to see how you can piece together a very complex story with such accuracy. Everything is recounted in public in the presence of hundreds of other people and what one informant has forgotten another has surely remembered. The women and children stood around us as an attentive crowd. The women were from another age, exactly the way Barth had found them a century ago, clothed in indigo colored robes and heavy brass anklets with a coiffure studded with red and yellow beads and bits of decorated metal. There was something very biblical about their appearance and they moved and reacted the way you would expect extras to perform on a Hollywood set depicting a story directed by Cecil B. DeMille.

We visited every hut and examined all of those who were still ill with smallpox. A great crowd of people followed us. There, near the desert, hundreds of feet can move across the sands in almost utter silence. All you hear is the swooshing sound of clothing rubbing on itself and the tinkle of brass anklets and beads. In many ways, it was like visiting a battlefield several days after the siege. I felt the emotions of the leader of a relief expedition. If only I had gotten there earlier. People stood in the limpid shadows of their huts and had that look common to those who have just come out of some great distress. The children had never seen a white man before and I am sure that they must have viewed me as a part of this whole terrible nightmare. Indeed, I later learned that some of them thought I was the evil genie come to Lellehoi in person to make my peace with the village.

People with smallpox were in huts all over the undulations of this great dune. Some cases were just beginning as barely perceptible rashes of small red spots and others were at their terrible peak. People had swollen faces and oozing limbs which had been covered with cow dung and urine. The stench of decaying flesh and the buzzing of thousands of flies filled every hut. Mothers covered their sick children with small soiled rags to prevent the flies from getting into the pussy wounds and fanned their bodies to drive out the smell. Some people were already half way into death, so hideously transformed that only the outline resembled anything human. This was not the first time that I had seen a smallpox epidemic at its peak, but I still felt helpless when confronted with people so sick that their survival would be in doubt even if they were in the finest hospital in the world. One little girl had pocks in each eye, over the pupils. She would live, but the pocks would leave her blind for the rest of her life. She would never see a sunrise again,

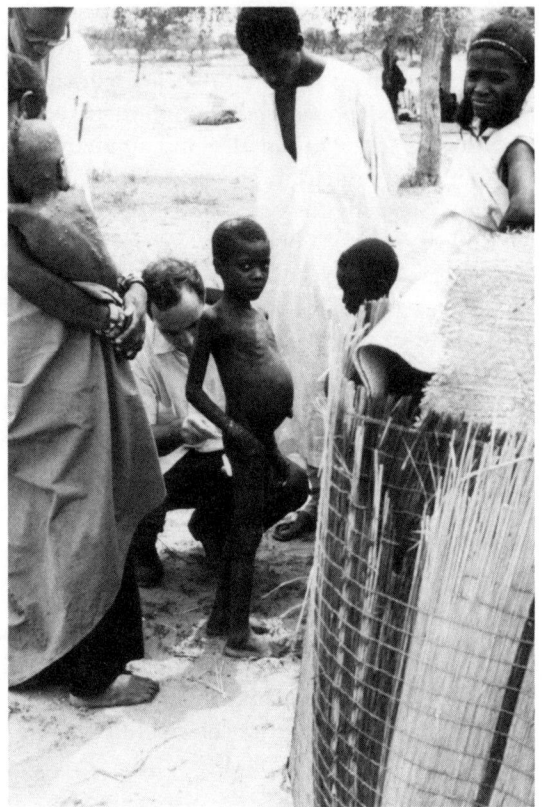

FIGURE 3. Dr. Imperato treating secondary skin infections in a young boy recovering from smallpox.

nor the river, nor the desert during the rains. She would spend the rest of her life in darkness.

The old men took me to see a little boy who they said was dying. He was lying on a straw mat in the center of a large hut not far from a fire which puffed out heat and smoke and made breathing difficult. I remember now that as I sat on a stool next to him I knew he was going to die. He wasn't more than four years old, at the beginning of his life, and yet he was dying. He turned his head and gazed at me for a long time. When I looked down into his submissive face I saw his resignation to death and my own defeat. We came from two different worlds, he the unschooled boy of four and I the physician and yet in this affair he knew as much as I. And when I looked up at his parents,

I saw their despairing conviction that the infirmiers and I who had come to heal the sick and stop the epidemic were as the marabouts and elders, helpless in the hands of destiny. Yet, when we vaccinated the village and stopped the epidemic, people believed in us and understood why I had come. Although I told them that I had come to Mali to stop smallpox, measles and many other diseases, among themselves they expressed this in their own terms. They said that I had come to stop what was in the wind.

Chapter II

Looking Up the Facts

Springtime is a delightful time of year in Atlanta, especially after an afternoon cloudburst when everything is bathed in sunlight and steam and the air filled with the exciting aroma of rejuvenated pines and pollinating trees. My thoughts should have been about spring and the rolling green hills of north-eastern Atlanta and their flowering tulip beds. But they weren't. I had just volunteered to go over to West Africa for the United States Public Health Service's Center for Disease Control and had come to Atlanta in order to receive my country assignment. So my thoughts were about Africa.

My involvement in this venture began in a very casual way one afternoon in a parasitology laboratory at the School of Public Health and Tropical Medicine at Tulane University in New Orleans where I was studying for my degree in tropical medicine. As my classmates and I studied our malaria slides beneath our microscopes, we chatted about what we were going to do after graduation. Some were returning to medical missions in Asia, others going to take up academic careers in universities and some going back to their native lands to take up responsible positions in public health. I had already volunteered to go into the United States Public Health Service in order to do my two years of military service and was being processed for assignment to a research project in Uganda. As we spoke, one of my classmates mentioned that he had just heard of a new program which the Center for Disease Control would be administering over in West Africa. -It was a smallpox eradication-measles control program which was being financed by the United States Agency For International Development, an agency of the State Department. The program was scheduled to be operative in twenty countries and had as its goal the complete eradication of smallpox by 1972 and the permanent control of measles. Congress had already appropriated fifty million dollars for the five years the program would be operative and President Johnson had officially announced the program to the press from the Texas White House.

The Center for Disease Control was in the process of recruiting physicians. Although I was being processed to go over to Uganda, I decided that the West African program would be more to my liking and so that evening I wrote a letter expressing my interest to Dr. D. A. Henderson, the program's director. A few days later as I sat listening to a lecture on tropical medicine, I was called out of the classroom by the dean's secretary. There was a long distance call for me from Atlanta. When I picked up the receiver, Dr. Henderson's voice came on. He invited me to fly up to Atlanta.

"Why smallpox eradication and measles control?" was one of my first questions when we met. Dr. Henderson then explained in great detail the World Health Organization's plan to eradicate smallpox from the globe by 1975. It was a disease which caused much human suffering and death in Africa and against which we now had effective vaccines which remained potent even under the high temperatures found there. Thus it was possible to vaccinate the rural populations of Asia, Africa and South America and eradicate the disease from these areas. Once the disease was eradicated, then routine smallpox vaccination would no longer be necessary. As it was, the medical risks from the complications of vaccination were greater in places like the United States and Europe than the risk from smallpox. But still routine vaccination was being performed because of the potential danger of the disease being imported from abroad. The United States supported program in West Africa was to be one of the most important parts of the world fight against smallpox, for West Africa was one of the few remaining areas where the disease was still epidemic.

Measles in West Africa, he explained, was a very serious disease, carrying a mortality of fifty percent in small children. The disease causes serious complications such as encephalitis and blindness and so weakens children that they become easy victims to other infectious diseases such as malaria. In order to eradicate the disease, one would have to vaccinate most children before they reached the age of one year, a difficult task because of the immensity of the African bush and the logistical problems that poses in reaching children on a regular basis. There were simply not enough funds, health personnel and vehicles in West Africa so that a vaccination team could visit every village once a year. The most that was hoped for was for a health team to visit every village at intervals of two to three years. Under these circumstances we could not eradicate a disease as contagious as measles, but we could control it.

I sympathized with Dr. Henderson in his job of launching a fifty million dollar aid program of this degree of complexity. This was to be the first large international program which the Center for Disease Control had ever undertaken. It couldn't fail. He went down the list of countries. This one would be a snap, that one posed no problems; these were a breeze. Thy all had good health services and no complicated ethnographic problems. There wasn't much for a person like me to do in these places. At any rate, this is what I was told. Inevitably the pitch had to come. He cleared his throat.

"Well you see Pat." There was a pause. "Well, you see, there is this country I've been thinking about. It's a tremendous challenge, rough terrain, thousands of nomads moving all over the place, health services not fully developed. You know what I mean. It's just the place for you."

I've always been suspicious about places which have been described as "just the place for you." It usually means that they have been someone else's headache and the someone else is anxious to rid themselves of the "just the place for you."

"If you can get the job done in this country, there's no reason for it failing anywhere else."

The first part of Dr. Henderson's offensive evolked my sympathy and appealed to my sense of duty. The second I thought was a friendly *coup de grace*. It was then explained to me that this country was just the place for me because I had already spent some time in Africa, was fluent in French, had a degree in tropical medicine and because I was an amateur anthropologist. While all of this disccusion was taking place, I had narrowed the possibilities down in my own mind to two countries, Guinea and Mali. It turned out to be Mali. Of course I could refuse to go. No one was going to force me into accepting the assignment. "But it would be unfair to send a less-experienced man to such a difficult place." And with that, Dr. Henderson convinced me to go to Mali for a two-year assignment which eventually evolved into a five-year stay.

I didn't know much about Mali at that time, but having been a student of African affairs for many years, I did know that Mali's political complexion was distinctly Marxist and socialist. I asked about this, and those who during the discussions had been so talkative were suddenly very quiet. Finally, someone said, "Oh, it's not too bad. They just have a left leaning government."

"Then you mean they're Communists."

"Not quite," came the answer. "They're Marxists and socialists."

There followed a session in which medical doctors expounded on the differences between Communism and Marxism and in the end both they and I were so thoroughly confused that we were happy to drop the conversation.

"You can do it old man! No question about it. We've got absolute confidence in you."

When I asked for a few basic facts about Mali everyone looked very ignorant. "You'll have to look up the facts," said Dr. Henderson. I tried to look up the facts and found to my dismay that the local libraries carried little more on Mali than that contained in a few paragraphs of the various encyclopedias. The New York Public Library and the Library of Congress weren't able to contribute much more. The sad fact was that there had never been a single book written about life in Mali. There were bits and pieces here and there in travelogues, but these, as I now know, were written by the "passers through" and were for the most part superficial and inaccurate.

The news of my going to Mali was first announced with some hesitancy to my Uncle Harold and Aunt Marianne who lived out in Decatur, Georgia. Uncle Harold held doctorate degrees in both English and Jurisprudence, but that didn't stop him from saying, "You're going where?"

"Mali," I said in a matter of fact way, as if it were a place one went for the weekend.

"Never heard of the place!"

My aunt was very concerned. "Do you have to go?"

"Not really, I sort of volunteered you might say."

That remark jolted my uncle's mother, Grandma Smith. She put down her horoscope reading and looked at me as if I were crazy. She had nver heard of Mali either, but according to the horoscope all sorts of horrible things would happen to me if I went there. When Uncle Harold told her I was going there to fight the Communists a revised version was produced.

"What will your family say?" asked my aunt.

My family had a great deal to say, but fortunately for me, the fact we were talking long distance distinctly limited just how much they could say. What wasn't said on the phone was followed up in voluminous correspondence. Why didn't I come back to New York and open up an office like the rest of my friends. "You've done enough. Let someone else do it." The advice was well meant, but the challenge to the altruistic leanings of one's nature of this enormous job in Mali was irresistible. I decided to take it.

Dr. Henderson finally managed to find an interesting document called a *Post Report*. Such reports are written by embassy wives who are dedicated to the cause of making their post, as the embassy is called, sound worse than the Black Hole of Calcutta. These members of the gentler sex are not so much interested in getting pity as they are in helping their husbands earn more money. The Mali Post Report had obviously been done by a very experienced editorial crew who didn't have to do too much exaggerating to convince the State Department that Mali was a hardship post. Every government employee assigned to the post was given twenty-five percent more of his salary, known in government parlance as the Post Differential. There were also allowances for the education of children and to cover the high cost of living.

The women had prepared this report with great care and had included a photograph of the embassy, taken either on a cloudy day or else with a very bad camera. At any rate, the net result was a building which looked one step removed from a shanty. Housing in Mali's capital of Bamako was much inferior in quality to that in other West African capitals. The ladies made the most of this, including a picture of the interior of a typical house which looked like a trappist monk's ideal of an uncomfortable cell. The climate was dealt with in depth, special emphasis being placed on the dangers of heat exhaustion and sun stroke. For the benefit of women states-side, insects, rats and snakes were dealt with in depth and recommendations made for bringing an enormous supply of rat poison and insect spray from the States. Cockroaches merited an entire paragraph, taking second place to rats and mice which were treated in two. One got the impression that American males spent their evenings at home in sweltering heat, defending their wives and children against the incessant raids of hoards of insects and rats.

Mali was given credit for growing fruits and vegetables, but these were described as being of inferior quality. One look at the map, showing Mali tucked up under the Sahara, is enough to convince any reader that there couldn't be much in the way of these things in Bamako's markets. It was strongly suggested that canned fruits and vegetables be shipped over as even Malians preferred these. To be on the safe side, I followed most of the recommendations and went out on a shopping spree determined to buy enough clothes, shoes, toilet items, canned goods and soap to last several years. I never regretted once that I did after arriving in Bamako. On this subject, the authors of the report were right because aside from poor quality meats and vegetables there was very little in the way of food products for foreigners in Mali at that time.

Speaking from the authority of experience, I can say that it takes a bachelor about a month of concentrated effort to get all of these items together. That takes into consideration his lack of experience in setting up a household, the help of a mother and three sisters and the wise cracks of two brothers, all of whom thought that any American physician who was going to a place where he had to take life supports necessary for several years deserved a free trip to a psychiatrist. Frankly, I never calculated how much toothpaste I used in a year, but everyone from store salesmen to friends were helpful in suggesting estimates ranging from a tube per week to a tube per month. Although most of my friends didn't know anything about Mali, they all had definite ideas about life in Africa. One friend advised me to take along at least fifty rolls of toilet tissue since I was sure to be down with dysentery most of the time. I became a delightful curiosity in department stores. Sales people were eager to share me with their co-workers. I also got to be shared by the other customers, whose suggestions ranged from a diet of sunflower seeds to automatic weapons. It was revealing to discover how many veterans of the North African Campaign had become salesmen in New York department stores and that they thought that their war-time experiences qualified them as experts on all aspects of life on the African continent. Even if people had never been to Africa, they surely had friends or friends of friends who had been. Anyone and everyone who had been within a few hundred miles of the African coast felt duty-bound to pass on to me what they considered to be invaluable advice. One old woman who had been to Cairo in 1936 told me not to take any blankets as the desert heat was so unbearable at night that I would never use them. I took several and huddled beneath them during the cold season. Sales people didn't feel obliged to restrict their advice to their line of sale. A shoe salesman told me to watch out for "those native girls." "They're infested," he added with emphasis as if he knew and I gathered he wasn't talking about lice.

It was difficult to buy large quantities of things without drawing a query from a salesman and my sisters and mother were only too eager to fill them in on the details. In fact, they would fill them in even if they weren't asked to. I then took to shopping with my brothers which was certainly less embarrassing, but not very satisfactory since they were firm in their view that I shouldn't go to Mali. My brothers were finally won over, through pity I think, and suggested I get hold of a wholesaler's catalogue of canned goods and order from it. When the delivery truck dumped it all off a few weeks later the order filled four hundred and twenty cases. They stood neatly packed in the celler next to the twenty five boxes containing everything from toothpaste for several years to an alarm clock. Before the huge van was sealed I thought of two more items and put them in. That umbrella and American flag have been put to good use ever since.

Most Americans have never heard of the Republic of Mali and they are not ashamed to admit it. In response to a blank expression, my next statement is that it is in West Africa. I've learned through experience that this strategy is best. It eliminates the possibility of their saying, "Why, of course, Malaya!" and then firing off a host of questions about Singapore and Kuala Lumpur. By the time you get a chance to put a word in edgewise, they're embarrassed and you're frustrated. Predictably, the conversation follows one of two courses. One group will think you're talking about Malawi and ask you about Hastings Banda and the neighboring Portuguese colony of Mozambique. The other will say they've never heard of the place. You then tell them that it is the former French Sudan and their eyes will show a glow. "The Sudan of course." That quick response lets you know that they're thinking about the former Anglo-Egyptian Sudan and so you brace yourself for questions about the Nile and Khartoum. "It's where Timbuctoo is located." This is a last ditch attempt to place it for them. For those who know that Timbuctoo is a real city, the battle is over. For the others who think it is an imaginary place, your problems have just begun.

Mali is a landlocked country which lies like a tilted hour glass in the heart of the West African bulge. The French who governed this area from the late nineteenth century until 1960 called it the Haute-Senegal Niger and later the French Sudan. *Bilad es Sudan* in Arabic means, the land of the black people. Like all other territories which made up former French West Africa, Mali was lost on maps and in geography books in an amorphous blotch of blue which represented all of the French possessions in Africa. Only places like Nigeria, Ghana, Gambia and Sierra Leone, standing out as they did in British red, attracted visual recognition as distinct countries in American geography books. When the country became independent in 1960, its leaders chose to call it the Republique Soudanaise. This caused no end of confusion since there was already a Republic of the Sudan. The world was probably willing to accommodate two Congos, but two Sudans was asking a little too much. Senegal and the Sudanese Republic joined together in a federation whose physical figure was as unappealing as the political alliance was awkward. They called it the Mali Federation, after the Manding empire of the fourteenth century. When the federation finally split up in September of 1960, Mali kept the name.

There has always been a difference of opinion as to what the name Mali means. Some linguistic authorities maintain that its original meaning was "where the king resides." The more generally accepted meaning is hippopotamus. Mali covers 1,200,000 square kilometers, about the size of Alaska, or as big as Texas, Oklahoma and New Mexico combined. The country is composed of three distinct topographic zones, the Sahara desert in the north which covers 360,000 square kilometers, the *sahel* (semi-desert) which covers 250,000 square kilometers and the savanna in the south which covers the rest of the country. The *sahel* is a transition zone between the desert and the savanna, characterized by sandy soils and thorn tree vegetation. It is the sap of these thorn trees, known as *gum arabic,* which has been used for centuries in the textile industries of Europe and America. The savanna is heavily wooded with a variety of trees, baobabs, shea butter, silk cotton, tamarind and sycamore. It is in the savanna where intensive agriculture is practiced by several ethnic groups using traditional agricultural methods adapted to prevailing conditions imposed by soils and climate. The short handed hoe or *daba* is a clumsy agricultural tool. But, it has been argued by some experts that it breaks up the soil more satisfactorily than deep ploughing which lays open the subsoil to erosion and rain. The sedentary farming peoples practice shifting cultivation wherein the fields are left fallow for many years and bush burning practiced to restore fertility. Fertilization is arranged for by having nomads pasture their herds on the fields.

The staple food cultivated is millet of which there are several varieties. Cotton and peanuts, which are cash crops, are also grown. Unlike many countries in Asia, Mali has more than enough land to support its peoples. However, in recent years there has been an annual hungry season due to poor harvests which resulted from inadequate rainfall. The growing season is short, from June to September and during the months of July and August, cereal shortages occur due to an exhaustion of the previous year's reserves. The United States government has been carrying Mali over this grain crisis for several years by supplying several million tons of surplus maize annually. Factors aggrevating the decrease in cereal production have been the diversion of farmers to cash crops and the overall rural exodus of the younger generations.

The population of Mali is 4.8 million of whom three quarters are subsistence farmers and traders. Approximately one quarter are pastoral nomads. The population density of the sahel and the desert where most of the nomads live is sparse and that where the agriculturists live is 11.6 per kilometer on the average. The nomads consist of three distinct groups, the light skinned Tuareg and Maure and the darker Peul, who are thought by some to have orginated in Ethiopia. The Tuareg and Maure are divided into several large clans and move with their herds through the sahel and desert in search of grass and water according to centuries old patterns. The Peul, who live in fixed villages for part of the year, move with their herds through the savanna and the sahel. Although the herds of the nomads constitute an enormous potential natural resource for Mali, they have scarcely been exploited on a commercial scale. There are as many cattle in Mali as people, twice as many sheep and four times as many goats. The chief impediment to the commercialization of livestock is the nomad's traditional attitude towards his flocks. They are viewed as symbols of wealth, the source of a man's prestige in society.

In contrast to this, the fish resources of the Niger are being developed with modern techniques by the itinerant Bozo fishermen. The Niger cuts through Mali for 1,400 kilometers, like an archer's bow, flowing in a north-easterly direction towards Bourem where it bends and then flows southwards towards the sea. Fishing is an important industry along the middle Niger where the river forms a vast inland delta of flood plains, lakes and streams. Several million tons of dried fish are exported each year from the riverine town of Mopti which is the commercial capital of the inland delta. Although much of this fish is exported to the coastal countries of Ghana and the Ivory Coast by truck along a modern road called *la route des poissons* much of it filters along the traditional trade routes in Mali. This consumption of fish protein accounts for the absence of protein deficiency syndromes which are frequently found in neighboring states.

The gross national product of Mali is about three hundred million dollars annually and the average annual per capita income is sixty dollars. What do these figures imply? Most obviously very low incomes for most of the people. The meaning of such statistics becomes more obvious when they are compared to those for other countries. The GNP of Mali is less than that of the Borough of Queens in New York City and a third of that of the Ivory Coast, Mali's neighbor. This disadvantaged ratio exists for exports, roads, railways and electrical capacity. If progress in Africa is meant to mean movement toward the material standards and social conditions of the societies of Europe and North America, then the coastal countries are far in the lead ahead of Mali. Not well endowed with minerals nor with suitable conditions for producing lucrative export crops, thinly populated, land-locked, and as a consequence obliged to pay the high cost for transport to ocean ports on which modern commerce depends, and disfavored by climate, Mali faces more problems and obstacles than her coastal neighbors. But it was not always so. For centuries, caravan routes across the Sahara were the main highways by which trade goods and new ideas filtered down into West Africa from Europe and the Arab world. It was in the Malian sahel that Ghana, the first great African empire, emerged in the seventh century. The power and wealth of this empire lay in its role as a great market place for the gold from the now exhausted mines of the Bambuk which are in the south-western corner of modern day Mali. The empire of Mali, founded by the Mandinka, rose up in the thirteenth century in the savanna surrounding the source of the Niger. It was in this ancient Mali that the trans-Saharan trade prospered, enriching the country not only with material goods but also with the theological, legal and scientific ideas of medieval Islam. Ancient Mali controlled the gold mines of the Bambuk and Boure and when in 1324 the Malian emperor, Mansa Moussa, traveled to Mecca to make the pilgrimage he astonished the Moslem world by his rich entourage and conspicuous expenditure. In the fifteenth cenutry, the Songhoi empire of Gao arose in eastern Mali and brought under its control the cities of Timbuctoo and Djenne which were then the centers of trade and learning in this part of Africa.

Although this impressive past constitutes a composite historical consciousness for Mali's political leaders it does not do so for the average citizen. At best they are familiar with those segments of it to which they can relate because of tribal affiliation. One group's heroes are often another's enemies, making it difficult for modern politicians to engender a sense of national unity through the appeal of the past. The Bambara, who comprise a quarter of the country's population and who are Mali's largest ethnic group are proud of the animist kingdoms of Segou and Kaarta which are viewed by the moslem Peul with disdain. The Malinke are the descendants of the old Mali empire and thus their *griots* (minstrels) sing of its glories and the greatness of its leaders. But neither the Bambara nor the Malinke sense any connection to the Songhoi empire of Gao. The present day Songhoi do, of course, and consider that their conversion to Islam in the thirteenth cenutry gives them reason to assert superiority over the predominantly animst Bambara and Malinke. They are keenly aware of their descent from the ancient Songhoi empire and attach great important to its capital, Gao. Surprisingly, they consider Timbuctoo and Djenne, cities which the ancient Songhoi conquered, to be of less significance. They are very perplexed

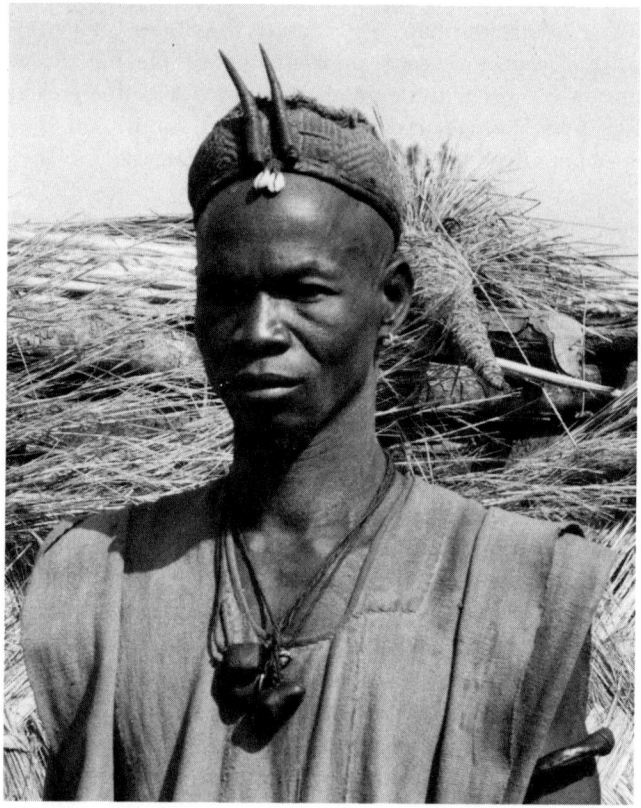

FIGURE 4. A Bambara hunter from the cercle of Kolokani wearing a typical hunter's hat decorated with the horns of an oribi and cowrie shells. The leather bags around his neck are Koranic charms known as *sebe,* and the leather arm band a Koranic talisman.

why so many Europeans and Americans visit Timbuctoo rather than Gao. That historical perspectives are different is difficult for an ethnocentric people to comprehend. Similarly, it is incomprehensible to the Bambara, Peul and Malinke why foreigners would want to visit Timbuctoo when there are such important ancient cities like Segou, Hamdallaye and Kangaba to be seen, their respective ancient capitals.

The modern day descendants of the Ghana empire are the Moslem Sarakole. They are among the foremost traders and merchants of West Africa and have left their bleak homeland up near the Mauritanian frontier in large numbers in order to settle throughout the rest of Africa. They operate large commercial enterprises which virtually exclude individuals who are not Sarakole. They are fanatical moslems who have spent much of their time stamping the sterile grounds of theological legalism. As a group they identify less with modern Mali than any other ethnic group and this coupled to their material success and ethnocentricity have earned them the intense dislike of other Malians. Because the Sarakole are Moslem they profess no association with the ancient animist empire of Ghana and have as their substitute heroes a pantheon of religious leaders who lived in the past century.

If the past does not completely unify modern day Mali, the country's diverse ethnic composition does even less towards achieving unity. How then does the country stay together in the face of such strong currents of tribalism? There are many reasons why tribalism has never been a great problem in Mali. There is a minimal degree of friction between various groups. On the economic level, they complement one another rather than compete. The Peul are herdsmen, the Bambara and Malinke farmers, the Sarakole merchants, the Bozo fishermen. On the political and social levels, they have not infringed on one another's vested interests. In a country as large as Mali, there are no population pressures on the land, eliminating the possibility of tribal conflict over land rights. The slow islamization of the population serves as a strong unifying force because Islam is adopted not only as a religion but also as a way of life. Although a high degree of syncretism is present, where people profess Islam without renouncing animistic beliefs, traditional laws, secret societies and initiation rites, enough of the practices of Islam are adopted to unify peoples from diverse ethnic groups through a religious denominator. Islamization is gradual, extending over several generations wherein Islam is phased in and animism phased out. Islam doesn't confront animism as does Christianity. Rather, it accommodates to its presence and gently displaces it. Because of this, it is difficult to characterize the Malian population as being so much the one and so much the other. While official statistics list the population as being seventy percent Moslem, it must be remembered that many Moslems still practice animism. Because of Islam's stabilizing and unifying effects on the population, the French colonial administration promoted proselytizing and built mosques in many parts of the country. Simultaneously, they discouraged Catholic and Protestant missionaries as much out of anti-clerical motives as from fear of their divisive effect on the population. Working to hold Mali together then is Islam and the absence of those forces which historically tend to pull young nations apart.

Mali's early post independence years witnessed the development of a one party state under a leadership which had been shaped by radical Marxist ideologies from overseas. The Union Soudanaise, as the party was known, established a secular state, but presented Marxist egalitarianism to the people as a Moslem responsibility. The imposition of the socialist option on Mali was not an easy task because it came into conflict with the vested interests of almost every level of traditional society. One must properly term it an imposition, since most Malians had no idea of what socialism meant when they voted the Union Soudanaise into power. Initially, the development of a socialist society was brought about through an emphasis on collective decisions and on broad popular activity at the grass roots level. There was a conscious effort to reconcile sectional differences and to build national unity. The confiscation of foreign owned businesses was hailed as a victory for African independence. But when the regime began to nationalize African-dominated sectors of the economy, Malians reacted very differently. Gradually, the government established state-owned enterprises which took over the economic life of the country. The private merchants who up to that time contributed enormously to the gross national product fled the country in desperation. A new non-convertable currency was issued in 1963, it being printed in Czechoslovakia. In 1966, a customs inspector accidentally discovered that an entering Czech diplomat had several suitcases full of Malian money. Apparently, the Czechs had been printing up a private supply for themselves. So, that year, the Malians changed the bills, having them printed up in London instead. Foreign exchange dwindled, agricultural productivity decreased and the exiled merchants turned their genius into smuggling activities which drained the country of the few exports it had. Farmers took their cereals over the frontier into Upper Volta and the Ivory Coast to avoid selling their crop to the government for what was a very low price. The nomads likewise fled with their cattle and even the Tuaregs who trade in the Sahara salt resources smuggled their salt from Taoudeni to Niger and Upper Volta. In an attempt to stop this mammoth outflow of the countrys precious few resources, the government set up a formidable system of road blocks, customs checks and frontier patrols which did not acomplish very much.

Because the country had little foreign exchange and a nonconvertable currency, there were severe restrictions on the importation of most consumer goods. Since imports and exports had to pass through the state owned import-export society, SOMIEX, this policy was easily implemented. These restrictions resulted in empty stores, high prices, and a flourishing black market. People talked about the black market as if it were a physical location and in many places it was. Housewives didn't talk about the weather and their children when they met on the streets. Rather they talked about the presence or absence of butter, sugar, salt and scores of other consumer goods. The ninety Americans who lived in Mali at that time managed to survive this shortage by bringing most items with them from the States or else by ordering them from Danish export houses where they paid forty percent extra for shipping costs. This "food order" as it is still called used to be sent out once a month in the ambassador's name and took about three months to arrive in Bamako. The two thousand Frenchmen in Mali weathered the storm in a similar fashion, the ones with diplomatic privileges doing all the ordering for the others so as to avoid the excessive customs charges. Many Eastern Europeans living in Bamako fell into very bourgeois habits by ordering goods from Denmark. The several hundred Russians solved the problem in a clear-cut direct fashion. They simply had an Ilyushian-18 fly supplies into Bamako periodically. I generally knew just when this plane came since my Russian neighbors religiously celebrated the occasion with boisterous parties. The thousand Communist Chinese technicians in the country managed to survive on the local market.

This lack of consumer goods affected the Malian population as much as it did the foreigners. Salt, sugar, rice and coffee are as much in demand in African households as they are in European and their absence caused a great degree of discontent. Malians were told to smoke locally manufactured cigarettes and to use locally made textiles even though they were of inferior quality. The government appealed to people's patriotism by saying these products, while inferior were nonetheless Malian. The Malians responded by smoking black market foreign made cigarettes and by wearing black market imported cloth.

It was abudantly clear by 1967 that Malians were weary of socialism. Instead of improving, conditions of living steadily deteriorated. This was a sharp blow to a people who had been taught that their pre-independence misery was due to French colonial exploitation. Even the basic necessities were scarce and long lines at government-run stores a daily facet of life in the towns. Although the economic privations severely tried the patience of the people, it was the subsequent repressive and dictatorial nature of the regime which proved intolerable. President Modibo Keita had initially been a very popular leader, responsive to the needs of the people. But over the years he and his leadership clique drifted into that self-deception with which absolute power often narcotizes its holders. In order to counter the syndrome of mounting discontent, President Keita came up with an imaginative and temporarily self-saving remedy. On the twenty-second of August, 1967, he launched a "cultural revolution" modeled on the one which had just run its course in China. The national assembly, which had long since become a rubber stamp, dissolved itself, entrusting its powers to the "infinite wisdom" of "the enlightened guide" and "the supreme guide of the revolution" as Modibo Keita was thereafter called. The National Committee for the Defense of the Revolution became the supreme advisory body of the president. Local committees for the defense of the revolution were formed in the city blocks, at the district level and in the villages. Mali's version of the red guard, the popular militia, was re-vitalized and enlarged so that it equaled the army in strength. Its ranks were swollen with social misfits and ex-criminals, who, armed with unlimited powers and Marxist indoctrination were set loose on the population. The popular militia became the private army and police force of Modibo Keita and under his direction terrorized the population into meek submission. The green uniformed militiamen became omnipresent in Mali, watching, searching, arresting and torturing thousands of individuals, most of whom were innocent of any crimes. Those arrested were the scapegoats for the faltering regime or individuals who raised their voices against the system.

It is often the instinctual tendency of failing political regimes to give themselves an added extension on life by launching appealing public campaigns against corruption, thereby demonstrating to the citizenry a tangeable cause for the political and economic ills of the country. In most countries, it is usually possible to uncover government officials who have embezzled state funds. And so Modibo Keita re-directed the popular discontent with his regime against those whose corruption he conveniently chose to expose. The long harangues over Radio Mali delivered the same repetitive message for popular consumption. Mali's plight was due to the corruption of exposed officials and the sabotage of western imperialists. Charmed with this circus and bludgeoned through fear by the militia, the population rapidly fell into line. People's security lay in cooperating with the regime. Thus, most attended the prescribed weekly Marxist indoctrination sessions, reported on their friends and relatives and were conscientious about displaying a bitter antipathy towards westerners. Mali rapidly became an African Haiti with a socialist veneer. For westerners, life was a continuous disagreeable ordeal in which the Malians saw plots being hatched behind every hedge. The expertise of inflicting petty harrassments fell easily to them. Some of these were humiliating, others frustrating, but most were simply aggrevating. Everyone suffered their misery in silence, creating a tranquility which gave birth to a bold and absolute despotism. The cult of personality was promoted in which Modibo Keita's praises were sung over the radio to traditional music, his thoughts printed in the newspaper and published in book form and his photograph hung on thousands of walls.

So convincing was this delusion to Modibo Keita, that he ultimately committed what proved to be his fatal mistake. He prepared to move against the army, whose junior officers out of instincts of self-preservation moved against him first. The coup d'etat of November, 1968 swept away not only a political regime but also a whole way of life.

What kind of a nation did Modibo Keita bequeathe to the army officers? On the positive side, they were a people who had a remarkable sense of national identity, seldom found in other African states at that time. If nothing else, Modibo Keita had vanquished tribalism. His successors also inherited an enormously proud people. It was a pride born not only out of a consciousness of past greatness and achievement, but also out of a regimentation with a catachism of self-praise and ethnocentricism. It is this pride which so impresses visitors today, most of whom erroneously attribute it solely to that historical consciousness of which only they themselves and the elite Malians are aware. Superficially, this pride is an admirable thing to behold. But it is also a self-destructive characteristic because it prevents many Malians from learning anything new. So great is this pride that they cannot bring themselves to make that self-admission of not knowing which is essential to learning.

Economically, the country was in ruin, a situation which has been steadily repaired over the years. In the wave of the fresh breeze of freedom which swept the country after the coup d'etat came rising expectations, both economic and political. The militia disappeared, the prisons were emptied of the innocent, private enterprise was re-born, the markets bustled once again and above all the oppressive yoke of fear and intimidation was removed. But beneath this greatly-improved exterior lies the basic and difficult to cure problems of underdevelopment and a young cadre of proud intellectuals whose books during their formative years were not Aristotle and the Koran, but the teachings of Marx. It is their whispered opinion that socialism did not fail, only Modibo Keita.

Chapter III
The Crocodile City

The Russian Ilyushian-18 descended ever so gradually, like a conservative old lady, down over the square mud roofs of Bamako. The powder blue of the Atlantic was a thousand miles away, behind endless stretches of parched bush, which rolled with a regular monotony into the four horizons. There were only seven passengers on the plane, eleven altogether, including the Russian pilot and his crew. The other forty three seats were empty, a mute reminder as to why Air Mali was loosing several thousands of dollars per week at that time. There were first and tourist classes, an unexpected oddity on a Russian plane serving in a socialist state.

Western journalists and visitors were often abrasive in their evaluations of Air Mali because it was an African airline operated by Russians. This was, in their view, credential enough for it being both unsafe and inferior. But compared to the French-owned airlines which service this part of Africa, Air Mali has more comfortable flights (the seats on the Ilyushians not only tilt back, but also have bottoms which slide forward), gives more courteous service and better meals. In recent years, they have added a Boeing 727 and an American crew to their fleet, thus competing with their French rivals who have given up cramped Caravelles for DC-Eights.

The Niger crawled into view out of a scintillating backdrop of opaque heat waves, a wide brown sluggish stream, twisting and turning in lazy loops and dead-end channels as if in no particular hurry to go anywhere. The engines were throttled down and we began to descend, the plane's pliable shadow gliding up and down over the rounded tops of the Manding Hills. The City of Bamako, which in Bambara means "Marshland of the Crocodiles," sprawled out along the left bank of the river, a dusty hot mosaic of varying shades of browns with white colonial era buildings, banked with clusters of trees sprinkled in here and there. The Malians had said they were looking forward to welcoming me to Mali and indeed I was looking forward to the day of my arrival there. The plane roared down through a choppy layer of hot down drafts and made a perfect landing on the simmering tar strip. We coasted up to a big red barn of a building which was the terminal. The door swung open and a gush of hot dry air inundated the cabin within seconds. I stepped out and from that moment onward for five years had the dubious renown of being unique as the only American physician in Mali. A delegation of two had come out from the embassy to meet me and they were the only people standing in the hollow empty building. No Malians were there. We drove off into town, past the rows of *banco* (mud) buildings and the architectural vestiges of the French colonial past, down the tree lined streets and into a quarter called *Quartier Fleuve*. The Quartier Fleuve runs along the river bank, shaded by mango and mimosa trees, an area of several square blocks, sheltering plain but cozy cement block homes. Most are built in a modern tropical design flanked by flowering gardens which are kept alive through tenacity, an unbelievable amount of water and a few prayers. The quarter has several swimming pools and is replete with the usual accessories of the ex-patriate ghetto, blonde headed kids riding their bicycles down the broken tarmac for fun next to Africans who ride theirs out of necessity, black nannies walking their white charges and pampered dogs and cats dominating the verandas with an arrogant air of ownership. This was Bamako's version of the European ghetto which exists in virtually every capital city of West Africa. They're more often than not white reservations, built on the top of the highest hill, across the river, on an island, on the other side of the road, anywhere which is physically, mentally and culturally away from the Africa they're in. They used to be occupied by colonists, but now they're lived in by more acceptable foreign experts, who while they have a different name, still possess some of the old ex-patriate habits and attitudes. There was even a time when the only Africans allowed into such quarters were servants. No one else had a good reason to be there.

With credit to Bamako and Mali, the Quartier Fleuve is a rather poor rendition of the standard ex-patriate ghetto. There are a good many Malians living in its twenty-one block area. Besides boasting cozy homes and swimming pools. The Juartier Fleuve has a lumber yard, a soft drinks factory, a body and fender shop, two noisy iron works, the equipment yard for the Public Works Department, the stretch of the Niger used for washing clothes and dredging sand, three schools bursting at the seams with several thousand Malian children, the offices of the ruling Military Committee of National Liberation, a local produce market, an occasionally used Chinese exhibition hall, the biggest open sewer in Mali and the homes of the American, Israeli and Yugoslav ambassadors.

At given times of the day, the streets are filled with boisterous school kids, balancing books on their heads, picking mangoes off the trees and killing bats with sling shots. They are joined by a few black and green Willys jeeps, carrying American embassy personnel and school children home, jerking Deux Chevaux and sleek Mercedes bearing license plates marked C. D., Corps Diplomatique in green and black paint. Most children walk home from school. Others, however, are shuttled back and forth in land rovers and Volkswagon mini buses bearing official government plates and the blue wreathed UNICEF insignia on their doors.

The Quartier Fleuve is also called home by the trucks and tractors of the Genie Rurale. It has always been my personal theory that the Quartier Flueve was originally meant to be an industrial park, until someone changed their mind, but not quite in time. It used to be called the Quartier Brasserie in honor of the brewery which no longer turns out beer but state produced Gazelle soft drinks. The Malians have two different names for this quarter — *Banantou* which is Bambara means "the place of the kapoc trees" and *Quartier Toubabou* which in French means "the white man's quarter." Both are appropriate considering what is found there. The kapoc trees provide plenty of shade and cozy corners which make this quarter a favorite rendez-vous for lovers and a pick-up area for unattached couples.

The homes and bungalows in this quarter don't measure up to the standard of those found in coastal cities in West Africa, but they are liveable and comfortable. Contrary to what one might think, the Americans in Mali did not live in the finer houses. They were for the most part less extravagant in their living habits than many other foreigners and occupy houses which are sub-standard even for Bamako. The majority of houses in Bamako are owned by Lebanese merchants, absent French landlords, and occasionally by Malians. The low cost of labor and building materials in Bamako enable these landlords to recoup their investment within three years by renting houses to diplomatic missions at inflated rates.

Americans who arrive in Bamako to take up official duties at the embassy walk out of the hot airport and into a home freshly painted, carefully cleaned and furnished, the refrigerator and cupboard full of all the necessities of life. The beds are made, the air conditioners churning and everything from the pillow cases to a can opener left in its place in order to help the new arrivals along until their household effects are dragged up on the railroad from Dakar. To my knowledge that has happened to each and every American who has come to Bamako to take up official functions with the exception of two, myself and the first consular officer who opened the diplomatic mission in 1960.

I pushed open the door of what was to be my home and got a couple of pieces of flaked off white wash on my head for the effort. The rooms were done up in ecologic natural, my description of a decor which includes empty rooms with fine red dust weeks old over the floor, ceilings and walls. Even the white wash had lost its tenacity to hang onto the walls. The furnishings consisted of two electric light bulbs of Russian make which didn't work, a French sink with no water running out of the faucet, an American made john which didn't flush, an English shower which didn't work, gaping holes for windows with no screens, tailor made for everything to enter from bats to mosquitoes, and enter they did, and finally an electric ceiling fan right out of an Edgar Rice Burroughs story, which didn't do much except round out the normal ecology by creating a miniature dust storm.

When I asked about the furniture, someone said the administrative officer was responsible for having it put in. But since there wasn't an administrative officer at the time, no one was really sure who was supposed to have it put in. It was later explained that I, being a member of the United States Public Health Service and not of either the State Department or the Agency for International Development, was not really an official member of the embassy. Although it wasn't said, I gathered that I didn't qualify for the usual reception.

It was close to lunch time and everyone left, saying that the Minister of Health and the Director General of Health wanted to see me in the morning. They also said the embassy nurse was dying to meet me since she had lots of chronic medical problems. Sadie Rogers was a kind old motherly person whom you couldn't help love and we later weathered many a medical storm together in Bamako. But when she walked into my "home" that first night, I was the coldest thing there and I didn't defrost until many weeks later. Sadie left Mali seven months after I arrived and by that time the rains had flooded me out on just one too many occasions. Even the Edgar Rice Burroughs fans had given up the ghost. Sadie willed me her cozy little bungalow, tucked away in a cool grove of mango trees, and although it isn't pretentious, it is at least a place one can call home. My original home later became a Malian government office.

The following morning we drove up the hair pin drive to one of the twin hills behind Bamako called Koulouba. That hill was a very simple and direct appellation in Bambara. It means big hill. The Presidential Palace and many of the government ministries are located on this hill, high up in the currents of a steady fresh breeze, away from the stagnating heat of the city. Koulouba used to be Bamako's white ghetto, the place where the governor of the Sudan and all the high officials lived, away from the people and perhaps a bit away from the reality at the bottom of the hill.

The Minister and the Director settled down with us for a two-hour conference. We were in a certain sense old acquaintants, I having accompanied them on an official State Department tour of the United States some four months before. The health and welfare of my mother and brothers were asked for sandwiched in between a discussion about gasoline for the trucks and our freedom to travel around the country. The Minister said he was very happy to welcome me to Mali and looked forward to our working harmoniously with the Director General. The Director didn't say anything along those lines. He bubbled over in domineering profuse oratory about eradicating smallpox and controlling measles, mentioning what he had already done, but saying little as to what he was going to allow me to do. He had very fixed ideas about most things and treated me as if I were an adversary.

My office, like my house, was dust covered, but the Malians had done the Americans one better and had at least put a fresh coat of paint on everything from the ceiling to the floor. Like my house, there wasn't any furniture, but through the help of Peter Daniells, the Director of AID, a desk was borrowed and with that I was in business. Peter also came up with an open Willys jeep, painted a bright Kelly Green, with which to navigate around Bamako. I got settled into Bamako by osmosis, without ever realizing it was happening and the inundation of work didn't give me a second to sit and reflect on the adaptation process.

Bringing a wife to Bamako is a gamble, the chances are less than one in a hundred that she'll like it. With the men it's different since they have their jobs to keep them busy. But the women have to be inventive and design their own pattern of work and living. They have to find things to do which will take their minds off their discontent, free themselves from long hours of solitude and isolation from the world they're used to and prevent themselves from becoming an unbearable nag to their husbands. If they do become nags, their husbands will end up agreeing to everything they've said without ever having listened. If there are children to be taken care of, a nanny will do it, except if they're of school age, then the boy will do it. A few ingenious mothers don't have nannies or cooks and keep themselves happily occupied the day long as they would back in the States.

The American women who have lived in Bamako have been extremely adaptable creatures. Aside from some movie theaters which show out-dated films, Bamako has little to offer an American woman. There are no concerts, no plays (except those the American women put on), no libraries, no museums, no meetings to go to, no community programs to take part in, no television, no good newspapers, backyard fences to lean on, but no one to talk over to and no far-away weekend trips to be made. Official Americans are still not allowed out of a sixty mile radius of the city of Bamako without submitting a written request to the Foreign Ministry five days before. It wasn't rare during the old regime that these carefully prepared diplomatic notes were sent back by the Malians ripped in two meaning the request had been denied.

The women have had clothing drives for needy Malian children, giving the clothing to the Malian social welfare centers and were told they couldn't be present to see it distributed. Had they been allowed to participate in the distribution of the clothing, some Malian mothers might have had reason to doubt all of the evil things they used to say about the American imperialists. They took turns taking supper to the Point-G Hospital where Angelo, the Peruvian born Italian who works as an electrician for the Americans in Mali was sick with hepatitis. I sent Angelo up to the hospital with his own bed, since there weren't any empty ones left up there, knowing that they could scarcely refuse a patient arriving for admission with his own bed. The ladies agreed to take him supper every night, even though one remarked, "Who is Angelo?" I have only been at odds with this group once, when they asked that I play the role of an angel in their Christmas pageant and agree to be suspended with wires from a tree on the ambassador's lawn. I qualified they said on the basis of my cherubic face. Even though they had to do without their angel (he having conveniently flown off to the States) they did collect fifty dollars and gave it to me for buying medicines with which to treat sick Malians out in the bush.

There are many ex-patriates who come to places like Mali, not out of crusading desire to ameliorate the problems of the country, but rather out of selfishness. With a cold sense of detachment, they come in with a private company or a bilateral assistance program and pursue their greedy goal of amassing their overly inflated salary checks, many times more than what they could justly earn at home. These people were once called colonialists, but now they are referred to as foreign experts, technical advisors, which in the eyes of the African makes them more acceptable. Since independence, their ranks have been swollen by the addition of numbers from the Communist bloc, who enjoy living in places like Mali because it gives them a freedom they've never enjoyed at home. They say they love Africa, but what they really mean is that they love the life they enjoy in Africa, a life they would never merit back home, a life which has its roots not in the altruism of giving, but in the crass pragmatism of taking. One old French ex-patriate who had been in Mali for twenty years put it all into a nutshell. "People like us are not scholars; we're not missionaries, in fact most of us aren't even interested in the least in the African. We're here because it gives us the chance of eating steak for dinner every night instead of chicken and beans back in France."

There are some Frenchmen who have stayed on in Mali for decades. One finds them in almost every major town in the bush where they form a peculiar sub-culture all unto their own. They are the local *broussards,* the man who came in 1918 looking for crocodile skins or the family which arrived at the turn of the century. Some of the men have married with Africans, placing themselves in a cultural limbo between the African and the European. No matter how one looks at it, all of these people are escapees from their own cultures, escapees which even Africa will not have room for forever.

Descriptions of Bamako have varied from that of a dumpy tropical town to the Paris of the savannah. The latter term while exotic and inventive is misleading, unless it refers to the Paris of another century. The truth like Mali's old political inclinations lies somewhere in between, but more towards the less complimentary side. Bamako is both physically and mentally a traditional sudanese town. The influence of the continuous French presence from 1883 until 1960 lingers on as a faint far whisper in the white birthday cake architecture of official government buildings, built interestingly enough by Chinese laborers at the turn of the cenutry, in tree-lined avenues, in the language, habits and tastes of the evolués, in the ponderous bureaucracy where everyone from the head of state down to the local gas station attendant has an impressive looking stamp, in the pallid remains of the French restaurants and shops and in the *depassé* sporting clubs which have long since lost their luster. But Bamako, unlike Dakar, was never so French that it would seem incongruous to find beggars, donkey carts and lepers, by the score, the latter thrusting their stumped hands out at passers by. They have the city divided into territories, so the same lepers are found on the same street corners all the year round.

If French influence is faint, it's because French investment in the Sudan was also faint. There wasn't much done even in a town like Bamako, and what was done was primarily for the convenience and facility of the French living in and administering the territory. There weren't many schools and most of those which one sees today in both

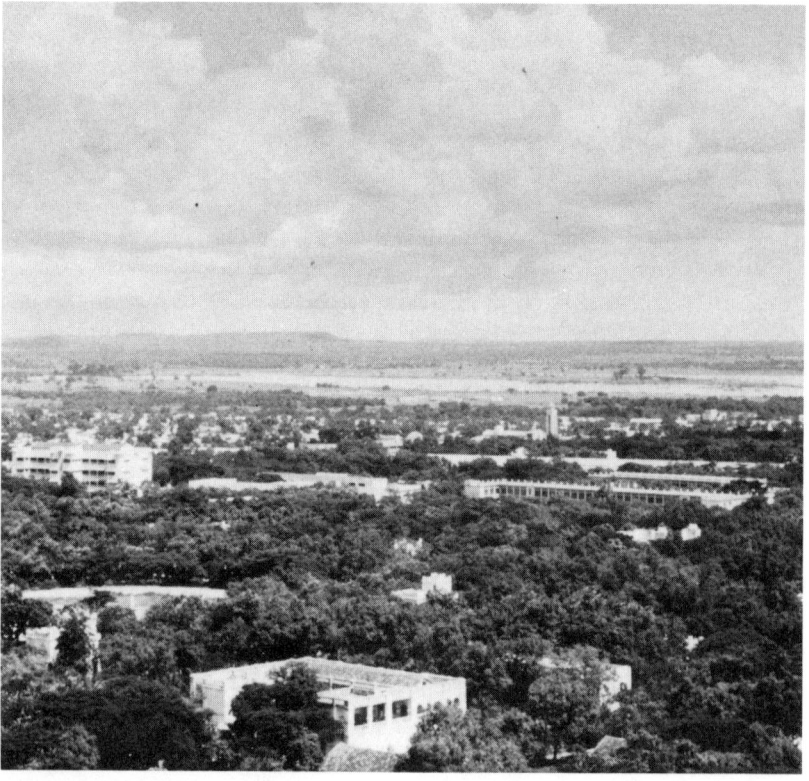

FIGURE 5. An overview of Bamako from Koulouba. The Niger River can be seen in the background.

Bamako and the bush have been built since independence. There was never a university, but the Ecole Normale which glistens in glass and steel on top of the hill across the river in Badalabougou is the seed of what will someday be Mali's university. The illiteracy rate is still ninety-five percent and in some districts in the bush the only literate men are foreigners to the area who have been sent in to administer affairs for the government.

There was no industry, no modern hospitals, no good roads, two important bridges, no rural development. Compared to Ghana and the Ivory Coast, Mali is what those countries were a half-century ago. The French rightly argue that they had their hands full just administering this enormous territory and that there was little in it which could be developed. They placed their emphasis on agriculture and developed a gigantic irrigation scheme on the middle Niger called the Office du Niger. But in spite of the impressive fields of cotton, rice and millet which stretch from horizon to horizon in the canal-fed office, the scheme has never paid for itself.

There was no rash of building in Bamako, no glistening white towers thrusting their heads against the sky, except the seventeen story Hotel d'Amitie which the Egyptians built. There was a ponderous sameness as if everything were suddenly stiffled and stopped in its tracks at an arbitrary point in time. The battle seemed not to build anew, but rather to prevent what was already there from falling into decay. Buildings crumbled, paint peeled, fences fell and windows cracked. The signs of a slowly creeping decay used to be everywhere, in the traffic lights which had long since ceased to give anyone directions, in the rusted road signs which told you nothing except how old they were, in the gardens interred in silent barrenness and in the paved streets full of holes and without names. Some of this has changed since the 1968 military take-over. At least the traffic lights now work and major pot holes in the streets are filled in. Even the airport now has its full complement of landing lights, a comforting sight to those of us who once landed in almost absolute darkness.

This lack of building had a philosophical basis which evoked more admiration than the white towers of Abidjan and Dakar. The Malians were committed to a course of independence, self-reliance and dignity. White towers would be built they said, but when they could afford to build them themselves and when Mali and Malians had need for them. This self-imposed austerity was said to be nothing more than living within one's own means, avoiding indulgence in artificial luxuries, doing things on one's own and in one's own good time. In principle, all of this is more admirable than stacks of skyscrapers built for and by the Europeans or shops full of fancy European imports which only the Europeans can afford to buy. Foreigners always considered Bamako to be a city undergoing decay in both physique and function. In a sense, they were right. The admirable principle of austerity became tarnished when it was found after the coup d'etat that the funds for the city's upkeep were always there, except in other people's pockets. The city continus to grow without the guiding hand of urban development schemes so that in the next decade Bamako will become a large city with all of the problems inherent to haphazard synthesis.

Many have called Bamako the city of nameless streets, because the streets often have no names and those which do lost their signs during the independence celebrations. People who live in Bamako manage to navigate around by following complicated instructions. If you're invited somewhere, your verbal instructions might be to turn left down the third street after passing over the little bridge which crosses the big sewer running between the two big kapocs. It's the small blue house with the white shutters, standing under three big mango trees and if you have trouble finding it just look out for my car which will be parked out front. If the car isn't out front, you're in for trouble, but usually invited guests are given a map as a precaution.

Visitors used to complain about the garbage piled up in big round mounds on the streets, the open sewers with smoldering fires consuming their debris, the mosquitoes and the flies. The Malians being sensitive people were insulted by these accusations and took them to heart. I told them that most West African cities have open sewers and there are few lacking in flies and mosquitoes. As for the garbage piled high on the streets, the visitors were right. It used to be collected sporadically by the Voirie who made their only predictable visit at Christmas time, not to collect garbage, but to collect undeserved gifts. The rest of the time it piled up on the streets and was either burned or sold for three hundred francs a bundle to local farmers for compost. Now the city has an excellent fleet of garbage trucks and collections are made three times a week, more than what is done in New York City.

The city boasts an excellent water purification plant which not only filters water, but also chlorinates it. But the city's pipes are old and often break, and since the water has to travel clear across town and up to the reservoir on Koulouba and then down again, the state of purity is questionable by the time it comes out of the tap. Most Malians drink water in Bamako which comes out of wells dug in the center of their family compounds. These *concessions* or courtyards may have half a dozen families living in them sharing a common well and a common latrine. Many of these wells are contaminated by nearby cesspools and this makes diseases like polio, typhoid fever and infectious hepatitis endemic in the city. The European Development Fund intends to give Bamako a new water supply system which is to cost some five million dollars to construct.

The earth around Bamako is brown, the houses in twenty of the twenty-one quarters are baked brown clay and there is brown dust covering everything in the dry season, even the trees. From a distance, the quarters look like excrescences on the earth's surface, produced by some quake, ready at any minute to fall back inside again. In the rainy season, the rains wash the mud away and smooth walls become pocked and scarred like eroded channels.

The air is acrid in the dry season, a peculiar combination of the scent of flowering mango trees and smoldering fires. It's both sweet and enchanting, but beneath it there is a hidden harshness which one cannot see nor touch, but which one intuitively feels. Fires are always burning in Bamako, not as huge roaring infernos, but as smoldering columns of belching white smoke. It seems nature always provides something to burn. If there aren't leaves, and that's rare, then there are the long sausage shaped pods of the acacias and when both of these are lacking, there is always a supply of garbage.

Cooking fires burn throughout the day, but it's only towards five in the evening when the inversion phenomenon sets in that one becomes aware of them. I've often climbed up on the hills behind Bamako at sundown, a thousand feet above the city, and watched the white smoke glide up until it hit the solid layer of cold air, and then spread out in milky horizontal sheets clear across the river. In January and December, the truly cold months in Bamako, the temperatures fall down to fifty degrees Farenheit and lower after sundown. The sun sets at six instead of at seven and people build fires in the concessions to keep themselves warm.

The *guardians* throughout the town lie on their low bamboo beds, wrapped up snugly in their white wool Macina blankets, a small fire smoldering less than a foot away. By morning, the city is blanketed with a thick white veil which brings tears to the eyes of the least allergic and cold and pneumonia to children and underfed bodies. Only when the sun comes out does the layer of cold air and smog lift.

But on some days not even the sun can break the grip of the cold air blanket and international flights head for Dakar and departing flights out of Bamako are grounded. The cause of this air pollution problem stands at the back of the city, the Manding Hills. They surround the city on three sides, the twin hills of Koulouba and Point G thrusting themselves like trapping fingers forward into the town, preventing any breeze from blowing in and ridding the city of its own smokey wastes. Complicating all of this is the *Harmattan,* the dry air current which descends down over all of West Africa in December from the Sahara, bringing with it a permanent and stagnant atmosphere of dust.

The peaks which surround Bamako have names, but few foreigners know them. They are at their best during the rainy season, covered with a dark green coat, with far off storms swirling ovr their heads, sending down rays of diagonal precipitation like a holy gesture. The sun sets behind them, behind Ntekedokoulou, Kokakoutou and Nieklkoulouni and all of the other mysterious peaks which mark off in gray misty symmetry into Guinea, off to the far away Fouta Djalon. The sun finally sinks out of sight, throwing the twin mesas of Sebekoulou and Quinsinkoulou into bold black silhouette against a screen of changing fiery red. These hills have known their share of history; the great and the small have walked up and down their slopes. Sundiata Keita, the son of the Lion Man and the Buffalo Woman, rode over them with his soldiers in the thirteenth century to defend his Manding Empire of Mali from the Sorcerer King of Sosso. At any rate, this is what the *griots* (story tellers) say. Mungo Park, the British explorer, was the first white man ever to see the little fishing village of Bamuku from them in 1805 and in 1883 they felt the marching feet of Borgnis des Bordes and his soldiers who had just taken Bamako for France. Now the hills are silent, worn down and rounded with age, a bit tired, a bit weary. They are deep in their wisdom, mysterious in their silence, tranquil to say nothing of Sundiata and his men, unmoved to issue a faint far echo of Mungo Park and his sailors, and disinclined to remember Borgnis des Bordes and his marching men.

Bamako's colors, sounds, smells and joie de vivre change with a stunning dynamism difficult to believe for a place which is supposed to be tropical. The city is drowned in red bougainvillea and poinsettas in January, red Bombax in February, yellow cassias and lace-like mimosa blossoms in March, silk cotton trees and their snowball puffs of seeds in April along with the yellow flowers of the *Sinjan,* vibrant red flamboyants carpeting the town from the Niger to the Manding Hills in May and then in June the rains, turning everything an unbelievable wonderful green. All of the trees get new dust-free leaves in March, a time when the city is its greenest from above, but its driest from below.

The higher orders have their cycles also. The grasshoppers come out in January, the flies in February, ants in March, spiders in late April, cockroaches and thousands of white butterflies in May and crickets straggling in from March until June. Millipeds meander in around June and don't leave until December, marching up and down my living room floor in batallions, regiments and companies. My houseboy, Ahmadou, used to keep a truce with the roaches out in the kitchen by leaving stale bread out for them to eat. His reasoning was logical in a Malian sort of way — that way they wouldn't eat the other things in the kitchen. But the roaches violated the truce and not only ate the other things in the kitchen, but also started rummaging through my desk drawers and pushing for room in the bed at night. So there was an end to the truce and when the battle was over Ahmadou counted over three hundred enemy dead.

Mosquitoes in Bamako are four motored, biting on bony prominences, on knuckles, on the nose, around the eyes and on the forehead. They bite on bites and then bite on top of these just for the heck of it. They go through clothing like a hot needle through hard butter and bite on parts of the anatomy considered inaccessible and off limits to any decent insect. Bees and mud wasps come on the scene in February, the latter minding their own business and the former causing no end of trouble. I once came home and found that a swarm of bees had moved into my kitchen without prior consent. The eviction proceedings didn't go off without incident and I had a swollen eye the next day, just in time to be presented with it to the visiting Undersecretary of State for African Affairs. Another queen swarmed down over a pool one day where twenty Americans were bathing and gave her followers the order to charge. This incident was extremely serious since many of the children present had a dozen and more bites.

Downtown Bamako is one huge throbbing cacophony of human life and energy which will never have an end. There is babbling, shouting and singing whipped into a noisy batter of chugging Deux Chevauxs, buzzing Mobylettes, creaking bicycles, the clicking of hoofs on the choppy macadam and the roaring of monstrous Mercedes and Berliet trucks. Women glide by in yards of flowing cotton, blues, greens and reds, shimmering like debutants, their thin necks supporting enormous enamel basins filled with bananas, lettuce, carrots and fish. The married women wear *grand bou bous,* a delicately woven lace like chemise of tulle of shining Chinese silk, underneath which is tucked a youngster, inconspicuous even as a bump buried under so many yards of cloth. Younger single girls wear blouses of printed cloth and wrap arounds stamped with pictures of Kennedy, leading African politicians and such phrases as Mon Amour and Mon Cher. Their outfit is cut so that the phrases wind up on prominent eminences of the anatomy where I suppose their wearers feel they will have the greatest effect. Men wear long mother hubbards, *bou bous,* black tasseled fezzes, conical straw hats, and occasionally a western suit, but the latter is rare. The poorer wear torn shirts and, like the more affluent used to have, an amazing variety of Mao buttons attached.

Beggars cry for alms in front of the shops frequented by the Europeans, the blind are led through the streets by youngsters pulling them along by sticks. They chant versus from the Koran and ask for money from those whom the youngster manages to corner. Some blind people walk around together, singing versus from the Koran or else their own songs in which they ask for alms. In most instances, their families are fully capable of supporting them, but the infirmity is used as a means of increasing the family income through begging. Urchins pester motorists for a few francs to guard their cars against what they're not really sure. The beggars and lepers descend on Sundays onto the steps of the worn-out Catholic Cathedral for the ten o'clock service since all of the Europeans go to church at that hour. They pass up the eight o'clock mass which is attended mostly by Malians, knowing that their chances of collecting anything will be quite slim.

Anyone from the age of five years to ninety who has anything to sell from a mango to a pair of second-hand shoes is in business, either pacing up and down the crowded streets in a tireless fashion, bothering all the shoppers except the Chinese whom they know won't buy anything, squatted against a wall with an arm and leg thrust out as a barricade or seated royally in a fixed spot in one of Bamako's five markets. People aren't in business to sell. Even if they don't sell anything they're happy if they've passed the day in what we would call non-productive palavering and social intercourse.

The main market, located in the center of the city, looks like a Hollywood mock-up for a scene out of *Lawrence of Arabia.* You almost expect to find turbaned riflemen posted behind the red battlements and some evil looking pasha sitting on a heap of cushions inside. The French Foreign Legion should logically charge down the narrow streets, surround the fortress and take the pasha and his men into custody. This market is called the *Grand Marché,* an obvious French appellation, even to the non-Francophone. The Malians call it *Soukoba* which means "big market' 'in Bambara. Its counters used to run over with Chinese made hardware and kitchen utensils from Poland. Since the coup d'etat the quantity of items in it has doubled, the majority coming from France and neighboring African countries. Printed cloth drapes its way in zig-zags around one third of its outer perimeter, a bold motif designed by a very unconventional artist. The stalls inside are splashed with tables of woven cloth sold by shrewd Sarakole, sacs of red kola nuts hawked by the Dioula, corridors of squatting Hausa tradesmen from Northern Nigeria bargaining jewelry, cowrie shells and medicines guaranteed to cure everything from cancer to impotence and groups of women sitting in the middle of neat little heaps of exotic and common spices, incense and red chili peppers. For a few thousand francs you can buy a woman's wig in *Soukoba.* Malian women have long liked wearing wigs, the wealthier ones buying theirs in France. The less affluent have to settle for the horse hair creations made locally in Bamako and sold at the market alongside kola nuts and spices. The aroma of this market is always the same, acrid, exciting and pleasing. It never changes, being just the right combination of spices, incense and cooked grain foods, mixed up with a touch of freshly indigoed cloth and human sweat.

The Avenue du Peuple is appropriately named, it having more people walking on it per square foot than any other street in Bamako. It splashes your senses with bicycle parts, dried fish markets, straw mat markets, markets selling the black and white wool blankets from the inland delta region, outdoor photo studios where for a few francs you can have your picture taken by a turn of the century box camera equipped with a bottle cap as a shutter, and scores of *petitis commercants* selling Malian cigarettes on top of their little wooden tables and French brands underneath. Men scramble down this street in their Sudanese trousers, the *taba ladji* which are enormous sacs, but in spite of them manage to balance everything on their heads from cement bags to six foot long *capitains* (Nile Perch). And once I saw a man carrying a fully grown banana tree on his head upright, making them together about twelve feet tall. This area of Bamako is called *Dabanani* by the Malians wihch means in Bambara "the place of four streets."

Emaciated horses pull dilapadated wagons charged with everything from a score of weary passengers to freight boxes stamped with Chinese characters. These wagons are locally made affairs, an essence of used automobile tires and old crate wood. The big green and white buses of TUB — Transport Urbaine Bamako roar down narrow streets with tenacious patience and the little Peugeot tarpaulin-covered pick-up trucks known as *baches* in French and *dourodouroni* in Bambara fly with reckless speed, honking their way down the Avenue du Peuple, their passengers oblivious to their second-by-second escapes with a near accident. Everyone is on the move, by foot, on bicycles, on motor bikes, in buses, on top of trucks and some of the more affluent in cars of their own. The few American cars circulating around town not belonging to the embassy are the acquisitions of Malians who were formerly assigned to the Malian embassy in Washington.

The heterogeneous nature of Mali's population is reflected on virtually every street in Bamako. Stern-faced Mauritanians briskly walk the streets of the Bagadaji quarter, their heads wrapped up in blue turbans full of lice, their white food-stained robes covered with leather sacs containing taismans called *barah*. Hausa barbers shave men's heads underneath the stunted trees surrounding the main mosque and give their customers a choice of cut from the sample and hair styles painted on wooden boards. For the ex-patriates not willing to sample the adventure of a Hausa barber surgeon, there are three conventional barber shops in town. The Peul are fine featured people who drive their cattle and sheep through the narrow streets of the quarters in a wave of swooshing sounds and dust. You can almost set your watch by their arrival at a given spot in town every day. One of the largest herds in Bamako used to pass the USAID offices every afternoon at 4 P.M. and it wasn't rare that a conference had the pleasure of the presence of a horned head in the window. The Maures move with herds of sheep and goats and if you're not expert enough to tell the difference between a Maure and a Peul you might look at their sheep. Those of the Maures are always much bigger. The Peul and the Maures camp for the night on the dusty embankment of the best paved street in Bamako — the Avenue de l'Independence where their herds of sheep pass the night in rosette clusters with their heads bowed down together at a central point on the ground. These nomads spend the night next to the retired looms of the weavers and a group of men who make their living stuffing a unique brand of Malian matress.

Mixed up into this stimulus rich environment are White Fathers on motor bikes and White Sisters on bicycles. Russians ride by the half-dozen in the back of Gaz jeeps and the Chinese by the score in big windowed buses. The Russian women carry their big hulky frames in plain housedresses and their heads in bandanas which sort of makes you think they really belong on a collective farm in the Ukraine. On Saturday mornings they are all carted into town in a bus so that everyone can shop collectively and insure that their friends and neighbors don't get too bourgeois in their tastes. The Russian embassy has a commissary which is stocked with goods flown in from Moscow once a week. I usually can tell the day of its arrival by the boistrous parties thrown by my neighbors to celebrate the occasion.

The Russians and Eastern Europeans wear sandles, but with socks. The French wear sandles, but without socks and Americans rarely wear anything but shoes. Practically everyone goes to work without a tie and jacket except the Americans and the Germans, but then they work in air conditioned offices where such attire can't be considered the English madness practiced in Nigeria and Ghana where, air conditioner or not, *everyone* must wear a tie and jacket. The Chinese wear baggy cuffed trousers from the style of the thirties and waddle with flat-footed gaits by the threes or the dozen. The North Koreans and the North Vietnamese have women among their official personnel, but the Chinese don't.

The Americans and the French will talk to practically anyone, the Chinese to no one and the North Koreans and North Vietnamese to some. Americans did not speak to the Chinese, North Koreans and North Vietnamese. The Russians speak to the Americans, North Koreans and North Vietnamese, but not to the Chinese. The East Germans ignore the West Germans, the Israelis ignore the Egyptians and Saudi Arabians and the Americans ignore the Cubans.

Only the Chinese and the Malians used to wear Mao buttons and carry little red Mao books. Now only the Chinese do. Malians now keep the outer red plastic covers of these books and use them as wallets since they have convenient pockets in them. Lots of other people have both buttons and books, but keep them at home as curios to show relatives and friends back home. The Chinese and Eastern Europeans smell of garlic when you pass them close by. Interestingly enough, the French don't. The Russians are loud in both voice and manners, the Chinese mute and the Americans admirably just right. The Israeli women remind me of Molly Goldberg, the Egyptian men of sinister characters out of an espionage film and the Lebanese matrons of bossomy mothers just made for hugging babies and taking care of big families. Frenchmen take to wearing beards in Bamako, not big unkempt bushy affairs, but neat narrow picture frame types. Malians wear beards too, primarily out of necessity to avoid the agony and post shave acne from using poor quality razor blades. The older men wear them in adherence to Moslem custom.

Americans swim in swimming pools, the Russians in the public pool they built at the Stade Omnisport, the French in the Niger River at Sotuba where they get schistosomiasis and the Chinese not at all. The Americans and the French keep horses out at the riding stable, the French have a canoeing club and all nationalities, the Eastern Bloc included, participate in outings sponsored by the Friends of Tourism Club. These outings are headed by a Monsieur Dumont who drags his sturdy followers up and down cliffs, into pre-historic caves which surround Bamako, down rivers in rubber rafts and occasionally far out into the bush.

The Chinese embassy in Bamako scarcely looks functional from the point of view of carrying out normal open office procedures. Surrounded by a high yellow wall with cut-glass on top, and with a bright red and yellow gate in the center, it looks like a left-over from the shooting of *The Siege of Peking*. Close by are the dormitories used by the Chinese, dashed with Chinese characters, political slogans, pictures of Mao and various "hate America" themes. The USAID compound was flanked by an interesting array which included the East German Economic Mission, the North Vietnamese Embassy (just across the street), the Chinese Embassy and dormitories and the North Korean Embassy.

Mao buttons used to shine in unimaginable variety from polo shirts bearing such slogans as "Joe's Bowling Alley," "Vicks Vapo Rub," and "Boy's Club of America." Up in the north in the desert, Tuareg nomads made an anachronistic sight decked out with their swords, their faces covered with indigo veils, their little transistor radios blasting away and their Mao buttons in place. After the coup d'etat, the word got around that Mao buttons and books were no longer in vogue and so one rarely sees them anymore. On the other hand, the used clothing coming from the United States and Europe is catching on again, after having been prohibited by thef ormer regime. The Malians call this clothing *yougou yougou* which means "to shake out," in Bambara. The appellation refers to the practice of shaking each piece after renewing it from a tightly packed bale. This clothing comes into Mali from the coast, especially from Liberia, where it is imported and distributed by traders and various missionary groups. The missionaries bring it over to Africa either having obtained it free from charitable organizations or else having purchased it from wholesalers. It is sold to traders for a price which covers the initial investment and transport charges and these men in turn market it to retailers for about thirty dollars a bundle. When you see *yougou yougou* polo shirts bearing such slogans as Los Angeles Dodgers and Baldwin, Long Island Little League on children up in the remote Sahara you do a double take and then smile.

Mao's picture used to be ubiquitous in Bamako. One could find it on office walls, staring up at you from beneath glass covered desks, looking out from inside medicine cabinets and tacked to doors, windows and classroom blackboards. Chinese goods with such innocuous names as Great Wall Powdered Milk, Two Swan stencil paper, Red Flower bicycles, Chrysanthemum office pins, Hero stamp pads, Fan soap powder and Panda condensed milk used to crowd the little stalls all over Bamako. One can still find Chinese products, but the quantity has greatly diminished since Mali and France signed a new financial agreement before the 1968 coup d'etat. French products are gradually replacing them. The Librarie Populaire still has its counters smothered with Chinese propaganda literature, color magazines from Russia, North Korea and East Germany, Paris newspapers, right, left and center and both *Newsweek* and *Time*.

Few Malians can afford to buy an American newsmagazine, and fewer still can read English. But for the price of one American cent, most can buy *La Chine*, A Monthly pictorial magazine about China, and virtually all can look at the color pictures of massive Nuremburg style gatherings and be duly impressed. Radio Mali still relates American economic setbacks and race riots in the United States. At one time, hours of broadcast time were filled up with traditional music into which was put un-traditional political messages and praises for Modibo Keita, the former president. Nothing was said of course about the general discontent in the Malian bush, the repressive strong-arm tactics inflicted on the peasants when they didn't produce their government quota of grain, nor the indiscriminate arrests and detentions without trial which were rampant. The only newspaper, *L'Essor,* once the editorial of Modibo Keita's Marxist regime is now the paper of the ruling military junta. It used to be full of hazy ideological discourses written by sophomoric Malians. Now one finds an occasional complimentary article about the United States and advertisements for various products and services. The editorial policies of *L'Essor* are said to be non-aligned, but in practical terms it is often difficult to appreciate this since the west is rarely praised. While the newspapers of the world greeted the flight of Apollo 11 as the event of the century, *L'Essor's* correspondent criticized it as a waste of money. He thought that this money could have been put to better use by the countries of the *tiers monde.*

In spite of the revolutionary Marxist fervor which existed in Mali, the Mao buttons and the Chinese soap powder, the French were still able to drink their wine in peace and comfort and have a good meal at the only decent restaurant in Bamako, *L'Aquariam,* while listening to the music of the only juke box in the country. The French cooperation teachers still dance their Saturday nights away on the illuminated floor of the discotheque bar, *Le Village* and evolué Malians do the same at *La Savanne.* Conservative old couples spend quiet weekends besides the overgrown swimming pool and water falls of the *Lido,* the Grossinger's of Mali, tucked away in the hills where until a few years ago tsetse flies and African Sleeping Sickness still abounded. The proprietors of this establishment all have had sleeping sickness in the past. Some of the North Vietnamese frequent the *Lido* on Sunday afternoons where they sip beer and eat locally made ice cream. Whiskey and gin have always been available in Bamako's two night clubs — *Les Trois Caimans* and *Le Jardin,* but the only place where one could get a Coca Cola used to be the campement in Timbuctoo. Now Coca Cola is available in Bamako.

An overview of Bamako is not complete without a description of its climate. One could not really call it distressing, but many feel it is oppressive. If you go to bed tired at night, without the benefit of an air conditioner, you'll wake up tired in the morning. There is no delicious balm in the air during the hot season, vistas don't stretch beyond the nearby trees, the horizons are blurred by a sand fog. You never feel like throwing out your chest, taking in a deep breath and saying, "How great it is to be alive!" One might say, "How sweet, how fragrant," and fall into a comfortable chair while saying it.

During the hot season which extends from February to June, the temperatures climb over a hundred and twenty degrees during the day and rarely fall below eighty at night. It reaches its worst during the months of April and May when the mercury never falls below ninety and the humidity is dried down to a bare twenty percent. Appropriately, the French call these months, *La Grande Chaleur.* The dust and the Harmattan are at their worst, all of which makes one too content to sit and do nothing. A coat of fine red dust covers everything in Bamako from the dining room table to the leaves on the trees.

Only when the rainy season begins in June does the sky at last seem pushed up high, a deep blue, powdered with oval puffs of creamy clouds. The cool wet air pushes in from the coast of Guinea and drives the hot dusty air back into the lap of the Sahara. The span of the world is almost gigantic and one can take a deep breath and feel the thrill of life all around. The nights become cool and tangy, with the stars beating down like a cold rain. The bare hills which for months have burned in copper colored dust become green and refreshing, the quivering heat waves disappear and the airless savanna is transformed into a sparkling meadow dashed with blue and yellow forget-me-nots. As if brought about by some miracle, the horiozns stretch out as far as sight will go, in alternating patterns of blue and green.

This violent seasonal contrast can only be appreciated by those who live in Mali. Visitors and tourists generally come in the dry season when the upcountry sights are accessible. And they refuse to believe that the burned up countryside, trilling with heat, could ever be transformed into a scene out of a Scottish summer. The rains end in October and from that month until January, Mali experiences cool dry weather. This is the most delightful season of the year and the best one for traveling. Tourist companies the world over have long known this and drag in their sturdy lot of retired school teachers for trips to Timbuctoo and the spectacular cliff villages of the Dogon. The temperature during the day hovers around seventy and at dusk when the sun tumbles below the Manding Hills, the thermometer registers a cool fifty. On such evenings you can sit comfortably outside and watch the egrets and herons fly in silhoueted formations down to the Niger. There is always a breeze in the air, filled with the fragrance of mango blossoms at first and later on with the sweet aroma of budding mimosas. More than ever, the Niger is a silver ribbon, cutting its way through a world of cool darkness and shimmering constellations. At day's end, the crickets chirp a deafening chorus, the sun goes to sleep behind the Manding Hills as it has done since the days when suns began going to sleep, the trees whisper, the smell of the Niger rolls up into the town, the drums start beating and the marabouts chant.

Bamako's silk cotton trees throw pools of darkness across the narrow streets and shower down the monotonous tolling of doves, the whistling of weaver birds and the chatter of sparrows. The frogs send up an endless throbbing litany from the river and off in the distance you can hear the night train whistling its way in from Dakar.

Night doesn't come quickly in Bamako, but in slow pleasant degrees, each moment new and different from the last. There is a sense of relaxation, of profound awareness throughout, but the sounds, sights and smells, all alien to the day, change with kaleidoscopic speed. When darkness finally falls the world is cold and still and not even the air conditioners in the Quartier Fleuve groan and hiss their way into the chilly darkness. You can hear the far off chants of the marabouts rolling over the flat roofs of the city and the pleasant thumping of thousands of pestles at work grinding the millet for supper. There is drumming and singing mingled with the musical hymns of the birds and crickets, all rising up over the town with the gray puffs of smoke from the cooking fires. And perhaps off on the peaks behind the town the ghosts of Sundiata Keita, Mungo Park and Borgnis des Bordes look down on their Bamako and see both the familiar and the strange.

Chapter IV

Hard Times

The Director General of Health was far too emotional a man to be a mean and calculating villain. I always felt that the reputation for toughness he had in the rank and file of the health service to be a few sizes too big. One disliked him and yet one pitied him at the same time. For in a sense he was a victim of the times and the helpless prisoner of an imposed political system which demanded of him an artful hostility towards westerners. In this, he certainly overplayed his hand, but it was his nature to do so. He could be a delightfully charming and courteous person and had an admirable gift for glib and fancy oratory which successfully seduced the less perceptive. Yet beneath all of this was a lonely human being, waging his own eternal struggle for cultural identification, hating colonialism but still trying to be very French, leading a bourgeois life while proclaiming to all the world to be an ardent Marxist. He was all impressive show and unless you were adept it was hard to unravel him. In a sense he was a reformer, trying to push his way through corruption and incompetence with an iron fist.

His office was a high narrow canyon of a room shut off from the world by peeling walls. A musty odor hung heavily in the air and fine red Bamako dust was everywhere, slowing creeping through cracks in the walls and puffing around your feet whenever they hit the shredded rug on the floor. The desk was oversized and submerged beneath a pile of rainbow colored folders whose spines were patinated through sweat and wear. He was always behind the desk, sitting upright and rigid in his chair, very much defensive, trying as it were to thrust his round frame in triumphal height over the scattered piles of papers. The battle between the Director and his papers never ended and you almost felt that one day in total frustration he would burn the lot to ashes to appease himself for his failure. I can't say the Director ever kept me waiting to see him. It was as if he anxiously looked forward to our long and arduous meetings as a field engagement against imperialism from which only he could emerge the victor since everything was stacked in his favor. One came out of these encounters full of anger, frustration and despair, which was as he wanted it.

He was my operational counterpart which wasn't desirable since a Director General of Health cannot be a counterpart to a technical advisor even under the best of circumstances. As it was, he was greatly overextended, holding several titles and playing the appropriate role as the moment dictated. Meetings had to be requested by letter, something which other advisors from the Eastern Bloc didn't have to do. The letters had to be written on official embassy stationery in French and had to explain in detail what it was I wanted to discuss with him. A week would go by before I would receive a response and then suddenly an official telegram would arrive informing me I would be received at a given hour. The fact our offices were but a mile apart and the presence of a telephone system made a telegram seem more part of an Italian farce than of reality. Things started off by his correcting the French syntax in the letter, using a red marking pencil. Each red stroke seemed a sacrilege to me since the syntax wasn't mine but that of the ambassador's translator, Madame Parthenay, who was the sole surviving keeper of the King's French in Bamako. Once the letter had been corrected it was handed back as a sort of homework exercise which hadn't met the required standard necessary for a place in the Director's files.

He went so far as to send an official complaint to the embassy about my letters and my French, protesting against the United States Government's sending of advisors who spoke poor French. In the end, it was he who looked absurd since I was fluent in the language and Madame Parthenay the recognized authority on French grammar in Bamako. The rebuff wasn't taken lying down because a few weeks later he came back with the reckless accusation that I was suspected of heading an automobile smuggling ring in Mali which by any standards would have been quite an accomplishment for someone in the country less than two months. When we took him up on the accusation, much to his surprise, he backed down and said it was all a bad mistake. But at the same time, he reminded me that the last American physician who worked in Mali had been asked to leave.

During my first month in Mali, he prohibited me from entering any of Bamako's hospitals, making a point of the fact that I was in Mali to eradicate smallpox and measles and not to treat sick people. But when I asked for permission to go out into the bush to investigate epidemics it was denied. My requests to leave Bamako were always handled the same. The stalling game was neither complex nor inventive; it consisted of saying that my request was under consideration by the local administrative authorities and in sequence by the local political and medical authorities. The process took the long months necessary to discourage anyone from pursuing the issue any further and as I found out later was a figment of the Director General's imagination. Many months later, when the Director General had left his post, and when the Malian security police were satisfied that I wasn't a CIA agent after all, I got to the sites of all these former outbreaks. There was an outpouring of complaints from the local medical authorities, the Director General having sent them impotent vaccine to fight their epidemics. He had also told them that I had refused to come out and investigate the epidemics or to allow American vaccine be used to fight them.

The Director General sought refuge for his actions behind the vague provisions of the project agreement which had been signed by the United States and Mali for this program. According to the letter of the document one couldn't say he was wrong, but finer men would have interpreted it in its spirit. He, however, had been its chief architect and it reflected his skill in composing double meaning phrases. The agreement was always before him whenever I walked into his office and I think he must have found great pleasure in checkmating me and in seeing his devious and crafty provisions finally at work. The first time I ever made a request to leave Bamako to investigate a smallpox epidemic he quoted the document, "smallpox cases will be investigated as soon as possible and reported to the project office." On the surface this looked fine, but his idea of as soon as possible extended to one year. "And of course," he added, "it doesn't say anything about you Dr. Imperato investigating these cases." The cases were reported in due course to the project office which for him wasn't my office but headquarters back in the States. And so, many months later these strange reports would arrive via sea mail in the States where no one knew what on earth to do with them.

I can't say I expected this extreme obstructionist behavior from the Director General. We had once spent a month together touring the United States with the Minister of Health on an official State Department tour before I had come over to Mali. I was bewildered at first and tried to humor him and I weighed and calculated every word before uttering it. But none of this worked and the Director went on his way not oblivious to the fact that I had no intention of passively playing the role of the favorite dog for very long.

In the Mali of those days, a westerner felt very much as if he were in a vice, being pushed on from all sides. It was only your internal strength which in the end preserved the integrity of your being. I could feel my gentility waning as I became hard and suspicious, tending to be on the defensive against everyone. Under such circumstances, your suspicion mushrooms beyond control and is no longer a calculated affair but an emotional one which operates on instinct. You are careful about what you say on the phone because it is tapped, and shifty-eyed in restaurants and bars because there are always a pair of informer's ears not far away. Even your trusted servants move in and out of the eclipse of suspicion.

In those days, my house used to be watched by green uniformed militiamen who were posted beneath the trees on the other side of the road. I think their job must have been very dull because nothing out of the ordinary ever took place at my house. Their main occupation was to copy down the numbers of all automobiles coming to my house and to obtain the names of those Africans entering on foot. They made no secret of doing this and I often walked out and told them, "Don't bother copying that number down. You already have it."

They never smiled, nor replied except the time I walked out with my unloaded camera and told them to hold still so that I could get a picture of them for my CIA files. They smiled at that and ran off. At the embassy, the affair was more clandestine, some local employees being in the service of the security police. It was their job to find out the names of the Malians entering the building. Malian government employees were prohibited from going to the American embassy unless they had permission from their superiors which in most cases was denied. At the Service d'Hygiene where I had my office two people were assigned to watch me and the dullness of that routine must have been too much for them because they went on to report that I was getting state secrets from a Malian health engineer who had done some training at the University of Oklahoma. This created a flury which lasted about a week and in the end the Minister of Health had to intervene and show it all to be a farce. Those who had their car numbers taken down were summoned to the security service and warned not to visit an American's home again and if they worked for the Malian government their jobs were threatened. One never knew who worked for the security service and so one quickly learned to trust no one. For the Malians it was a life of continual fear in which superiors were intimidated by their inferiors and people afraid even to be seen in the presence of an American.

I rapidly lost most of my Malian acquaintances. I can't say that many of them were my friends in the true sense of the word, and it wasn't totally because of the political situation of the times. Under most circumstances, it is difficult for a westerner to establish a true friendship with a Malian and it is not because one doesn't try. Rather, it is that the great economic gap between you and they puts you both on such unequal planes and it is this which makes true friendship difficult to achieve. This doesn't mean to say that this is a problem unique to Mali. Even in American and European society, friendships between persons coming from markedly different backgrounds of economic affluence are the exceptions rather than the rule. Then there is the natural inclination of many Malians only to form close bonds outside of the family and clan circle for the purpose of utility and gain. Their need for the virtuous aspects of friendship are amply satisfied in the close matrix of the extended family. They don't have to go outside of that setting in order to fulfill this need. The westerner finds out after experience that the Malian's concept of friendship and his own are vastly different. Sooner or later it becomes evident that the relationship is profitable in one direction only. Were the requests reasonable perhaps the acquaintanceship would weather the stresses and mature into a friendship of sorts. But unfortunately they are not. It may be a loan of a thousand dollars today and a request to pick up a spare car motor for them on your weekend trip to Dakar tomorrow.

The unseasoned idealist is not used to this concept of an exclusively utilitarian friendship and comes over to Africa with a true desire to make what Thomas Aquinas calls, "friends for virtue." The orientation and advice which he often receives before coming over is frequently given by people whose expertise in African affairs stems from continuous involvement in the subject at home but who lack prolonged experience in Africa itself. They are scarcely in a position to tell him something which has to be learned through years of living in Africa. Thus, in the beginning, this fellow will accede to the requests because he very much wants to be friends with the Africans and sees it as the duty of an egalitarian. But eventually he catches on and sees that while from his end it is friendship, from theirs it's a profitable business relationship. This all happens in the world of the long-term relationship where a man spends day and night with Africans. But those who oriented him in African affairs don't know this world. Theirs is the one sparkling with ministers and officials in fancy robes, the cocktail circuit, the casual contact.

If you use the right tactic in turning down a Malian's request he bears you no malice and if you do it frequently enough he will cease to bother you. Many westerners complain that Malians know nothing of gratitude and that it makes no difference what you do or do not do for them. It is the same. And when they begin to say no to the demands and requests they see that their relationships don't change. They are still acquaintances, never friends.

Westerners in Bamako have over the years been asked for many things by many Malians, but three requests stand out. There was the cabinet minister who no sooner had his foot in the front door of the house of an American official he had met only once before than he asked for a bottle of whiskey. An American ambassador was once whistled over to the curb by a policeman, and thinking he had committed a traffic violation he obliged, only to find out that the man wanted a loan of two hundred dollars. And then there was the chief of the security police who summoned an American official to his office with the greatest urgency to ask him for some free basketballs. It is always a sad awakening to realize you can't have Malian friends. In a way it's an alarming experience because it is contrary to our western humanistic instincts. You realize that for those who are not members of their families it is the same. They judge you not for what you are but rather for what you do for them.

When I first came to Mali, I spent a great deal of time in a hot tin-roofed warehouse, teaching forty vaccinators the technical aspects of a mass vaccination program. For the most part, they were raw recruits with only a a few years of schooling. Some were illiterate. Few of them had had any previous experience with medicine of any sort and most had only hazy ideas as to what they were going to be doing. The vaccinators were sheperded by a Frenchman, Monsieur Jean Lastouillas, a nervous but effective man who had been in Africa since 1941, and in Mali since 1956. Monsieur Lastouillas' official title was that of a technical advisor to the Ministry of Health but he did everything from being quartermaster for the Grandes Endemies Service — the mass preventive medical service — to playing house mother for the vaccinators.

The vaccinators were in the habit of working three months a year, a pattern established through lack of vehicles and materials. The rest of the time they camped in front of Monsieur Lastouillas' ramshackled office or else were given out to loan to the Hygiene Service for hunting mosquito larvae in the city. Monsieur Lastouillas and they lived a commensel existence as long as the vaccinators behaved and that wasn't very often. Retaliation took the form of roll calling.

"Maintenant, je vais faire l'appel," Lastouillas would scream from the top of his stoop as he drove out a bunch of vaccinators from his office. The infraction which they may have committed could have been anything from stealing menthol tablets from his desk to interrupting him on the phone.

Panic spread like wildfire and the word that Lastouillas was calling the roll raced out across the yard of the Service d'Hygiene and into the nearby quarters. Vaccinators rolled out of the backs of abandoned trucks, from behind trees, from beneath crates. They came running, panting, cursing, on foot, on hastily borrowed motor bikes and bicycles. Those who arrived late received a point next to their name, the significance and consequences of which not even Lastouillas knew. But that didn't stop Lastouillas from giving them out just the same nor the vaccinators from spending hours pleading with him to erase them.

Neither Monsieur Lastouillas nor the vaccinators had anything to do with the Service d'Hygiene, nor did I, even though we all occupied a large portion of their physical compound. By rights we should all have been across the street in the building of the Grandes Endemies, but there wasn't any room there since the space meant for us was taken up by people who really belonged in the Service d'Hygiene.

Jay Friedman, a former Peace Corps volunteer from Sierra Leone came out to Mali with me. Our immediate job was to train the vaccinators in the practical job of carrying out a mass vaccination campaign. This meant teaching them how to use and repair the automatic jet injectors which would be used to give the shots, how to take care of fragile vaccines in the bush where the ambient temperatures are 120° F, to vaccinate villages, to keep records and scores of other technical points. Jay and I spent many hours in the sizzling warehouse trying to imbue the vaccinators with a sense of professionalism. The afternoons were specially languid and the perspiration would roll down in uncomfortable hot trickling sensations over the forehead, back, arms, legs and fingers. One felt as if his entire body were slowly dripping away from him and being soaked up by the ground.

Most of the vaccinators became quite accomplished in the technical aspects of their job. I think though that we failed to make them a better

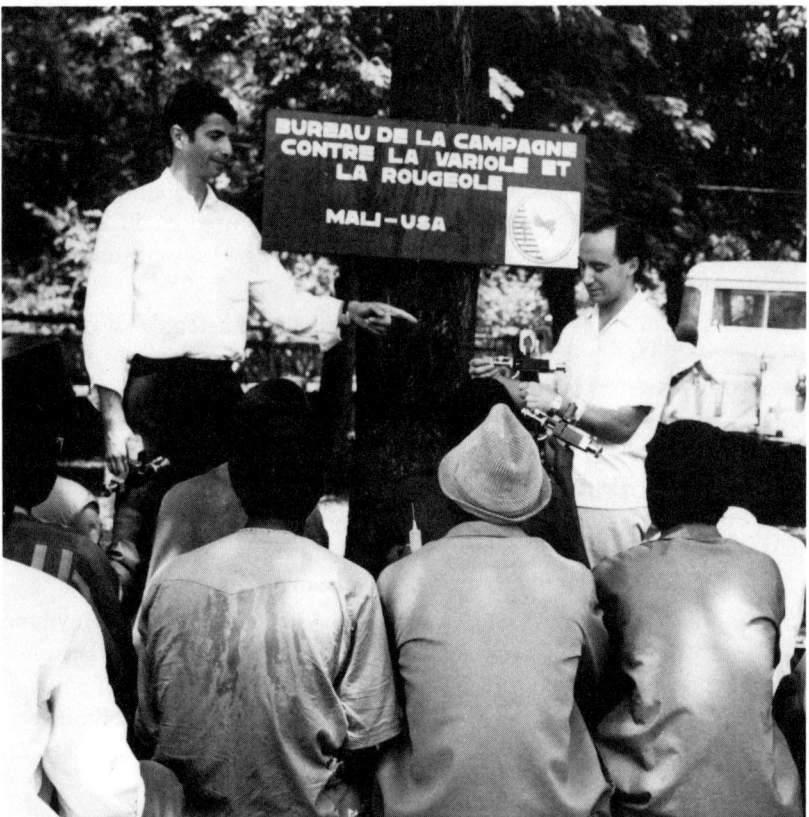

FIGURE 6. Jay Friedman *(left)* and Dr. Imperato *(right)* conducting a training session for vaccinators in the courtyard of the Service des Grandes Endemies.

group of men. It wasn't our job to do this, but it was something I always felt very strongly about. They lacked professional integrity, had no espirit de corps and in general were a complaining and demoralized lot. They were underpaid, receiving the equivalent of fifteen dollars a month and had taken the job because of their inability to find any other type of work. In spite of the draconian measures which Jay and Lastouillas took to prevent things from disappearing, thefts always occurred in the warehouse whenever the vaccinators walked in. They didn't consider this to be immoral because it was a question of their own survival which in their hard pragmatic subsistence society had to come before the welfare of the whole. I can't say that I ever became upset by the petty thefts, reasoning that they went towards the good of some unfortunate human being anyway. But one had to always keep petty theft in check else it would mushroom out of control and in the end completely paralyze the whole operation.

The drivers who stole gasoline and the vaccinators who pilfered medicines and camping equipment rationalized their acts on what they considered to be pressing personal need and the ownership of what they stole by an impersonal entity — government. They were fast sizing us up and it only took them a few days to figure out just how we were and how much they could get away with. Inherent in all of this was the sober calculation, equationwise, of how much hurt we could potentially do them and their degree of impunity. Since they didn't work for us directly and it wasn't we who paid their salaries, there did not exist the mutual relationship of employer to employee in its African context of master and client. So they didn't have to give us the allegience one would expect of a member of one's household. Over the years I was able to establish this relationship with some of them, but with the others it never amounted to anything more than a detached contact.

Complicating our relationships with these men in the early days was the political atmosphere. They all went to indoctrination sessions several times a week and many of them were former militiamen and civil guards well versed in the art of informing the secret police. Had I had direct administrative power over them things might have been very different, but as it was I was filling the vacuum created by the absence of a Malian superior without having any of the authority required to implement change. In principle, the Director General was their immediate superior, but he saw them but once a year and as a result they were without discipline. Perhaps he preferred it was this way because in those days in Mali people such as he in high positions were always at the mercy of the lowest men in their service. Even a minister could be brought under fire through the false accusations of a disgruntled laborer. In a sense, it was a system of mutual blackmail also in which people thrived and survived on knowing the evil doings of everyone else. It wasn't that they would take corrective action on uncovering theft and corruption, but rather that the knowledge would be kept for a rainy day and brought out against a future accuser.

The vaccinators respected me, but I can't say that they overly liked me. I was firm and just and for this in Mali you are rewarded with respect. Had I been easy going I would have been liked but not respected. One had a choice between the two, but one couldn't have both.

I remember we were training them during the Moslem fast period of Ramadan and most of them had to go to the door of the warehouse every few minutes to spit out their saliva. It seemed anachronistic to me at the time that people so fastidious about religious practice could be also so dishonest.

We trained them to use the jet injectors in about three week's time. These are capable of delivering a thousand injections per hour and can deposit vaccine either in the skin or underneath it. The vaccine passes through a small hole in the gun's platinum head and so no needles are used in the vaccinating operation. For a massive undertaking such as ours, they were the ideal solution, and during the years we used them we never regretted the choice.

During the years I was in Mali, there was always a steady flow of equipment and material by air from Paris and Abidjan and by train from Dakar. In these shipments came twenty-three two ton trucks and their spare parts for five years, fifty jet injectors, motor bikes, refrigerators, camping equipment, tents, cots, stoves, needles, syringes, bales of cotton to wipe every arm in Mali, tools of every description, loudspeakers, batteries for the trucks, five million doses of smallpox vaccine and an equal number of doses of diluent and a million doses of measles vaccine. At some point a crate of pith helmets arrived, but it was an enigma as to who had ordered them. Pith helmets are part of the dated and romantic Africa of long ago and strangely enough they are now frequently worn by Africans. We managed to find good use for our pith helmets by giving them to the men in the tsetse fly control service, All of this equipment plus the administrative costs of the operation cost in the end some million and a half dollars.

After the vaccinators were trained, the Director General sent them off into the bush to vaccinate the Region of Bamako, a vast area which extends from the Mauritanian frontier down into southern Mali. The man whom he put in charge of this first vaccination campaign was the medecin chief of Secteur Numero Trois of the Grandes Endemies Service. In physical appearance, El Hadji was a synthetic mixture of a marabout, village elder and kola nut trader. He was tall and slender with a pair of deep set eyes piercing his empty facial expression. His saintly form was always draped in soft looking flowing white robes and a tasseled shawl which he tossed over his head on cold days. During the cold season, he wore a World War II army overcoat which fell down to his ankles and made quite a sight with the shawl thrown over it.

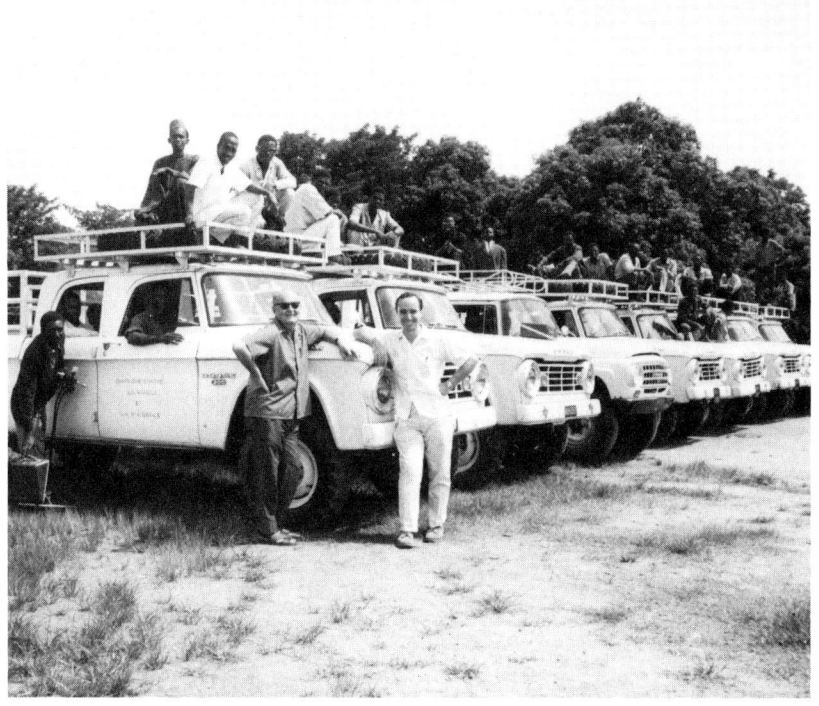

FIGURE 7. The vaccination teams of the Malian Smallpox Eradication-Measles Control Program prior to their departure for Koutiala. In the foreground *(left)*, the late Dr. Jiri Nedvideck of the World Health organization and *(right)*, Dr. Imperato.

El Hadji was a devout Moslem whose religious bent some people said verged on the fanatical.

His plan for the vaccination of the Region of Bamako was strategically one of dispersal which I thought appropriate since it characterized most of what he did. When the Director General rejected it, he came up with an alternative which in essence was the direct opposite of the first. El Hadji was kind and well meaning, but both his age and professional training stood against him in the running of a large scale mobile medical program. Encounters with him were always abortive, mainly because he would say "Weh Weh," his way of pronouncing "oui," to everything said and then go off and do the opposite. Advisory sessions with him were carried out under very trying conditions. His office squatted in the center of a veranda-encircled building around which people sat, argued, discussed and slept. This building was called the "Trypano," — sleeping sickness building because under the French all cases of sleeping sickness were taken there. In spite of the superficial disarray of uncoordination many things did get done due to the conscientious infirmiers who worked at the Trypano treating patients suffering from various infectious diseases. El Hadji's office was a tangle of dilapidated steel furniture, dust and un-read medical journals several years old which slept beneath a cover of undisturbed red dust. An hour's meeting in this office used to be taken up by fifty minutes of interruptions which is slightly more than average for most Malian offices. Even though El Hadji might be conferring with someone, people would barge in simply to shake hands and exchange *ca vas* which covered everyone from one's grandmother to the family livestock herds. Sick people came in complaining, relatives dragged in family disputes for mediation and vendors basins of smelly fish and calabashes of milk which had been soured with a dash of human urine.

It is often said that privacy is a luxury in Africa because people by reason of cultural tradition crash in anywhere whenever it strikes their fancy, to say hello and exchange *ca vas*. Hands are shaken until they almost fall off and you must resign yourself to shake the same person's hand at least four times a day. The defenders of tradition maintain that all of this is culturally acceptable to the Malian, which it is, but it cripples efficiency. One is unable to escape the responsibilities of the extended family and its problems even while at work because there is always an old auntie or uncle, brother or cousin who knows where the office is and unafraid to walk in and take up half the day. Private family affairs may in fact consume that much of a civil servant's day and additional time is taken up afterwards discussing the problem with the office colleagues.

There was a telephone in El Hadji's office as unbelievable as that may sound. Like many Malians he didn't speak over the phone; he shouted and the farther away the call came from the louder the decibels in the belief that voice volume had to increase proportionally with distance. His telephone conversations while conducted in French were a Bambara form of discourse in which only the individual words were French. The accountant at Secteur Numero Trois didn't have the necessary funds to pay the telephone and electric bills and there were many who suspected that they had been embezzled. While Energie du Mali may have been a poor ureliable supplier of electricity and five months late in sending their bills, they were fast to cut the electrical supply of non-solvent customers.

Watching El Hadji's vaccination program from my imprisonment in Bamako was like being an eyewitness to an inevitable disaster. I saw all the ingredients for failure the day the teams left for the bush, although El Hadji didn't. He had dug up a list of the 1,678 villages in the Region which had been made up ten years previously and was either unaware or unconcerned that in the interim many villages had moved, new ones had been established and old ones abandoned. Then too the sequence in which he ordered the teams to vaccinate the villages approached no logic I know of, African or otherwise. Naturally the second village on a teams' list should have been the one closest to the first, but not so on El Hadji's list. The second village was always a score of miles off in the blue and the third an equal distance in another direction. Ignoring the enormous waste of time and gasoline this approach made for, it was chaos at its best. The infirmiers who headed the teams finally threw their lists away and fell back on their own resources and made up their own programs. Since El Hadji had made no provision for the teams to report back to headquarters, within two week's time all of them were lost in the bush and no one knew where they were, least of all El Hadji.

The old man made several aborted attempts to find them, but it was always the same — no teams. He once asked me if he could borrow my binoculars to help him in locating the white trucks in the bush. In the midst of this disaster it was amazing to see the peculiar impression of security and calm which El Hadji conveyed. He was always courteous and gentle and would smile and nod even in the face of receiving such news that all of the trucks were broken down in scattered areas of the bush. In this there was a certain consistency in his nature produced I think by a total religious acceptance of things as they were. I could never become angry with him. It was like dealing with a well intentioned saint whose integrity and devotion are beyond reproach, but who moves through the world oblivious to the crude facts of life, set in his beliefs and resigned that they remain unchanged. I don't think El Hadji's lean noble head ever retained anything I said because anything of worth to him had already been perceived and absorbed many years ago.

He once told me how he had come on a team broken down on the banks of the Niger in an area where there were impassable rapids.

He was on the opposite bank and powerless to do anything to help them except shout over a few words of encouragement. When I asked him why he didn't drive a few miles upstream where one could cross the river, he simply replied that it wasn't on his program to cross the river that day.

It was against my nature to precipitate crises, but it slowly dawned on me that if I didn't, things would go on to their disastrous end. In all of this I was hesitant to hurt El Hadji because it was like beating a venerable old man. But El Hadji was incapable of surprise and when the day came that I struck back at the Director General he took it in stride, as if it were a matter of course. The mise en scéne of our confrontation came about quite accidentally although I must admit

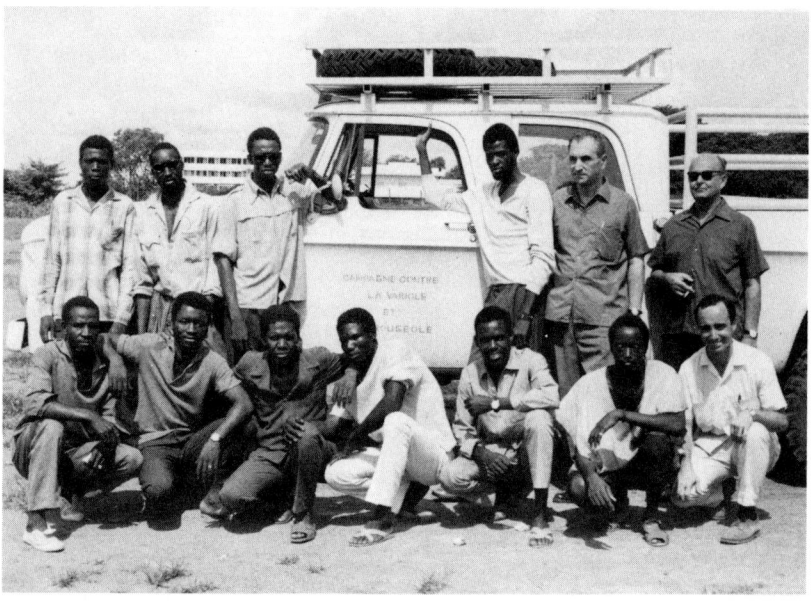

FIGURE 8. Some of the drivers of the Smallpox Eradication-Measles Control Program with Monsieur Jean Paul Lastouillas and the late Dr. Jiri Nedvideck *(standing, rear)* and Dr. Imperato *(kneeling, front)*.

I had been looking for an excuse to have a showdown for several months. Pessimism is always a fatal state of mind and try as I could, there was no way to rationalize our going on much longer. We had still not gotten permission to go out and inspect the work of the vaccination teams and the sorry spectre of El Hadji taking himself over river and dale in a vain search for them had become a tragic comedy. But all this gave the Director General the political security which came from toying with us while standing behind the comfortable protection of a diplomatic document.

Africans take a certain amount of pleasure in announcing disasters and one of our vaccinators was only all too happy to tell me how my office had been entered and a bottle of measles vaccine taken out and used to vaccinate the child of a governor. The other forty nine doses stood in the vial on my desk, now useless because they had rested most of the day in the heat which slowly killed the live virus of which the vaccine is made. The governor's wife unquestionably felt herself important enough to warrant a private vaccination session for her child, even after it was explained to her that once a vial of vaccine was made up it had to be used or else it would go to waste. When the vaccinators turned her down and told her that there would be a vaccination session in her town the following week, she went to see the head of the Service d'Hygiene who said he could do nothing since it wasn't his affair. But this woman was persistent and she finally called the Minister of Health on the telephone. In the end he ordered the head of the Service d'Hygiene to vaccinate the child. The remaining forty nine doses presented an embarrassing problem once her child had been vaccinated and to solve it the head of the Service d'Hygiene sent an infirmier, Dramane Samake, out to round up forty nine children. Dramane came back with two possibilities — the children of the post office employees and the children at the North Korean Embassy. It was very much a mixed bag and as it turned out neither group was vaccinated since the post office children couldn't be rounded up in time and the North Koreans were scarcely candidates for American vaccine given to the people of Mali. In retrospect it was amazing that the North Koreans actually wanted their children vaccinated with American vaccine, they making only one condition, that it not be administered by an American.

Under any other circumstance this vaccine incident would have been regarded as an administrative accident and as such it would have been dismissed. But in our microcosmic stalemate with the Director General I saw it as the issue over which we had to precipitate a confrontation. I sent a letter of protest to the Director General of Health in which was outlined the violation of the project agreement, the financial cost of the vaccine now lost and the fact that as a result forty nine bush children would be deprived of protection against measles. For what I wanted to achieve such a letter wasn't sufficient since it didn't touch on the really important issues. The Malians had to make up their minds whether or not they wanted us and what we had to offer. With this in mind, the director of AID went up to Koulouba to see the people at the Ministry of Plan and explained to them all of the problems we had been having since our arrival in Mali. He made it clear to them that all of this obstructionist behavior meant to us that they didn't want this vaccination program and if that were the case we were prepared to leave.

It was distasteful for me to have to put the Minister of Health in an awkward position. He was greatly respected by everyone and in my dealings with him I had always found him to be an excellent physician and fine human being. But as I saw it unless all of these problems were taken up to the level of the Minister we would soon be forced to leave Mali out of sheer frustration. Piecing things together a few years later when we could all talk jokingly about the affair it came out that the Minister was called in to see the Minister of State for Plan. He was asked why AID found it necessary to protest about problems which seemed to them the product of illogical spite. The Minister was somewhat bewildered by all of this because up until that time he didn't know of the obstructions which had been created by the Director General.

The Minister's secretary called me on the phone the following morning and said that the Minister wanted to see all of us that afternoon.

"Nothing important," he said, "just to discuss some routine matters."

When I arrived for the meeting I found that most of the principal characters were there except the Director General of Health who had found it necessary to make an emergency trip into the bush and Dramane Samake who had been sent out of town on some ambiguous mission. The Minister looked both serious and uncomfortable.

"Your letter has been read with great interest," he said. " It really wasn't necessary for this matter to have been taken all the way up to the President. He is a busy man with many problems on his shoulders."

He explained his side of the vaccine story, indicating that the head of the Service d'Hygiene had assurred him that there were forty nine other children already waiting to be vaccinated. He had also been led to believe that we were aware that the child was to be vaccinated and that we had in fact concurred. The Minister then asked the head of the Service d'Hygiene to explain what went wrong. He started his defense by saying that he had not had anything to do with vaccinations in the city of Bamako in over five years and, therefore, didn't feel responsible for what had happened. Not even the Malians present followed this reasoning, but everyone heard him out.

"Dramane Samake told me that forty nine children from the post office were on their way. How was I to know that they would never come."

"But you told me that they were already there, lined up," interrupted the Minister.

"Maybe I did say that, but what I really meant was that they would be lined up."

To me it all looked like an unfortunate misunderstanding and I wasn't interested in pinning blame on anyone. The Minister asked if anyone had any questions and seeing that no one did, expressed his opinion that it was a question of misunderstanding emanating from Dramane Samake's vague allusions to forty nine children who never materialized. In the end Dramane was blamed for the incident.

"Dramane is responsible for this," said the Minister with comfortable ease.

"Yes it is Dramane," echoed the head of the Hygiene Service in tones reminiscent of the memorized lines of a high school play.

"Weh weh," whispered El Hadji not wanting to be left out on the kill. In turn all of the others joined in, pouncing on poor Dramane who wasn't there to defend himself.

The Minister then went on into a long monologue about his concern for the poor peasant children of the country. Certainly he didn't think that a governor's child was worth forty nine poor village children. In Mali no one received preferential treatment, not even the family of the President. After a long discussion of these points we passed on to the crucial issues concerning the program.

The Minister's secretary started off by saying that all foreign experts accredited to the Ministry of Health were given passes to circulate all over the country in connection with their work. He himself was responsible for getting these passes stamped into the passports at the security service.

"Why didn't you ask me for the pass," he demanded as if we never had.

"We have. We've asked the Director General many times and he told us to write to the Ministry of Foreign Affairs."

There was a short uncomfortable silence and then the Minister, evidently embarrassed spoke and apologized for all that had happened. This was quite a concession on his part, knowing that rarely will a Malian admit he is wrong.

It was the purposeful design of things that El Hadji was left until last. Perhaps it was because the Minister already knew that no matter what he said to the old man the result would be the same. There was nothing ferocious nor headlong about the Minister's discussion of El Hadji's shortcomings. And for his part, El Hadji was calm, the picture of a noble saint from the far away world of mosques, and minarets and burning incense and Friday prayers. The atmosphere of the meeting had changed; it was the period of the post storm calm. The old man was as immobile as an ancient idol sculptured in yellow patinated ivory and didn't say a word. Even the Minister found it hard to be angry with him. It was like trying to desecrate a sacred shrine. El Hadji didn't have it in him to counter the accusations and defend himself because as he saw things he had done nothing wrong. At the gateway to his world, the wonders of modern man and the accessories of an efficient administration disappeared before fate and the will of God.

This confrontation between an Islamic holy man and a modern cabinet Minister was not part of the embroidery of the traditional scene. In El Hadji's world of intermediaries and *porte paroles* such differences were never discussed directly let alone in the presence of strangers. One didn't throw out curt remarks even at a despised adversary no matter how great the bitterness and contempt. As if by some pre-arranged and understood ceremonial men were civil and polite face to face and argued their differences through the emotionally detached lips of their intermediaries. In this way the issues were settled dispassionately without ever jeopardizing the interpersonal relationships. It was an effective device which avoided feuds and which made eventual mediation by force a remote possibility. El Hadji finally spoke, transforming himself in a single gesture from a lifeless icon into an obsequious and gentle old man. He didn't have much to say in an encounter of this kind conducted outside the rules of his Koranic world. He had tried his best and the rest was left to God.

It took a year's time to push away the veil of suspicion which surrounded us in Mali. It was a calculated and thoughtful process on our part which required months of diplomatic maneuvering, the essence of which was a daily demonstration of sincerity. Full acceptance was not achieved and it was never my hope that it would be. But we managed at least to establish an atmosphere of mutual understanding in which there could be a free exchange of ideas. You had to be gallant in such an affair because improbable and inexplicable reactions emerged from Malians and left one bewildered. A reconciliation had to take place between your inner dedication and sincerity and your being trusted only so far by the other side. I never expected, thanks to be forthcoming where full trust was wanting. The most I ever hoped for was cooperation and tolerance. The job of building bridges of understanding never ended because my work brought me into continuous contact with new officials all the time.

Their greatest need was to survive as best they could in a world where political idealogy was practiced with the fervor of those whose religious orthodoxy is under continuous inquisition. Contact with a westerner was just as heretical as a verbal pronouncement against the regime. I could sense their panic whenever they learned I was an American. They made a conspicuous effort to have third parties document and monitor everything that went on between us. There was a certain amount of blundering and awkwardness on their part because their reaction to me represented a mingling of fear and courtesy. I was never at ease with them, nor they with me. In my dealings with them I felt like an untouchable moving in a world of eternal condemnation, somewhat disgusted and despairing.

Our work was greatly facilitated by the departure of the Director General and by his being replaced by a young Malian physician just out of a school of public health. He was very different from his predecessor and gave us a free hand to do what we thought best to rid Mali of smallpox and measles. Up until that time no one possessed any precise knowledge about smallpox or measles nor about how they spread. People said they appeared out of nowhere with the wind during the dry season and then vanished when the rains fell. Somewhere in all of this was the belief in the dark shadow of a sorcerer or evil genie, moving underfoot without clamour or witnesses and unleashing magical powers during the night, unintelligible murmurings, making smallpox a tragic gesture of the supernatural. The problems of magic are always insoluble to those who believe in it. Nobody really searches for solutions because magic is the terrifying weight in the balance of men's lives. There is no indignant outburst against it when it inflicts harm. It has an indisputable right to exist; it is a necessity in the order of things. One seeks therefore to live with it, to survive its angry incursions, to use it to advantage.

Chapter V

A Miracle Is Born

The plan of operations to eradicate smallpox took a year to produce. It began taking shape in my mind as I traveled all over the country investigating smallpox epidemics and launching the *fire fighting* operations to stop them. The striking thing about smallpox in Mali at that time was its almost exclusive occurrence in the central part of the country in the inland delta of the Niger. Here live thousands of nomads, the Peul, a people who previously had rarely been reached by the health services of the country. Most of them were unvaccinated and it was they who principally kept smallpox alive in Mali.

The inland delta is one of those unusual topographic formations which the doubtful must see with their own eyes before they will accept that it really exists in a country as arid as Mali. It is a complex zone the size of the State of Maine, composed of seasonal swamps, flood plains, rivers, lakes and ponds. During the rainy season, it is a refreshing panorama of blues and greens in which idle lakes reflect the group flights of white egrets and rivers twist with grace and silence around high hillocks which are crowned by mud and straw villages and tall stately dolm palms. There is an uplifting breeze in the air, an endless view of green *borgus* grass swaying away in three feet of water off into the blue horizon like the ripples of a calm sea and the deep reflective sense that you are in the midst of some magnificent and overpowering creation which is eternal. In the dry season the Niger River falls, the water on the flood plains dries up and in place of a great swamp there is a world reminiscent of the dry flat fields of western Kansas. The water recedes in a centripedal fashion so that the lost areas under water are those closest to the river. The falling crest also moves downstream leaving the last large accumulations of water in the region of

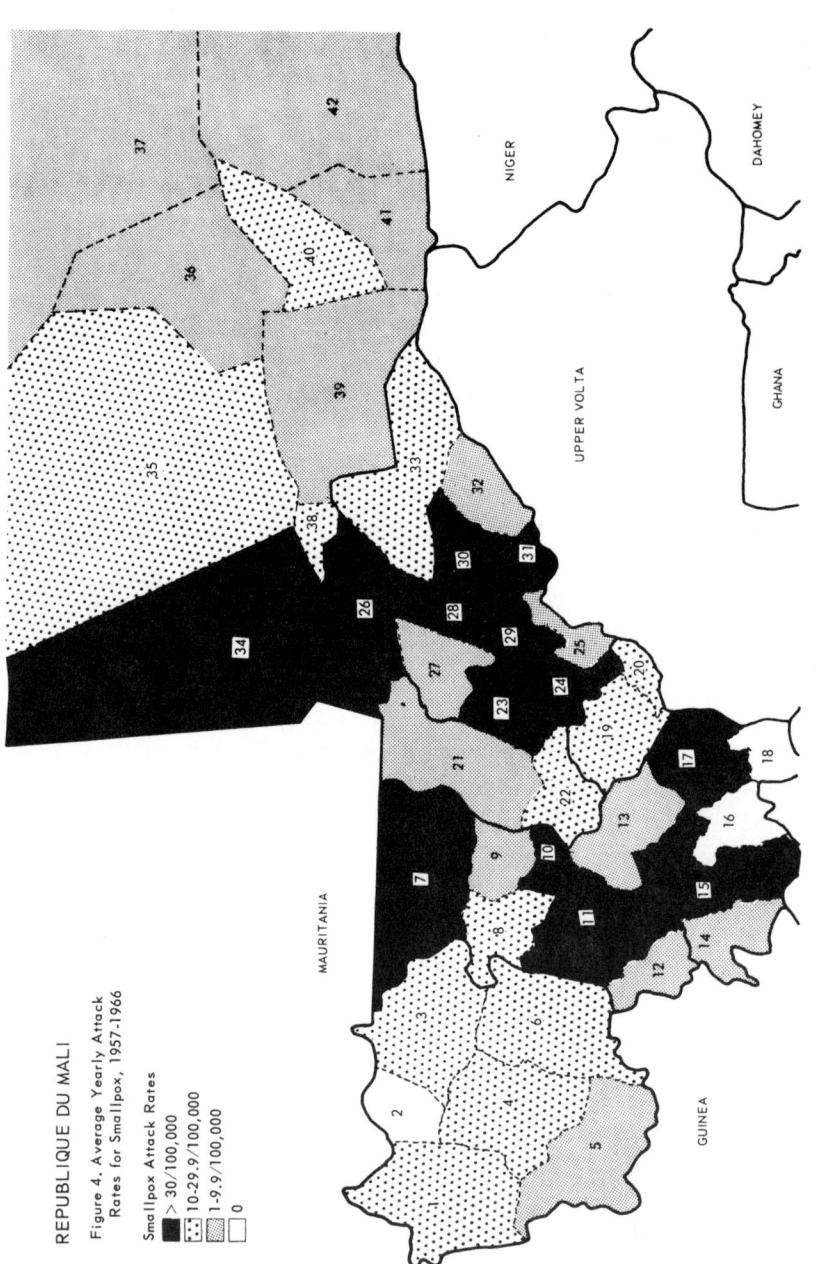

REPUBLIQUE DU MALI

Figure 4. Average Yearly Attack Rates for Smallpox, 1957-1966

Smallpox Attack Rates
■ > 30/100,000
⋮ 10-29.9/100,000
▒ 1-9.9/100,000
□ 0

Lake Debo which is a great spidery mass of water between Mopti and Timbuctoo.

Nature's seasonal symphony long ago shaped man's habits in the inland delta. When the river begins to fall, the itinerant Bozo fishermen ride the lowering crest in search of migratory fish, the Peul herdsmen come down into the plains from the high rocky Bandiagara Plateau and the dry northern sahel with their millions of humped backed cattle, goats, sheep, donkeys and camels, merchants flow in from as far away as the Ivory Coast and Ghana to buy the never ending supply of dried fish which inundates the town of Mopti in January and seasonal workers come to work in the rice fields.

I am neither a geographer nor a professional anthropologist, but I knew that if a detailed study were not made of life and human society in the inland delta we would lose our battle against smallpox and measles in Mali. It was never my intention to come up with a sophisticated scientific document, but simply to obtain an outline of information which would permit us to vaccinate the majority of people who lived in the inland delta. I can't say that my knowledge of this area was ever complete. As with all such studies of this kind, there was always the frustration of gaining new knowledge and of simultaneously realizing the immensity of my own ignorance. In a way I was venturing into the unknown because the hard facts were not published anywhere. Even if we surmounted the complex difficulties posed by seasonal topographic changes and the mass displacement of cattle nomads, there was no guarantee that once found they would accept what we were offering. I had to find out such basic things as how they moved, their numbers, where they came from and where they went. Was it a haphazard movement dependent on individual whim and fancy like that of the gypsies or was it an organized and regular pattern which didn't change from year to year. Did they move as a hoard, as large groups or as family units. If the movements were organized then I had to talk to the people who directed them. I knew that even if I found the answers to all of these questions there was no guarantee that a program aimed at nomads would be successful. I also had to learn about their attitudes towards modern health services, towards administrative authorities, probe into their notions about smallpox, about vaccination and then design an overall psychological approach which would win them over. In the end, it turned out to be an enterprise which required the patience of a saint, a general's imagination and the tenacity of a zealot.

Many people believed that smallpox could never be eradicated

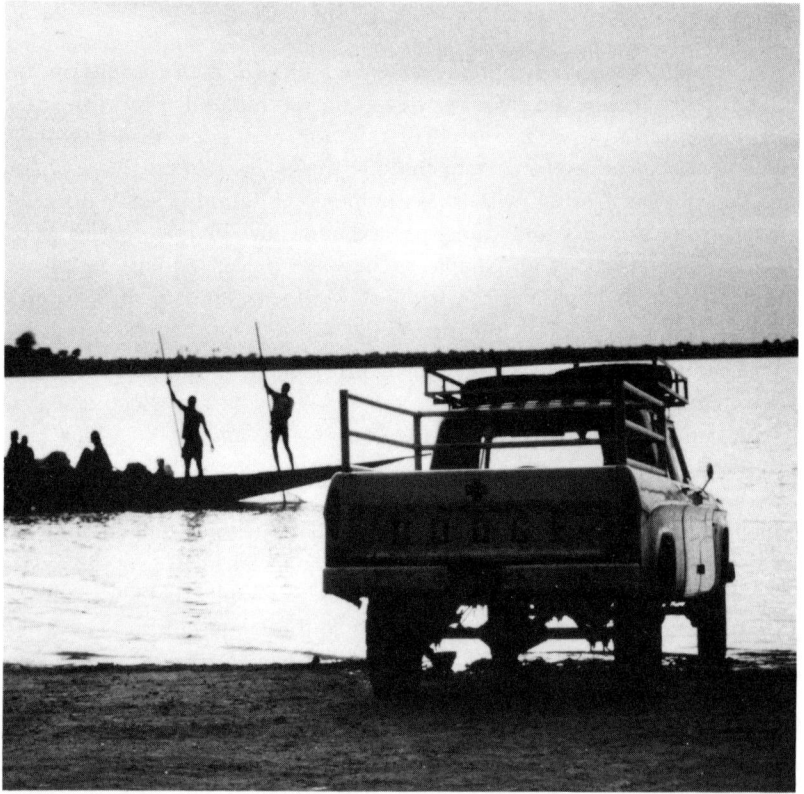

FIGURE 9. On the banks of the Bani River in the inland delta of the Niger waiting for the barge to ferry us over towards the track which leads to the town of Djenne.

because it was there through God's will. In a sense, then, I was wasting my time whenever I made an appeal to the reason of some Moslem health officials in the bush by showing them a plan of operation. Few among them were able to grasp its significance because among them reason had long since been dwarfed by a blind faith in predestination and the role of God not only as a prime mover, but also as the proximal cause. Although Islam implies the peace of God gained through submission to His will, in Mali it produces at its best a dispassionate acceptance of fate and at its worst complete passive fatalism. In such fatalistic societies, neither man nor anything he does appreciably alters the divinely determined course of events and so it is considered pointless and even sinful to challenge destiny by introducing a feeble man made force into what is God's exclusive design. This leads men to sleep in the inertia of fatalism where they don't attempt to alter events, but rather allow events to run their course and eventually determine their lives. God is given credit for many of the unhappy things and failures which occur in life and Moslem Malians are quick to attribute their failures in life to Him. However, when it's a question of personal achievement or gain, they tend to leave Him out and take credit for themselves.

It always amazed me that Moslem officials listened with deference to what I had to say. I don't think this was an expression of understanding, but rather of tolerance. It was an admirable thing to witness how they could sit for hours listening to what they considered to be in principle irrelevant. Strangely enough, they followed my advice, not because they believed in it, but out of politeness. As one can imagine, it required tremendous patience to work out a feasible scientific strategy, confronted as I was with all of the complexities of the inland delta and this Moslem mentality. It was never my hope that they would associate the disappearance of smallpox with the plan so the matter of its success or failure was never taken into consideration. When smallpox finally disappeared it would be God working His very special miracle among Malians.

During the early months of my work, I met by chance the *imam* of the mosque of Djenne. The mosque at Djenne is the largest mud mosque in Mali and stands in a city which for centuries has been a center of Moslem religious and intellectual life. I had gone to the old Peul capital of Hamdallaye and found the imam there supervising the construction of a cement block building over the tomb of the first Peul emperor, Cheikou Ahmadou. This was no feverish building operation but more of a meditative exercise in which the laying of every block was an event of great dimension. The old imam glided around the building site in soft white robes followed at a respectful distance by a retinue of venerable looking marabouts. It looked like a consistory of cardinals, debating and pondering some grave moral affair of the faith. The imam possessed a unique magical sway over his laborers because with a turn of his head or a whispered word he could completely change the pace and direction of things. The laborers for their part didn't say anything and unlike most I have seen in Mali kept a clear and attentive eye on their work and their construction foreman. It all had the appearance of a sacred religious ceremony and so I didn't interrupt until a murmur from the imam stopped the work and sent the laborers off into the shade of a shea butter tree.

I don't think that the imam had ever met a white person who was able to move through the ruins of Hamdallaye with an air of knowledge and discuss the happenings of another century. It didn't unnerve him to confront a white doctor stepping out of a vaccination truck who could greet him in Bambara and then suddenly launch into a discourse on Peul history in the inland delta. Rather, he was warmed and pleased that someone unknown could unexpectedly drop into his quiet and inward looking world and suddenly begin to utter the names of its heroes and saints and recite its great events with intellectual comfort and security. When the retainers drew close, they put away their prayer beads and moved diplomatically into the conversation. They were careful not to contradict the imam nor to eclipse the first among equals position he enjoyed. None of them ever asked me why I had such an intense and praiseworthy interest in their horizons. Although I told them voluntarily that it was because we wanted to vaccinate all of the people living in the inland delta, I don't think they really believed it because that was too simple and banal a reason. "C'est le Dieu!" they murmured among themselves and so like all else in their world I too became an inexplicable phenomenon of God. This had its advantages because I could move among them fully accepted and discuss and challenge, agree and contest every standard and fact in a friendly spirit.

We spent the day in one another's company, climbing over the old stone fortress and battlements and walking across the broad plateau which dominates this section of the flood plain from an advantageous height. These men had a very friendly relationship with time. It was not there to be efficiently used and so it played no important dominating role in their lives and was held to be of little consequence. It didn't compress the verbal expression of their ideas nor enslave them to succinctness and I for my part didn't try to hurry them along in their narrative. For them, time was simply there.

I viewed our conversations as a foundation on which a more complicated superstructure of knowledge had to be built. By that time, I could recite important names, places and events which told them that I was knowledgeable. Certainly their knowledge was greater than mine, but I think they over-estimated how much I really knew and viewed my failure to say something not as ignorance but as the strategy of a learned man. In assessing me, they saw me as someone like themselves, a man who did not divulge the whole store of his knowledge all at once. For knowledge in their world is the key to prestige and influence and a learned literate man must always be capable of relating something new and different which has never been heard before. Throughout our unpretentious conversations ran an admirable safeguard for accuracy. They viewed me as informed and so they dared not waver from the truth as they knew it for to do so would lay them open to criticism and loss of prestige.

Before I left, I pressed two thousand francs into the imam's hand. "It is to help with the construction of the tomb." The others looked on with attentive approval. He recommended me to several griots whom he said could tell me what I wanted to know about the social organization of the Peul and about their history. My own conviction at that time was that I had to understand these oral traditions in order to understand the Peul of today. And so over the next few months I spent long hours with the griots, taking a walk back into history where today's enigmas became historically reasonable and the seemingly confusing a real symphony of order and harmony.

You have to be a good and patient listener in West Africa in order to collect information, someone who likes hearing a story told. You can gather up an enormous store of data simply by listening to people talk. What they say may be embellished and somewhat distorted, not from any dishonest desire to deceive you, but rather because the oral tradition they know has not been immune to the risks incurred in generation transfer. One is truly impressed by the traditional minstrel's ability to explain happenings with astonishing accuracy and to relate his story in a meaningful way so that few will ever leave until the whole is told. Africans of course are wonderful listeners and they can sit for hours, enraptured by the guitar music of the griot. These guitars have only four strings, but they can carry a story through romances, battles, into the depths of sorrow and up to the heights of victory. Their monotony is almost hypnotic and they draw their listeners into the story such that people actually feel that they are participants.

Whenever we, the outsiders, listen to these narratives we almost automatically begin to analyze what is being said, search out the essentials and cast away the unnecessary details. This is because we, unlike the African listener, are interested in using the information for some practical purpose. What separates us from the Malian listener is that for us what is being said is more important than the experience of hearing it said. When you live in Africa for a long time you have the opportunity of hearing the same account retold many times. It is then that you can become like the African, divest yourself of the compulsions and anxieties inherent to intense and rapid data gathering, and sit back and relax and in doing so have a very meaningful experience. You have to live in Africa for many years before you develop the ability to sift out the essentials in any kind of account. This is because in order to do so you must have many common experiences with Africans and discover what they have to say about them. You are always astonished that they have retained not only the important facts, but also the small details which you sub-consciously discarded even while the experience was taking place. But for them every detail and essential is given equal weight, everything is equally important. This poses many practical problems because it is you who must take on the burden of deciding what is important and what isn't. Depending on how you look on such a challenge it can be either high adventure or nagging frustration. So, in being presented with a surprising combination of facts, you must not only be capable of making a wise judgement, but also be patient with those whose judgement it should have been.

I remember once that one of our drivers came to me in the middle of the bush and said, "My truck is broken down and I had to reach you on someone else's.

"What is wrong with it?" I asked.

"The side window on the left doesn't roll up all the way."

A less experienced listener would have lost his temper and sent the man off on his way. But I knew that I had to ask what else was wrong, especially since the driver had traveled to see me in another truck. When he told me that the front axle was also broken in half it was not with any dramatic emphasis. There was obvious sincerity in what he said, a firm belief that both the broken axle and the malfunctioning window were equal in seriousness. The key to success then lies not in forcing people to make this judgement for to do so may gain you a lot of useless detail and in the end you will have missed out on the high points. Rather you must learn to be a patient listener, a fastidious collector of facts and an experienced judge. The more questions you ask the less good information you obtain because in being overly interrogative you tempt an African informant to do what is his natural inclination, to please you by telling you what he thinks it is you want to hear.

I knew that I could never apply statistical formulae to the data the Peul gave me nor placate those for whom truth was only found at the end of a mathematical equation. But it was possible to test the validity of what I heard by hearing the same facts recited by different minstrels in numerous localities. In the end, I traveled thousands of miles and heard of the same happenings, told perhaps with differing abilities of dramatic skill and clothed with different details. My study became a great pleasure and I cannot recall that a single dark moment of doubt or distrust ever crossed my mind. I realize now that it better enabled me to cope with the political complexities of socialist Mali and the officially pronounced hate feelings against Americans. Among the rural Peul such things were not at work.

Most griots begin their story in the fifteenth century when a Peul chief, Maga Diallo, moved out of the west and built a village called Dia next to a pond whose name was Macina. Today you can still see Dia, a small village of gray mud quietly asleep beneath the swaying shadows of the dolm palms in a far off corner of the flood plain. Maga Diallo's descendants created a small kingdom called Macina which was eventually annexed by the Songhoi empire of Gao. When the Songhoi empire was destroyed by the Moroccan invasion of the sixteenth century, the Peul revolted and fought the Moroccans for thirty years. The Moroccans finally withdrew from the Macina, not because of the superior force of the Peul, but because they were defeated by malaria. They recognized Ahmadou-Amina II as Ardo or king. The title "Ardo" in Fulfulde, the language of the Peul, originally meant "warrior," but it later became synonymous with "king" and pastoral chief. Ahmadou-Amina died in 1663 and the minstrels say that between that date and the year 1725 there were seven Peul kings, but little is known of them except for the last, Guidado who began his rule in 1706.

In 1715, Biton Coulibaly, the most famous of the Bambara kings of Segou, conquered the Macina and made Guidado his vassal. This Bambara domination of the inland delta of the Niger lasted for almost a hundred years, until 1818 when a Moslem marabout usurped the throne and in so doing brought an end to the four hundred year reign of the Diallo dynasty. He freed the Macina of the domination of the Bambara animists and set up a theocratic state in the flood plains.

This marabout, Cheikou Ahmadou, was born Ahmadou Hammadi Boubou in the Peul village of Malangal which is situated some twenty miles from the present day town of Tenenkou. He spent the early years of his life under the influence of local Koranic teachers and by the age of twenty was recognized as a marabout of exceptional quality. He then traveled over a thousand miles overland to Gobir in Northern Nigeria where he came into contact with the Fulani Moslem reformer, Ousmane

Don Fodio. Full of Don Fodio's zeal for reform, Ahmadou returned to the Macina with several followers and launched a religious crusade against the animist practices of the Peul, against the domination by the Bambara whom he regarded as inferior fetish worshipers and against the Moslem religious establishment. Obviously, Ahmadou's self confidence must have been running high for him to have taken on at once all of the religious and secular powers in the Macina. His preaching brought him into immediate conflict with the marabouts of the mosque at Djenne. They retaliated by prohibiting him from entering the mosque and with the help of the Ardo imposed other forms of persecution which in the end won for Ahmadou the sympathy of a population long tired of Bambara rule. Ahmadou next began preaching open revolt against the Ardo and in time was able to muster an army of forty thousand men against the Ardo. It is debatable whether or not he had that many men, but he did manage to defeat the combined army of the Peul king and the king of Segou at Noukouma in March of 1818. In a very generous way, he did not kill the Ardo, but simply deposed him and allowed him to retire to a far end of the inland delta.

Cheikou Ahmadou then undertook to build a new city, called Hamdallaye, whose ruins now lay some twenty miles to the south-west of the city of Mopti. He destroyed the mosque at Djenne, the griots say, because its beauty distracted men from prayer. But those who are less inclined to aggrandize Ahmadou say that it was an act of revenge against the marabouts who had humiliated him by prohibiting him entry. According to griot tradition, Hamdallaye was divided into eighteen quarters and surrounded by a fortified wall pierced by four gates. The city was policed by seven marabouts and defended by ten thousand horsemen. Griots enjoy recounting in detail every aspect of life in Hamdallaye and no doubt much of what they say is embellished with details no serious historian could accept as credible. One griot spoke for hours about the health code which Ahmadou promulgated in the city. Urinating in the streets was prohibited and each family was responsible for cleaning the streets, their houses and courtyards. No dogs were permitted inside the city and those belonging to herdsmen were required to stay outside the city gates. This prohibition against dogs probably stemmed from a fear of rabies which is still a serious problem in the inland delta. Anyone bitten by a dog was required to have the wound washed seven consecutive times by a marabout. This was a remarkable health rule since today we recognize that thorough washing of such a wound is the most important measure in preventing rabies.

The selling of the meat of sick animals was punishable by imprisonment. Milk sellers were required to cover their calabashes to keep the flies out and urinating into milk as is done today to prevent it from souring was prohibited. No one was allowed to wear a garment which touched the ground nor to have sleeves which fell below the wrists. It was believed that long garments transported disease from one part of the city to another, and probably they did. There is no question that there was an astonishing degree of wisdom in Ahmadou's health code reflecting a remarkable insight into the role of sanitation in preventing disease transmission. The fact that these laws were promulgated over a hundred and fifty years ago before the germ theory of diseases was an accepted concept in Europe indicates what an unusual man Ahmadou must have been. Today his health code still lingers on in Peul villages where modern health teams have never set foot!

Ahmadou declined the title of Ardo and took that of Cheikou, meaning "spiritual guide." He was also known as Amir ul Muminina, or "commander of the faithful." But by whatever name he was known, he was in effect a priest king, a theocratic emperor. He divided his empire into six regions, Farimake, Kounari, Seno, Macina, Sebera and Pignari, and although these names appear on no modern map of the inland delta they are the ones still in use by the people who live there. They group clans together, possess sets of pastoral movements which differ and have individual traditional power structures. It was according to these traditional units that a health program in the delta had to be planned, not according to the modern administrative units.

Cheikou Ahmadou's laws diffused into every aspect of Peul life. Because many of the Peul were animist at that time, the early years of his reign were not peaceful. Many refused to convert to Islam and migrated to the east where today one finds their descendants in eastern Mali and the Niger Republic. At the inception of his reign, most of the Peul were completely nomadic with no fixed villages to return to during the rainy season. The problems of governing and taxing such a mobile population rapidly became apparent in Ahmadou and so he ordered the Peul to build permanent villages to which they would return during the rainy season. This first attempt at sedentarization of nomads in the inland delta was a success and today those villages built under Cheikou Ahmadou still stand on the *toggue* (hillocks) which lie scattered throughout the flood plain. He also reorganized the movements of the herds in and out of the flood plains, taking into consideration the available grass for the various clan herds and the threat of raids from

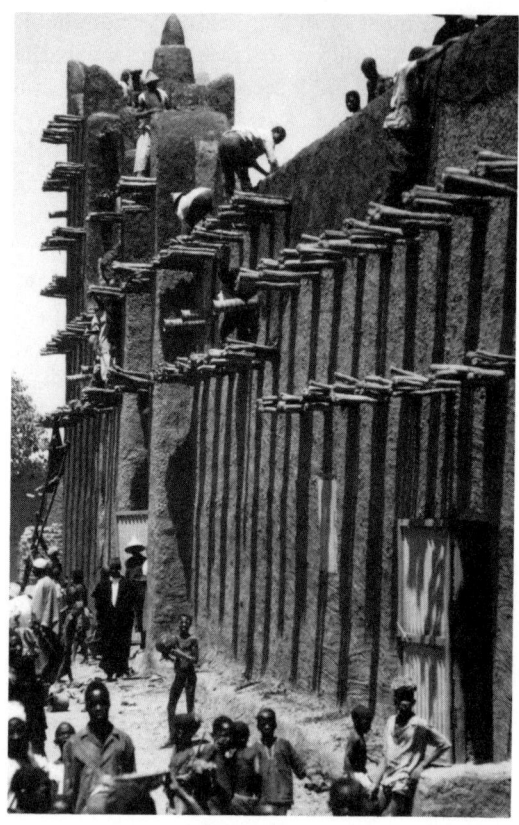

Figure 10. The mosque at Kona being resurfaced with mud at the end of the rainy season. All of the able bodied men of the town donate their labors for this annual task. The original mosque built by Cheikou Ahmadou, the Peul emperor, lies within the walls of the present structure.

the Bambara. It was the first serious attempt at range control in this part of Africa and the patterns established by him are still in effect in most parts of the inland delta. Since the time of Cheikou Ahmadou, both the French and the present-day Malians have tried to sedentarize the Peul and to alter the grazing patterns of their cattle. Neither of them were successful, perhaps because Cheikou Ahmadou's innovations of the last century have now become sacred traditions which have maintained a peaceful balance between groups of nomads who always live on the edge of survival.

Cheikou Ahmadou died in 1845 and was succeeded by his son

Ahmadou Cheikou who had a peaceful reign of seven years. In 1853, he was followed by his son, Ahmadou Ahmadou who continued the theocratic rule of his grandfather until 1864 when the rampaging armies of the Toucouleurs, led by a religious warrior, El Hadj Omar, launched a holy war whose aim was to force people to accept his brand of Islam. After destroying the Bambara kingdom of Segou, the Toucouleurs marched on Hamdallaye where their muskets and gunpowder brought them a rapid victory over the lance-equipped army of the Peul. Ahmadou Ahmadou was wounded in the chest and had his right arm shattered by a bullet. He retreated down the Niger in a canoe with his family and library of Koranic works. Near the present day village of Sindegue, they were intercepted by one of El Hadj Omar's lieutenants, brought back to Mopti and beheaded.

El Hadj Omar occupied Hamdallaye and built a *tata* (fortified wall) of clay around the city which you can still see today beneath the thorn trees. But his victory was short-lived. The Peul regrouped under the command of Ba Lobo, the dead king's cousin, and drove the Toucouleurs out of Hamdallaye. El Hadj Omar fled up into the Bandiagara Plateau pursued by the Peul army. At this point, versions of the story differ. The Peul, who are his arch detractors, assign him an inglorious death by being sealed alive in a cave. Others maintain he committed suicide, and some say he was killed by an accidental explosion of gunpowder stores. Westerners are often puzzled by the mystery surrounding El Hadj Omar's disappearance. After all, it is strange that the head of such an enormous army should just disappear. But, in this part of Africa, unusual personages such as he rarely just die. It seems more fitting that they simply vanish or fade away in a cloak of mystery. People seem to prefer it that way. Although Hamdallaye lay in ruins and the Peul empire in disarray, the echo of half a century of theocratic rule remained alive in the inland delta. Theocracy had left as its legacy a code of social custom and religious ethic and an ingenious design for pastoral organization.

Chapter VI

On the Trail of the Nomads

After I had obtained all of this historical information, I set out to see if tradition and the codes of Cheikou Ahmadou's theocratic rule had in fact survived a century of worldly realism. What was involved was an extensive trip of several thousands of miles through the inland delta. People said that such a trip was impossible during the rainy season, June through October. Rivers were in flood; tracks were either washed out or under a foot of water; villages were inaccessible except on horseback and the mosquitoes so thick the Malians said they would smother you if you took too deep a breath. Whether or not I liked it, and with a complete disregard for reason and prudence, this enterprise of mine was undertaken as Ahmadou my houseboy said, "By the will of God," at the height of the rainy season. At home, it was the season of summer vacations, beach parties, graduations and weddings. But, in Mali, it was the time of water, mud, mosquitoes and patience.

It would have helped matters a great deal had I been in good health at the outset of this long bush trip, but as luck would have it, I came down with a bout of severe dysentary two days before I was to leave. The laboratory in Bamako said I had amoeba in my stool, but this really didn't clarify things since they were always finding amoeba in people's stools except when they changed laboratory technicians and suddenly found that no one in Bamako had amoeba. I treated myself empirically, but this time the empiricist's intuitions didn't pay off. I did my packing in a dilapidated state of physical decay, full of a sense of duty and empty of physical reserve. In spite of my feverish state, I didn't overlook taking along several boxes of paperback books of the Nouveaux Horizons series put out by the United States Information Service.

My friend, Bob Baker, who was a USIS officer in Bamako at that time, always managed to put together a miraculous collection of a-poltical, non-controversial subjects which brought pleasure to readers in remote bush posts and avoided the suspicion of militant supporters of the regime.

It was always a pleasant event whenever I handed out the books to school teachers or other literate people. There was always a crowd of onlookers, eager to get a glimpse at the covers and the pictures inside. Had I known in Bamako that Ahmadou had decided to replace some books with extra rolls of toilet paper, I would have decried the precaution as unnecessary. As it was, I made the discovery of the substitution along with all of the local officials of a small town after having told them what wonderful books I had packed away in the box. Most of them had never seen toilet tissue before and so an embarrassing explanation had to be given covering both manufacture and use which in the end left me with a red face and put a crowd of eavesdropping children into fits of laughter. That I was caught in possessoon of such a large quantity of the stuff prompted a number of well-intentioned questions about the bowel habits of Americans. It was rather befitting I think that they should have thought me somewhat strange especially since I walked around under an umbrella when it rained (Malian umbrellas are for the sun and are not waterproof) and slept on a foam-rubber pillow. When a vaccination team passed through this town a year later, they were asked if they knew of the strange white doctor who walked beneath an umbrella which kept him dry, slept on rubber, and rolled his feces in long white paper and put it in a box to send back to America.

Long road trips into the Malian bush can be divided into three distinct phases. The first occurs before starting, and consists of arm-chair dreams of romance unbound by any horizon. It is a period of joyful anticipation, of uplifting fantasies, of imagined experiences devoid of physical discomfort which combine adventure with satisfaction. The second phase shatters the first because in place of idyllic experiences you are rewarded with an aching back, dehydration, desalination, dust, scorching heat, friction burns on your skin and an uncomfortable blotch of sweat on the back of your shirt as big as a serving platter. When a tepid shower fails to revive your spirits, you wish you had never come and swear you will never do it again . The third phase is when you finally get back to Bamako, to the relative comforts of a soft chair and churning ceiling fan. You reminisce and remember and realize that the unreal and unimaginable actually happened. There is an inward sense of satisfaction, of having accomplished something of worth and because this stirs your altruism and philosophical thoughts, phase two is accepted with resolution.

Malian road trips affect most people adversely, but there are a few stalwarts who enjoy them. Those who dislike such trips can support their argument by complaining of the heat, the hot wind blowing through the window, the monotony of the flat savanna landscape, dust, and the danger to life and limb posed by Malians behind the wheel. People like myself who enjoy bush trips are often asked why. I think it is because I always feel an immense sense of freedom in the African bush, develop an uplifted state of mind devoid of the pressures created by the necessities of a noisy and busy modern world, and feel in touch with what is infinite. In the bush, one sees the world as it was created, untouched by man's hand, where plains and mountains, river-beds and lakes and great valleys wander off into the horizon in an unchanging and eternal way and in great silence. Before you there is not a road nor a fence, a house nor any human creation for hundreds of miles. It is a world of powerful stillness, a place for those who prefer to listen and think rather than speak.

There is always a frightening awareness of loneliness running through you for in that immensity you feel yourself the least significant of creations. Often, when I look out over the unending spread of low thorn trees, across deep valleys and down the never-ending channel of the Niger cutting its way through the white dunes, I think of those famous men and the deeds they authored in this part of the world. It is all written in bound books stored in modern libraries and, yet, here in the wilderness where it took place, there is no trace, no faint echo telling of either their passage, their accomplishments or their destiny. The bush is unchanged, just as it was in their time. Here, no one remembers them and their passage and deeds have been muted by time and erased in a world where nature does not seem to allow change and itself only turns over in a perpetual and unchanging cycle.

Men are of no consequence here, simply passers-by who, after a time, move out of the scene leaving little imprint on things. It is a frightening experience for many to confront such an enormous creation knowing that it considers them to be of little importance to it. You know that whatever you do will effect no drastic change, leave no permanent mark, and like the works of all those who have gone before, be erased by the gentle hand of time. The good done lingers on where it is felt rather than seen, in the depths of men's hearts and only you and they know what it is and where to find it. But the ego-filled man leaves nothing behind and in return has his very existence nullified. The lonely landscapes of Africa invoke in him a terrible fear because they are adverse to man's ego, give it no comfort, make no recognition of its self-esteem, pay it no compliment. Such men fear the bush, dread its endless views and feel swallowed up and destroyed in its overwhelming size and power and for them the experience is a terrible nightmare. But, for others, here the communication of the heart is not with man and what he has created, nor with his busy and rushed world, but with the wind and the sky, the sunset and the stars, the flow of the river and the silence of the hills and through them with something which is greater and more powerful, which is seen in an unchanging immensity.

We drove out of Bamako and across the narrow Niger River Bridge. The sun had just begun to nudge itself up over the last low remains of the Manding Hills, and far down over the river the silvery crescent of a new moon hung high in the chilly air. The early morning air during the rainy season is full of a special intangible power which both stimulates and pleases. The countryside sweeps by you, a mosaic of high grass, light-gray baobabs and shea butter trees. A delightful chilliness flows into the truck and rushes your face which is an unexpected luxury in a hot and arid country. The dry season seems to deprive everything of smell, to sap nature of that extra reserve she needs to bestow this added dimension. But, during the rains, smells rush in on you, sweet grass and flowering shrubs, the tang of burnt grass, the satisfying aroma of a village fire. There is a peaceful blending of elements, of green land and blue sky, of patches of warm sunshine and sprays of drizzle from scattered clouds. You are more observant when it is cool and can better examine your surroundings uninhibited by the usual obsession with heat and thirst and a craving for the shade.

A large truck makes a great deal of noise and were you not to stop you might travel many miles with the conviction that the bush is full of silence. But when you stop, you hear the far-off rushing of a stream, the muffled noise of village life drifting through the trees, a bird declaring his happiness and whirls of breeze dancing across the grass. Everything you see makes for an immensity full of a noble resistance to being tamed. The trees dominate the savanna of West Africa, not in the graceful and supple forms of the Eastern African bush, but as twisted clusters of crooked trunks and branches whose struggle for survival has deprived them of the luxury of beauty. There are no long delicate branches humming in the breeze nor towering lines reaching up into the sky. Rather, it is a continuous monotony of rigid and heavy forms in which only the leaves vibrate in the afternoon breeze. All is conformity, a world of repetitive shapes where individuality is diminuitive like some unnecessary accessory which, if taken away, is not missed. Only the giant baobabs serve as landmarks in the savanna, their broad ponderous gray trunks rising up two-hundred feet into the weightless clouds. Their branches are massive, protruding from the trunk in a haphazard design which is abstract and when seen against the red glow of a setting sun look like giant goblins from an ancient fairy-tale. The whole baobab dances against the sky, a figure sporting many arms with fingers, twisted and formed into the meaningful lines of some great ballet. The fruit of the baobab is green like a giant pear and inside are thousands of pits covered with a white sugary wafer material. Long ago, people discovered that it was an excellent remedy for diarrhea and today it is used as such even in modern clinics in West Africa. The bark of the baobab is thin and smooth and rumpled into folds at the base of the trunk and where the giant branches emerge. You are apt to wonder why so giant a tree has survived the axes of the woodcutters. It is because the wood is pulpy and unsuitable for firewood. And so the baobab survives in the savanna where it attains great age and becomes a landmark. Great cavities often form inside of the trunk and long ago in Senegal, where the tree is the national emblem, the dead were buried inside of these huge holes. In Mali, the Bambara often hide their fetishes and their masks inside of the baobabs and invariably bees establish hives in the trees, making them unsuitable as a place to rest beneath.

During the rains, it is the shades of green and the blue of the sky with its mighty oval puffs of clouds which relieve the tedium. I sometimes think it strange that one could find the sky and the clouds of such immense interest. But, during the long dry season, there is no luxuriousness either in the heavens or on the land. One is hemmed in by horizons limited by dust and heat waves and made to bear the heavy burden of a leaden sky. So, a blue sky, and a floating procession of clouds sailing across it, become such a delightful change of character for the heavens that you cannot resist enjoying it to its fullest and taking in some of its vigor.

When I first began traveling in Mali, most of the roads were not paved. I learned to live with washboard corrugations, potholes and dust. Then they began building new paved roads over the old ones and my system had to adjust to the bumps and white powdery dust of the detours bulldozed out of the bush. Now there are a thousand miles of paved road in Mali and I have no cause to complain. The Dodge truck I traveled in was not built for comfort, but I was able to sit up high, and, through the broad windows of the crew cab, have a superb view of the countryside. I always accepted the bouncing, which went with the hard springs, as the price for this splendid view. Small Renaults and Deux Chevauxs glide over the bumps without shaking the innards of their passengers, but the view never rises above the level of the low bush. All of this bouncing over the years took its toll on my back and kidneys which suffered disabling after effects.

Although I am a keen observer of the countryside, I am also a back seat driver. This is a laudable quality to have in Mali and it has often saved people's lives. A Malian driver must never be viewed as the product of some sudden creative act, who, equipped with a license to drive, embodies all that is to be desired in perception, judgement and reflex. Rather, he is someone who possesses a self-styled and arrogant greatness and the comfortable conviction that his skill is so perfect as to preclude his learning anything new. Drivers receive their tutoring in an apprenticeship system where for a period of up to five years, they change flat tires, load and unload the trucks, and rarely get a chance to drive. During this time, they are paid about a dollar a month and are dependent on their teacher for food and lodging. After five years of tedious scut work, they present themselves for a driver's license totally unfamiliar with the wheel and lacking any real mechanical skill. Most fail the examination and finally pass through the pay-off system. Exploited as cheap labor for many years, they are finally unleashed on the roads where, like their teachers, they become an incredible menace.

No statistics are kept on road accidents in Mali, but if they were, one would see that they have already reached staggering proportions. There may be twenty or thirty killed when a market truck overturns. That the driver used poor judgement in swerving his five ton truck off the road to avoid hitting a chicken is never brought into question. "C'est le Dieu," the driver will reply, and, if he survives, the police will echo the same refrain. Paved roads in Mali are a nightmare of blind curves, narrow pavement, low shoulders and sudden contacts with speeding taxis and trucks, often on the wrong side of the road, without headlights, brakes or reflectors. Side and rear-view mirrors are often missing and hanging on the bedroom wall back home or else turned in so that the driver can spend long hours admiring himself. Drivers aren't concerned with anything which is on the side of them or behind. What matters for them is the roadway ahead. They sit hunched over the wheel as if in a trance and stare ahead aglow with that omnipotence which comes from having a powerful machine at one's command. Their arrivals and departures are a thunderous roar of unnecessary acceleration and swirling clouds of dust which ruin starters and carbureators but gain for them the admiration of female onlookers. The concept of maintenance is alien, submerged by Islamic fatalism, and so, vehicles die from a lack of oil, brake fluid and radiator water.

For the most part, road accidents in Mali occur as a result of speeding and encounters with obstacles which come from the side and behind. The roads are banked by ten foot high stands of thick grass and are full of goats, sheep, donkeys, cattle, ox-drawn carts, dogs, cats, birds and people walking, on motor bikes, horses, camels, bicycles and a host of other inanimate objects. Although I never lived in a rural area of the United States, since coming to Mali I have had ample time to observe the behavior patterns of most domestic animals on the road. These behavior patterns are predictable and so a driver with good judgement can learn through experience what is to be done when they are encountered. Goats are quick and alert and full of instincts and reflexes which send them off the road when they hear a vehicle coming. So, it is rare for them to get hit. It's disquieting, however, to encounter sheep because they are capable of running alongside the speeding car and of suddenly rushing across the road in front of you. Cows take notice of you, but stand their ground and donkeys take no notice of you at all. It is a terrifying experience to witness a Malian driver speeding down a road into a herd of cattle for you think that he should know as you do that they are not going to get out of the way in time. Then when the final few seconds are left he tries to slow down by breaking and forgets what you once told him about slowing the truck by shifting into lower gears.

In an Africa so endlessly big, you are apt to wonder why so many domestic animals are found on a narrow strip of pavement. It is as if fate is playing a nasty trick on you. But in Mali, the millions of domestic animals prefer to rest on the soft surface of the tarmac instead of on the hard laterite earth.

There has always been a fatal misunderstanding between vehicles and Malian pedestrians. It doesn't seem to matter whether they be on foot or riding a bicycle or horse. Their reactions are almost always the same. They loom up ahead of you on the road and you know that in a few moments the vehicle will be on top of them. If they turned their heads and didn't get out of the way you might conclude that they have taken notice of you but have no capacity to judge speed. But they don't turn their heads, and simply continue to move along in quiet harmony with everything non-motorized, getting out of the way with a frantic explosion of movement only when you are on top of them. So, whenever you approach them, you must slacken the rhythm of the motor, move the gears downward and put the brakes on so as to put yourself into a companionable relationship with them. I know that you can hear the combined noise of the Dodge motor and eight-ply tires for a great distance. It was only natural to wonder then why people didn't get out of the way.

"Don't they hear the truck?" I used to ask our drivers.

"They're too stupid," they would answer with certainty.

Others, who considered themselves privileged educated persons, gave less-complimentary reasons. "They're too savage yet, too primitive," they would say. "That is why they don't get out of the way." Had such remarks come from me or another foreigner we would have been accused of being racists. But, Malians could make such statements in their splendid uninhibited way, injure no one, and in all sincerity think that they had spoken the truth. If men learn through experience, then it seemed plausible to think that even people in the bush would come to know what had to be done in face of an oncoming car. It took me quite some time to find out why people didn't get out of the way. But the reason was very simple. Although their bodies were moving along the major arteries of the country, their minds were lost on the shadowy paths of daydreams. Jay tried to solve the problem by buying mountain bus horns. The manufacturer claimed that they could clear the road of anything animate. I had certain doubts about that claim, but the cattle did move and the sheep ran off and even the donkeys took notice of us. Although the donkeys didn't get out of the way, at least they gave us a blink of the eye and a few twitchings of the ear which was more than they did for anyone else. But our mountain bus horns never succeeded in shattering the continuity of a Malian daydream.

As we bounced along the twisting paved road to Segou, I wondered how we would all get along together. A long bush trip weakens both the body and the mind, strips them both of their usual defenses, and lays bare the underlying structure for what it really is. There were three other people in the truck with me, Modibo Keita, the driver, Djigui Diakite, the un-official dean of the vaccinators, and Boundiar, an infirmier. Modibo is a quiet person, generously endowed with honesty and loyalty and a strong inclination towards serious introspection. I have always thought that Modibo's long thin form could move with ease into the quiet shadows of some far off monestary and feel perfectly comfortable in its contemplative routine and detached outlook on life. He is a man of great principle and has a very keen sense of the rightness of things in life. I always thought he took things too much to heart and because of this was often hurt and depressed by it all. It was fortunate for Modibo that his desire to learn and improve himself, overshadowed his appreciable endowment of pride. This pride of his was not without some foundation because in the fading world of tradition he was a member of a Malinke chiefly family from Kita. There was much rancor in Modibo's heart about this whole matter and he gave it considerable thought. His greatgrandfather, Togunta, who was the strongman of Kita, signed the treaty with the French General Gallieni in 1881 which put Kita under the protection of France and opened the way to Bamako. The sword which Gallieni gave Togunta as a symbol of friendship now hangs on a wall in the family compound in Kita. Togunta was succeeded by his son N'Faly Keita whom the French appointed *Diamana Tigui* (paramount chief) of the then recently created cercle of Kita. When N'Faly died in 1941, the French administration upset the traditional succession in bypassing Modibo's father, Mamadou Keita, appointing instead a distant cousin whom they considered more cooperative with the colonial government. Modibo's father never forgave the French for denying him what he considered to be his birthright and the people of Kita still considered him as their leader. Emphasizing this point never quieted Modibo whose dislike for the French will be eternal. As he saw it, his father, who died in 1956, had been the victim of an injustice which was no longer reparable. With independence, the traditional structures were officially abolished, but continue today in the attitudes and inter-personal relationships of those who respect tradition. As things stood, Modibo's oldest paternal uncle now possessed the succession of family chieftaincy which would eventually fall to him.

Modibo never spoke much about all of this nor about who he was. I think it was because he possessed that inner confident sense of who he was and was convinced that everyone else was aware of it. He only had to speak his name and those of his ancestors to draw an obsequious reaction from other Malinke people. This gave him the complex of a princling. But, in spite of it, he was able to move into most settings with an enviable gift of tact and understanding. At a very young age, he had been sent off to school in Dakar which gave his character that added quality of discipline which his fellow drivers didn't possess. Because of his interests in mechanics, he studied this field in school, and, with the lowering of all class and caste barriers at independence, became a driver for the Ministry of Health. Modibo was still torn between the two worlds, somewhat resentful of what he considered to be the unfair course of history. By necessity, he was a driver and mechanic; by desire he would be a chief.

There is great consistency in Modibo's driving, sound judgement, perception and rapid reflexes. All of these qualities were greatly developed in him by Jay who, during a patience filled year, shaped Modibo into one of the finest driver-mechanics in the country. He

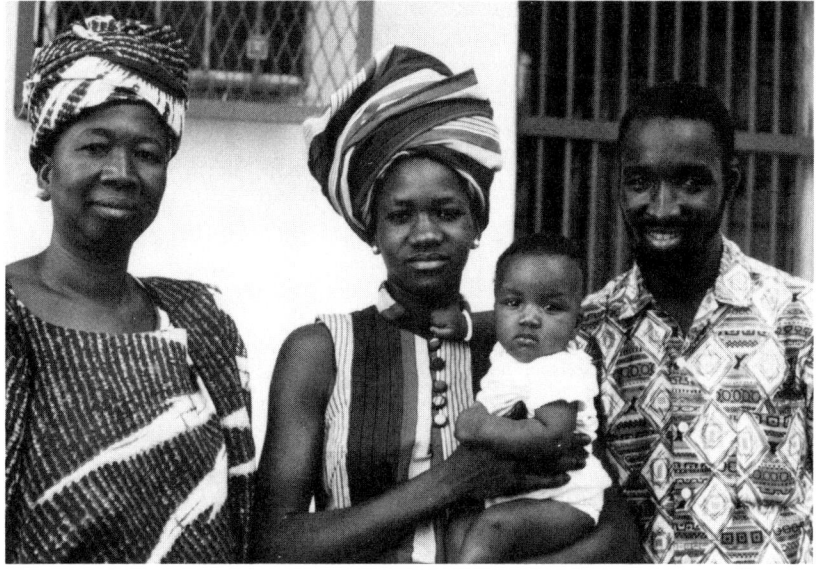

FIGURE 11. Modibo N'Faly Keita *(right)* with his wife, Astan Cisse *(center)* holding their first child Moussa, and his late aunt, Mari Diallo Keita *(left)*.

eventually took us over two hundred thousand miles of tracks and roads, open country, up cliffs and across rivers, through mud and sand dunes, and each time brought me back to Bamako safe and sound.

Boundiar was a man of fifty years who towered over six feet tall and who behaved like an aristocratic rogue elephant, convinced of his authority and superiority over all, yet to everyone else so obviously broken and defeated by time and the hardships of life. Boundiar had an uncontrollable love of fighting, like some trained and undefeated cock from the arena. He also had an unusual contempt for saying anything good about anyone else except himself and was always full of anger and indignation against any person or institution with which he had contact. Because Boundiar's criticisms were always vague and unfounded, lacking the luster of being true, they were never taken seriously by anyone. It was pitiable that Boundiar's old heart was still full of so much turbulent strife and anger when in the twilight years you would have hoped for equanimity and a soothing calm. I couldn't regard it as anything less than pathologic and respected it as I would the emotional ills of a patient.

Boundiar had been a trouble-maker all his life. But, because he was an irreplaceable asset, he moved through life under the protection of both a French and Malian policy which preferred to transfer its problems rather than fire them. Whenever Boundiar's trouble-making became intolerable at a given post, he was transferred. And, when I met him after he had done thirty years of service, he was unchallenged as the most travelled infirmier in Mali. Although Boundiar never lasted very long in any one place, his gregarious nature enabled him to accumulate an impressive amount of knowledge about local customs and attitudes. It always astonished me that someone so involved in disputes had the time to make such observations. But even in his descriptions of the various ethnic groups, Boundiar was neither benevolent nor endowed with the anthropologist's natural urge to defend and praise the objects of his study.

During one of Boundiar's brief assignments, this time in Timbuctoo, he became friends with a schoolteacher, Modibo Keita, who in spite of the name similarity, is no relation to Modibo our driver. Modibo Keita had been sent into exile to Timbuctoo by the French because of his political activities. Even though it was to be another twenty years before he would become the first president of Mali, Boundiar's cold instincts drew him into a benign friendship which for him was a singularly rare thing. Boundiar's explosive urge for trouble-making was channeled this time by Modibo Keita in a political direction. At first, the French administrators of Timbuctoo displayed tolerance, but when Boundiar's antics led to physical violence, he was transferred. His friendship with Modibo Keita, however, remained firm and in later years enabled him to get his way in any dispute.

Boundiar's claims of being a true Communist were obviously at variance with his incessant bragging about his noble ancestry. He often spoke about his father who had been a chef de canton in Kayes and of his mother who he said came from a noble Moroccan family. He felt that this background gave him a natural pre-eminence over everyone and so he never tired of talking about himself. In the end, you felt that you were dealing with two separate and distinct personalities, Boundiar as he was, and Boundiar as he *said* he was. He saw himself as a mighty and noble figure, triumphant by nature and great through genetic linkage and the hero of innumerable medical exploits. But in front of you sat a very insecure and unhappy old man.

Boundiar's appointment as my escort and guide was an expedient choice for the Malians. In his back offices at the Service d'Hygiene, he was causing too much trouble and it was time for a transfer. It seemed logical to dump him on me since other transfer locations were by this time virtually exhausted. Also it was certain that he would be contemptuous of seeing anything good in what I said or did and would hand the security police the kinds of reports they desired. He took enormous pleasure in later years telling people that I worked for the CIA. Hadn't he himself seen my diploma. Actually, what he had seen was an insurance certificate from the COA, the Commissioned Officers Association of the United States Public Health Service. It gave Boundiar prestige in Bamako to have been chosen as a watchdog for one of the most dangerous spies in the country. At least, this is what he liked to think people thought. He thrust himself into his dual role with enthusiasm and vigor. As he saw it, the success of Mali's fight against smallpox and measles hinged on his helping me, but in his dedicated vigilance lay Mali's internal security.

I never thought that my relationship with Boundiar would prove the exception to a rule remarkable for a half-century of consistency. It was a certainty that the unhappy moment of fatal misunderstanding would come. Such breaks usually left Boundiar delighted even though there was no doubt in anyone else's mind as to who was at fault. This time, Boundiar's inventory of libel would not be dismissed as mere bable. Malians are so generously endowed with splendid imaginations that they did not have it in them to resist believing Mali the possessor of a treasure of assets so important that a great power like the United States could afford not to send spies to uncover it. It fired their fancies and warmed their egos to think of me as a spy and added a wonderful spice of excitement to the usual routine of their lives.

Djigui rapidly became the unofficial dean of the vaccinators. In many ways, the role fell to him quite naturally. He had served as a sergeant in the French army for eight years during which time he passed through a kaleidoscopic series of experiences from falling in love with the French commanding colonel's daughter to having bar room

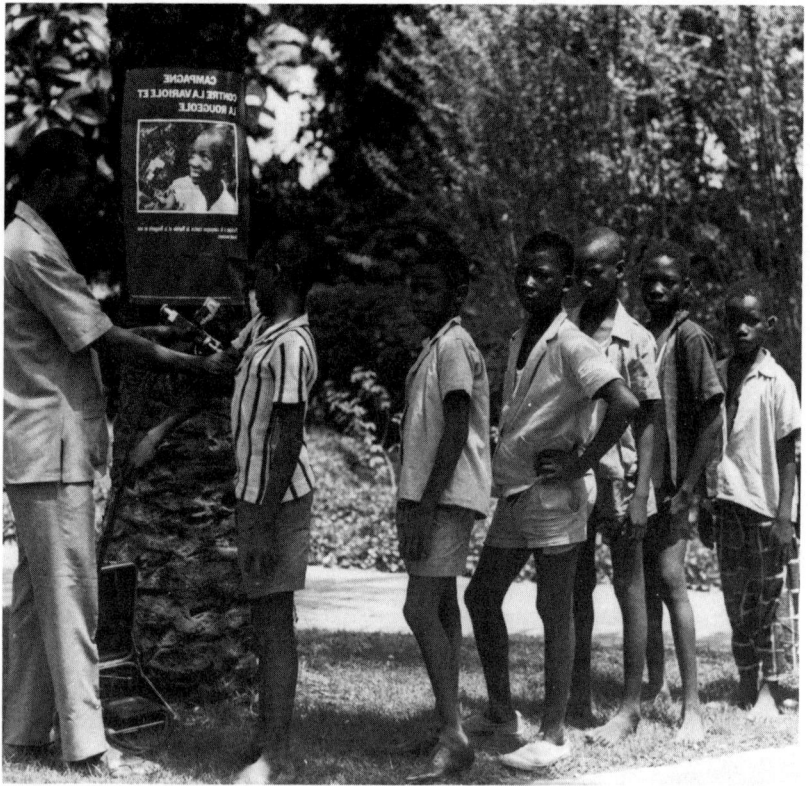

FIGURE 12. Djigui Diakite *(right)* vaccinating a group of young boys in Bamako. In the rear, attached to a tree is one of the vaccination campaign posters designed by Robert Baker of the United States Information Service, Bamako.

brawls with Foreign Legionnaires in Algiers. Had Djigui been born in Europe or America, he would have made a natural for the stage. People are greatly attracted to him, to his warm personality, joking manner, and ability to recount a story in all its detail without ever losing the listener's interest. He is a wise politician, a master at rhetoric who has a persuasive skill every confidence-man would envy. There is nothing malicious or devious about him and most of what he says is not pre-meditated in advance. For Djigui, smooth persuasive syntax is an unconscious quality which operates instinctively in just the right way under every imaginable circumstance.

If Djigui has a fault in his make up it is that he is easily led. I could never conceive of him as being partisan to a given cause or principle or loyal for long to any person. He is a bon vivant who sails with the prevailing winds. Because Djigui was only recently converted to Islam he was a member of all the Bambara and Malinke secret societies and had an encyclopedic knowledge of their masks and statues. It was through him that I was initiated into the *Komo*, the most secret of these societies. With his help as an interpreter, I was able to carry out an extensive study of the Bambara and Malinke secret societies, their customs, dances, fetishes and masks. It was wonderfully satisfying to be able to channel Djigui's great abilities into a variety of creative enterprises. The most obstinate village chiefs became models of cooperation under his sway and, thanks to his diplomatic skill, health services were delivered to thousands who otherwise would have refused them.

Djigui always felt that life had cheated him. When independence came to Mali, he was three years from retirement from the French army. Retirement would have brought with it a monthly pension, the equivalent of which now takes Djigui a year to earn. He would have been a wealthy *ancien combattant* (veteran), joining the ranks of the thousands of other pensioned Malians who served in the French army. But Djigui was charmed by the eloquent discourses of President Modibo Keita, urging every native son to return to Mali. Promised a position in the new Malian army, he returned, only to learn that all who had served in the French army were excluded from enlisting. He found himself without a job and no longer eligible for his pension. In desperation, he took the only available job he could find, that of a vaccinator in the Ministry of Health. Djigui was not bitter about the unfair blow fate had dealt him; he only thought it unfair.

It began to rain as we got to Segou, a light drizzle which barely fell through the canopy of Caicedra trees lining the main street. As you enter Segou there is a long file of massive cement buildings on either side of the road, red and cream-colored creations with moorish arches, turrets and battlements and massive verandas endowed with shade and gentle currents of air. There is something very functional in the design of these neo-sundanese creations, the thick walls and high ceilings, the encircling verandas arching their way around the perimeter with massive green drapes hanging limpid in the archways. Boundiar chose to ignore the beauty which lay behind the cool veil of drizzle and erupted instead into a fierce criticism of the French colonials who had forced the Malians to construct the buildings . These buildings were in a way very depassé, built by Frenchmen whose dreams of a sudanese Eldorado were full of cities of spires and turrets and sumptuous palaces of Moorish magnificence. When the French romantics came and found only the desolate bush and the small crumbling villages of baked mud, they themselves built what they had expected to find, what in their dreams they thought should be there. None of it served any urgent need. It only lessened disappointment and helped realize a dream.

We drove on to Koutiala, a delightful town which sits in a shallow valley in south-eastern Mali. The new paved road had not yet been built and in premature anticipation of its completion, the Travaux Publique had let the existing dirt track fall into decay. Puddles and red mud lined the way for two hundred miles. The truck twisted and swerved with the contours of the track and churned up a never ending spray of red mud. Normally, vehicles are not permitted to travel on dirt roads in Mali when it is raining. *Barrières de Pluie* are set up and not taken down until two hours have elapsed since the last rain falls. The system usually works except that occasionally there is a dispute between the watchmen and the truck drivers over when the rain actually stopped. A downpour may stop and an hour go by and then suddenly there is a light drizzle for five minutes. Truck drivers maintain that the drizzle doesn't count, but the watchmen at the roadblocks do and start counting time again. Generally, the end-result is a fist fight. Ministry of Health vehicles are permitted to pass rain barriers, but others who are cunning can sometimes talk their way through. I once traveled to Bamako from Mopti with André Szabo who was a fisheries expert for the United Nation's Food and Agriculture Organization. He insisted on taking his own car which I warned would never get through the rain barrier at San. I moved ahead in my Dodge and as soon as the watchman saw the red cross he rushed out and pulled back the bar. Szabo who was miles behind me finally got to the barrier and found over thirty vehicles piled up in a torrential downpour. But that didn't stop him. He drove up to the front of the line and shouted that the bar be removed. The watchman refused.

"Can't you see it's raining," shouted the watchman. "You can't pass." Szabo replied that he was on an important mission and that he had to get through.

"I don't care who you are and what you have to do," answered the watchman.

"Whether you are white or black, you can't pass." And to prove his point the man pointed to several Europeans sitting patiently in their cars. Szabo wasn't to be disuaded. "I'm the chief inspector for the Water and Forest Service," he said. "I'm here to inspect the flooding on the road ahead." Down came the barrier and Szabo was on his way.

Whenever we arrived at one of these barriers, the young watchmen rushed out from beneath their straw shelters and pulled back the bar. If for some reason they were too slow, Boundiar shouted at them, threatening them with ridiculous prison terms, such as twenty years at hard labor, for not being deferent enough to a high-ranking official such as himself. If it weren't raining most of the men would have laughed at Boundiar. As it was, they simply ignored him. Neither Djigui nor Modibo took Boundiar seriously at such moments. It was a remarkable phenomenon to witness how in between these outbursts the three of them in spite of their diverse backgrounds and differing personalities could fill up the time with a pleasing murmur of Bambara conversation.

All the way to Koutiala the air was cold and the grass dripping wet. From out of the soft drumming of the rain came the lonely calls of hornbills and the tranquil conversation of doves. Small rivers and streams swelled and boiled as foamy brown torrents and raced with tremendous speed beneath the small cement bridges which were a reminder of provincial France. Once the rain stopped, the stream beds were muddy and damp and the water well on its way to join the Bani and the Niger.

Koutiala is the logical place to begin a study of the Peul nomads in Mali. It is the southernmost point of their distribution and the place from which begins their complicated movements across the Mali-Upper Volta frontier into the flood plains of the Niger. In the rainy season, it is a high green land of rolling hills and deep lush valleys covered with fields of millet and cotton and accented with courts of baobab monarchs

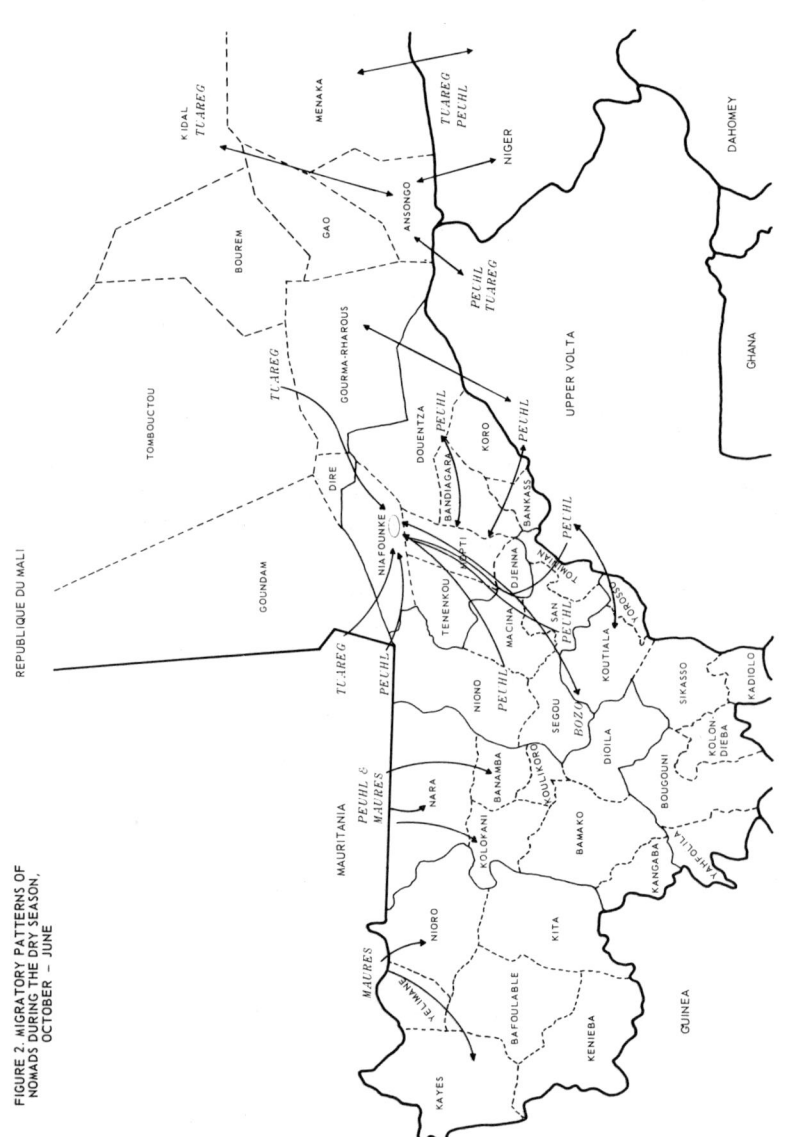

FIGURE 2. MIGRATORY PATTERNS OF NOMADS DURING THE DRY SEASON, OCTOBER – JUNE

and shea butter trees. This country doesn't belong to the Peul, but to the farmers who till it, to the Bobo-Ulé, Minianka and Bambara. The Peul are thought of as strangers, as people who pass through in transit, as men who hold no direct communion with the land. There are about four hundred thousand Peul living along the arching frontier of the Upper Volta. For the administrators, some are Malian and others Voltaics, depending on which side of the frontier they live on. But such classifications have no place in the Peul's traditional world, except that when taxes are collected in Mali, they all move to Upper Volta and if the government of Upper Volta begins to count their cattle for taxation prposes, they move to Mali. The Peul in this area live a very traditional life centered on their cattle. They call this frontier area the *Seno*, the high place, and from it move down into the flood plains when the rains stop and the waters recede.

It was my plan to move up along the Malian side of the frontier from Koutiala to Douentza, a distance of six hundred miles and in doing so make contact with all of the Peul clans who migrate into the flood plains. This was a very difficult undertaking since all of the tracks in the regon were a nightmare of water and mud. Modibo didn't look forward to what lay ahead. An unexpected complicating factor that year was the unusually heavy rains which imposed a new time sequence for harvests and nomadic migrations and made difficult the predicting of the direction nomad movements would take.

From where we camped for the first time, you could see a small stream which formed part of the international boundary between Mali and Upper Volta. It was the site of a very large wéré, a nomad camp, containing several extended families and several thousand head of cattle. The huts were arranged in a semi-circular fashion and made of dried ten foot high stalks of millet and built in the shape of an American Indian wigwam. The head of this camp was a middle-aged Peul by the name of Alfarou Diallo who was responsible for taking all of the cattle into the flood plain between the Bani and Niger rivers. Although Boundiar claimed credit for our being accepted into this camp, Modibo and I knew that it was chiefly because of Djigui's expert efforts.

Mornings in this camp were truly delightful. I would wake up and see a triangular piece of sky between the flaps of the roof window of the tent, deep blue and cool, and feel the wind as a gentle flury sifting through the canvas windows. You have to be up early in a nomad camp because the cattle begin to move at sunrise. When the first yellow rays of dawn break on the horizon, the valleys are full of a litany of crowing roosters and singing finches. Then you hear the muffled thuds of the women's calabashes, the soft shuffling of human feet, a baby's hungry cry and the soothing sound of water splashing up from a shallow well. Puffs of smoke from a cooking fire drift by over the west ground and off in the background you hear the steady crash of streams of milk falling from several teats into large hollow calabashes.

Once the milking was completed, the cows, bulls and calves moved out of the camp in a slow shuffling procession. They followed a path which went west toward an open plain down in the valley. It was a wide trail, well beaten and used, which skirted around fields of standing millet and ripened corn, detoured the villages of the sedentary Minianka farmers, and ended where there was only grass. The herdsmen walked up and down the column with their wrists dangling in a relaxed fashion over their shouldered clubs. They didn't shout or scream at the cattle, but moved them along with a constant cough like sound. Several small naked boys from the camp followed, their pot bellies and legs still covered with thin layers of red mud from the previous afternoon's play. They carried little sticks and jumped over the trail of steaming dung left behind by the herds. The few sheep and goats in the camp followed at a respectable distance, but the donkeys and their long-eared fuzzy colts stayed behind in camp. The herds pastured all day long under the watchful eye on the shepherds who took special care that the cattle didn't get into the cultivated fields. This is one of the greatest causes of disputes between the nomads and the sedentary farmers. But once the harvest is in, the problem never arises and the farmers are only too happy to have the herds pass over their fields and fertilize them.

The daily routine in Alfarou Diallo's camp scarcely changed from day to day. The women who stayed at home, ground corn and millet, churned butter, milked their own cows, sewed garments, plaited straw mats, made millet cakes and in the evening went down to the international frontier and did the wash. In the warm hours of the afternoon, the women and children crawled into the low doorways of their huts and waited out the heat spinning cotton and repairing their broken calabashes. Only when it was market day in a nearby village did the huts of the camp stand still and silent in the sun. The women always started off early in the morning, marching off single-file down the narrow bush paths with three or four calabashes of milk, butter and cream stacked on their heads. Some of the markets were over ten miles away and it took them many hours of walking to go and come for what amounted to a transaction of only ten cents. But the business side of things is secondary. Market day is a day off, a time to put one's finery on, to gossip, to meet friends, hear the news, solidify friendships and have fun.

It is hard for we who are the sedentaries of this world to accept the fact that people like the Peul can live indifferent to their surroundings. We develop attachments to places and find security in familiar things and settings. And so it is that we find it difficult to come to grips with a man's incessant search for new and unknown places. But for the nomad, security lies not in his surroundings, but in the herds, the family, clan and friends. Those who would sedentarize him try to attract him to the security a fixed habitat offers. That their offer goes unheeded is no surprise.

The Peul are a people who also have an inimitable ability to ignore strangers. One goes into their camps with the finest of intentions and comes away dejected. You are not greeted by a rushing crowd of eager faces and warm hand shakes nor by an effusion of friendly greetings. Instead, you receive a gentle distinterested turn of the head, an aloof glance, a shrewd evaluation, and nothing more. They are polite, never gay nor hospitable and you are not made to feel at home among them. Even if you go up to their huts you probably won't be invited in out of the sun. You look inside and it surprises you with its sturdy walls of plaited grass hung with calabashes and gourds and swords and spears. Soft skins and rugs cover the floor and the scent of Moroccan incense hangs delightfully in the air like a beautiful distillation of the luxury of another world transported across barren deserts and through hardships beyond imagination. Beautiful calm faces look at you from the darkness, you hear the shy giggles of the girls, the daring laughter of the boys, the growl of an annoyed dog. They may not come out to greet you, but if they do, the head of the family will touch your hand. No hefty handshake this, just a slight quick touching of the palms. But it is sincere, the hand touching the chest first to show that the handshake comes from the heart and afterwards to show that it is where yours goes. There is much protocol to handshaking in Mali, especially among the Bambara and Malinke where a young man must never give a hefty handshake to an old man. It is a sign of disrespect. Only those of the same age groups may give hardy handshakes. I remember once that a visiting physician from the Center for Disease Control traveled with me into the bush and gave a hard handshake to all those he met. It was while we were camped in a small Marka village that the old men came to me and said in Bambara, "Who is this man who dares to shake our hands so hard." I never told the physician anything about the matter since he was leaving the country in a few days. As it was, it had been a trying trip. But I made excuses to the old men, telling them that in our country it was a sign of respect.

It is easy to become exasperated with the Peul and your first temptation is to leave and let them be. And this is just what they want you to do. But I didn't leave and I didn't let them be and that is why they no longer have smallpox in their camps. I know that their stagnation and detachment for the outside world cannot last much longer. It will not be long before the aggressive and demanding economic needs of the country will break into their lives. There may be a few more years of blissful isolation to run out yet, but the upheaval is coming as a trickle out of the unimpressive straw hats where nomad children learn to scratch their letters with their fingers in the sand.

Like all Peuls, Alfarou Diallo was accustomed to the unexpected and fully equipped to deal with the unforeseen. The hills and valleys of the Seno were his domain where among the nomads he was a man of undisputed power, property and prestige, and so he had little reason to fear three Africans and a white man traveling in a white truck marked with a red cross. When he readily agreed to our staying in his camp I don't think it was because he had summed us up and thought us to be good men, but because he could not resist the adventurous experience our presence would bring. He was the *amirou-nai,* chief of the cattle of the Senekobé Peul who are the largest clan in the Seno. Looking at him in his patinated hat and tattered wool *sinyare* you would have never supposed that he was responsible for organizing and directing the movement of thousands of head of cattle into the flood plain. To appreciate Alfarou Diallo's magnificence as a human being you had to talk to him, hear him out, see him standing upright and firm before a group of his shepherds, and as he spoke, sense the respect which flowed from their grave faces as they listened to what he had to say. In him was a firm dedication to his own nature as a Peul shepherd. There wasn't anything assumed about his manner and nothing in him which was an imitation of what foreigners held in their world to be perfection. What he was had grown from inside and was nurtured and developed through conscious and disciplined effort. The young men thought of him as the ultimate expression of what a Peul shepherd should be because he embodied everything that history, race and tradition had set forth as the goal of achievement for Peul men.

When talking with me, his manner was always mild and deferent but in his passive face you saw the quiet pride and the self-assurance by which the Peul announces his indisputable superiority. The first afternoon we were in his camp he came over to my tent along with several shepherds and some youngsters carrying a calabash of milk. There was an overall rigid reserve about him and even when we exchanged thanks and endless counter compliments over the gift of the milk, his face never broke into anything more than a weak smile. He was not a man who spoke either freely or at great length but he showed much originality and frankness in whatever he had to say. Behind his calm exterior was a daring spirit and a high strung emotional core all held in check in a truly beautiful manner. Because he was a chief he had to show patience where others gave vent to anger, and mediate the conflicts which others had generated in moments of passion.

The people in Alfarou Diallo's camp were extremely handsome. The women were soft and delicate, light skinned and graceful with fine aquiline features and slender limbs. The men were tall, not husky nor heavy boned, but narrow and spare with lean smooth faces and deep-set eyes. There is great distinction in the eyes of the Peul. They are light brown and occasionally blue, set in a smooth and silky complexion beneath long black lashes. They have a way of staring at you with their eyes and in a few moments size you up and decide what you are. Their hair is straight, their lips thin, their whole form a harmony born of a hard and disciplined way of life. No one really knows where these unusual people came from. Some maintain they originated in Ethiopia or in North Africa and others maintain that they are descendants of the Jews who crossed the Sahara to Senegal centuries ago.

The Peul stand out wherever they are, not only on account of their physical appearance, but also because of their dress. The women glitter in a crowd, their coiffures being masterpieces of embroidery studded with silver coins, shining sequins, white cowrie shells, red beds, great tiarras of amber stones and gold rings. Those who know the Peul well have only to look at the women's coiffures and jewelry to know from which part of Mali they come. The men look more austere, especially the shepherds. Their tunics and robes are of coarse wool or cotton, white or else dyed a maroon color with the bark of the *nere* tree. They wear sandals and great straw hats rimmed with red leather and a coupola of the same. During the cold season, the shepherds carry intricately woven blankets known as *khasa* over one shoulder and wear turbans and mufflers.

Their rigid form of Islam, and austere way of life, has always

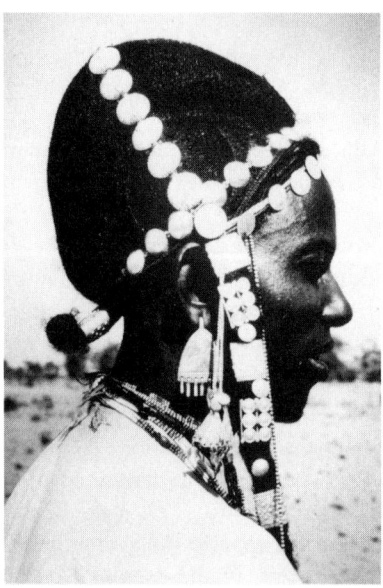

FIGURE 13. A young Peul nomadic herdsmen from the Seno wearing his finery for market day.

seemed to me to be out of step with the extravagance of their dress. You couldn't call the Peul an artistic people for they have not produced much in the way of a material culture such as sculptures or masks. Being Moslems they look down on such things and on the animists who make them. It is ironic that they should have intimate contact with those societies in Mali who have been the authors of some of the finest traditional art in West Africa, the Dogon, the Bambara, and Bobo. But I think their artistic impulses are there, thwrted perhaps by religious sanction, but diverted such that expression comes forth in personal beautification.

For the Peul, cattle are the center of life. It is the needs of these animals which shape and determine their way of life. The owner is the servant of the possession, the master the worshipper of that which supposedly serves him. There is no greater joy in the life of a Peul than for him to stand in the center of his herd, to watch them move off into the crisp morning horizon and to hear them shuffling back in the evening. His greatest passion is to count his cows and bulls, to hear their bellowing, to rub their sleek hides, to know everyone of them by sight, to see their greatest qualities and smallest defects, to see the dust and hear the roar of his passing herds, to have the scent of milk and manure in his nostrils, to be able to say that they are his. His whole emotional reserve is lavished on his cattle, his entire life a cycle of finding water and grass for them and of drinking their milk. Because of this, many say that the Peul are an unproductive society, their lives a pattern of hard work and inefficiency in which only the cattle grow fat and healthy and enjoy the comforts of life. But the Peul would have it no other way. They are resistant to the changes the government would like to introduce, reducing the size of their herds, improving their stock and increasing grazing. They are outside of the cash economy and seek little in the way of material possessions. But government is persistent and determined that all of this must change. An annual tax is placed on every head of livestock, two dollars for cows and a dollar for goats and sheep. People, too, must pay taxes and the government hopes that this will force the Peul to cull their herds and sell their cattle for the cash necessary to pay the taxes. But the Peul have developed counter measures to all of these taxes. They declare as little as ten percent of the cattle they own, pronounce grandma dead for the tax collector and deny that the last six children were ever born. But a gentle pressure is forcing the Peul to sell some of their cattle to the government buyer and the fine work of the veterinary department has begun to put relations between nomad and government on a plane of mutual understanding.

It would be wrong to saw that cattle represent wealth for the Peul. On the contrary, they are wealth, the bank account, the stock certificates and real estate all rolled into one. Political alliances are made with cattle, marriages contracted, disputes settled, wrongs made right, debts paid and gifts bestowed. If the rains fail or if the fields of the farmers are ravished by locust, there is no famine among the Peul. There is always milk, great calabashes of it, fresh or curdled, churned into butter or made into cheese. Peul cattle would take no prize at a fair for their milk production, but they produce enough to sustain those who need it.

Several days after our arrival, word came that one of Alfarou Diallo's shepherds had been arrested by the police and was being held in the gendarmerie in Koutiala on charges of having allowed his cattle to trample a field of millet. The irate Minianka farmer managed to chase the cattle off, but not before they had ruined his field. Then he began hurling insults at the Peul who in turn took offense and began hurling the insults back, starting with the man's mother and father and ending by saying that the Minianka were fetish worshippers who ate the meat of dogs, donkeys and pigs. While all of this was true, the manner in which it was said led the Minianka to draw his sword. The Peul let fly his club, first knocking the man across the knees and then giving him a blow over the back of the neck. The farmer fell to the ground convulsing and twitching and the Peul was about to let him have a few finishing blows when he was overpowered by some villagers. It was fortunate for the Peul that Koutiala was near by, for if the incident had taken place deep in the bush no one would have bothered to walk him to Koutiala for justice. He would have been punished on the spot. When the injured farmer finally recovered from his cerebral concussion he cried out for retribution, not for the trampled millet but for the insults. The Peul countered that he had been insulted first and was only defending his family honor. And such was the situation when word came to Alfarou Diallo.

While the story was being told, I stood by uncomfortably because I didn't think it was any of our business. Boundiar didn't lose any time in meddling. "Those Minianka are stupid," he bellowed. "It's all their fault, those dog eating idiots." Alfarou Diallo didn't voice any opinion and said that he wanted to hear things first hand. But Boundiar was as persistent as a tsetse fly. "I know the commandant in Koutiala. I'll have those worthless Minianka in prison for twenty years." The one thing I admired about Boundiar's justice was that prison terms were always handed out in rounded dimensions of tens which certainly would have made bookkeeping easy for any prison director.

Alfarou Diallo asked me to take him into Koutiala in the truck. I agreed, but told Boundiar that he would have to remain behind in camp. He protested violently and said the case would be lost without him. My own feeling was that with him there would be no case, not for the Peul at any rate. He would have turned the whole affair into an enormous mess, dragged in everyone and in the end so exasperated the commandant that he himself would have wound up in the gendarmerie. I decided to take Djigui along instead, realizing that he would be an asset if Alfarou Diallo asked us to intervene. When we finally left camp, Boundiar was pouring out his groan of protest into the ears of some sympathetic old men in front of my tent.

When we got to Koutiala, I dropped Alfarou Diallo off at the commandant's office and went to the Grandes Endemies dispensary where I had some business to do. But from down there I could hear the noise of the process of justice going on in the commandant's office. The meeting was the usual pallmall of shouting and screaming with everyone talking at once and no one listening to what the others had to say. People got so lost in tangential arguments that the original problem became an almost forgotten affair. It finally took some shouts from the commandant to restore order. What had started as a misunderstanding between two men had now become a struggle between two peoples. When the fury died down, the commandant pronounced the verdict. The Peul had to pay a cow to the Minianka for the damages done to the field. And then he stepped out into the yard and arbitrarily picked out a cow from the impounded herd. Such a pronouncement of justice might have settled a dispute between people in Bamako. But in the matter of a conflict between nomads and sedentary farmers it takes a deft politician's hand at coming up with a solution which leads both sides to think that they have won. The commandant didn't have it in him to manipulate such a tricky affair. He had been born and raised in Bamako and had only recently taken up his post in the bush after having served for several years as Mali's ambassador to Paris. He embodied the refinement of the *evolué* and had a French cultural reference and a liking for Bach and French cuisine. In talking with him, you saw the acquired politesse of the schooled diplomat and a thoroughly western non-Malian system of logic which had taken root in primary school and which matured at the Ecole William Ponty in Senegal. For this man, Mali was the Bamako of the educated elite and so he was thoroughly out of his element in a bush post like Koutiala. For the first time in his life, he faced the real Mali on a day-to-day basis and had come to the sad realization that the wishful place he had often described to foreigners in Paris was a fanciful dream. This left him both frustrated and angry, but he was unwilling to compromise his dream and during the years I knew him he was never able to understand the real Mali nor come to terms with those who knew nothing of Molière.

There was an instant uproar from both sides as soon as the commandant announced his decision. The Miniankas broke out in long wails of protest. They wouldn't accept the cow. She was thin, sick and old and sure to die on the way back to the village. The Peul couldn't restrain themselves from answering the implied insult. They cried out passionately that this cow like all of their cattle was healthy, beautiful, well-fed and sure to bear many calves in the future. Old men coughed out their asthmatic arguments, toothless old women chimed in their quiet opinions and the young men shouted one another down until the yard was a cacaphony of bitter remarks, insults and threats. The cow in question was pulled, poked and rubbed by both her admirers and detractors and scrutinized at a distance by a fast forming crowd of onlookers. It appeared that the whole of Koutiala was being drawn into the dispute. There is of course nothing in the affairs of men which holds the interest of Malians so well as a cow. Offices will be closed, weddings postponed, funerals delayed and sickness denied for the sake of cattle. Even though most of those present had nothing to do with the affair, they felt morally obliged to give their opinions and see things through to the end. In most Malian litigations, the plaintiff generally has the sympathy of the crowd. In my own mind, I thought that because of this the Peul would come out second best in the settlement.

The commandant told me later that he was not used to such indelicate scenes. His face twitched, he bit his lip, wrung his hands and looked longingly off into the distance as if the answer to his dilemma lay among the flocks of white egrets crowding the trees. During this uproar, Alfarou Diallo remained calm and never lost his self-composure at the height of the emotional crisis. Finally, Djigui spoke to the commandant who was visibly calmed by what he had to say. The man who had lunched with DeGaule at the Elysée willingly accepted the wisdom of a former army sergeant. When the fury died down to the soft hum of everyday conversation, the commandant told the Miniankas that they could pick out any cow they wanted in the herd. Such fair play was rare among the Minianka so the proposal left them dumbfounded and threw them into suspicious silence. They eyed one another nervously, chattered a great deal and finally came to the conclusion that it was all a clever trick. Where before they had seen only deficiencies in the commandant's choice, now they saw the prize of the herd. They figured that the Peul didn't want them to get this cow, that was the reason for the generous proposal. But they were bent on outsmarting the Peul and they opted for the original cow. While all of this was going on Alfarou Diallo didn't say anything, but left it to others to put their thumb print on the paper argrement with the Minianka.

Chapter VII
The Thoughts of Mao

I learned through Alfarou Diallo that half a million Peul move through the inland delta along traditionally fixed paths called *burti.* The main herds known as *garti,* are organized into convoys of up to fifteen thousand head, the *egguirgol,* which are supervised by an *amirou-nai.* From the time the trek begins, the *amirou-nai* travels with his wives and children, but the other shepherds move alone, leaving their families to follow at a distance of five day's march with small herds of milking cows called *benti.* Once the women and children reach the flood plain they join up with the main herd and continue on with them for the rest of the season. Some of the old people stay behind in the villages along with some adults and children and don't take part in the transhumance trek. For the most part, the cattle are not the property of the shepherds who herd them. Cattle owners are usually the affluent men of Peul society and rather than herd their own cattle they hire men to do it. The shepherds are remunerated either in cash or in cattle. Shepherds combine themselves into convoys on the basis of calm affiliation and move along the *burti* long since established by Cheikou Ahmadou.

After the last heavy rains, the convoys begin forming and then start the long slow march down the plateau through a hundred miles of farmland to the edge of the flood plain. At the same time, similar convoys begin to descend from the dry sahel so that in effect there is a vice-like convergence of nomads on the flood plain. The forward advance has to be gauged according to the availability of grass and water on the plateau and by the status of the harvesting which is usually going on at the same time. The overwhelming consideration during this march is the optimal use of all available water and grass between the starting

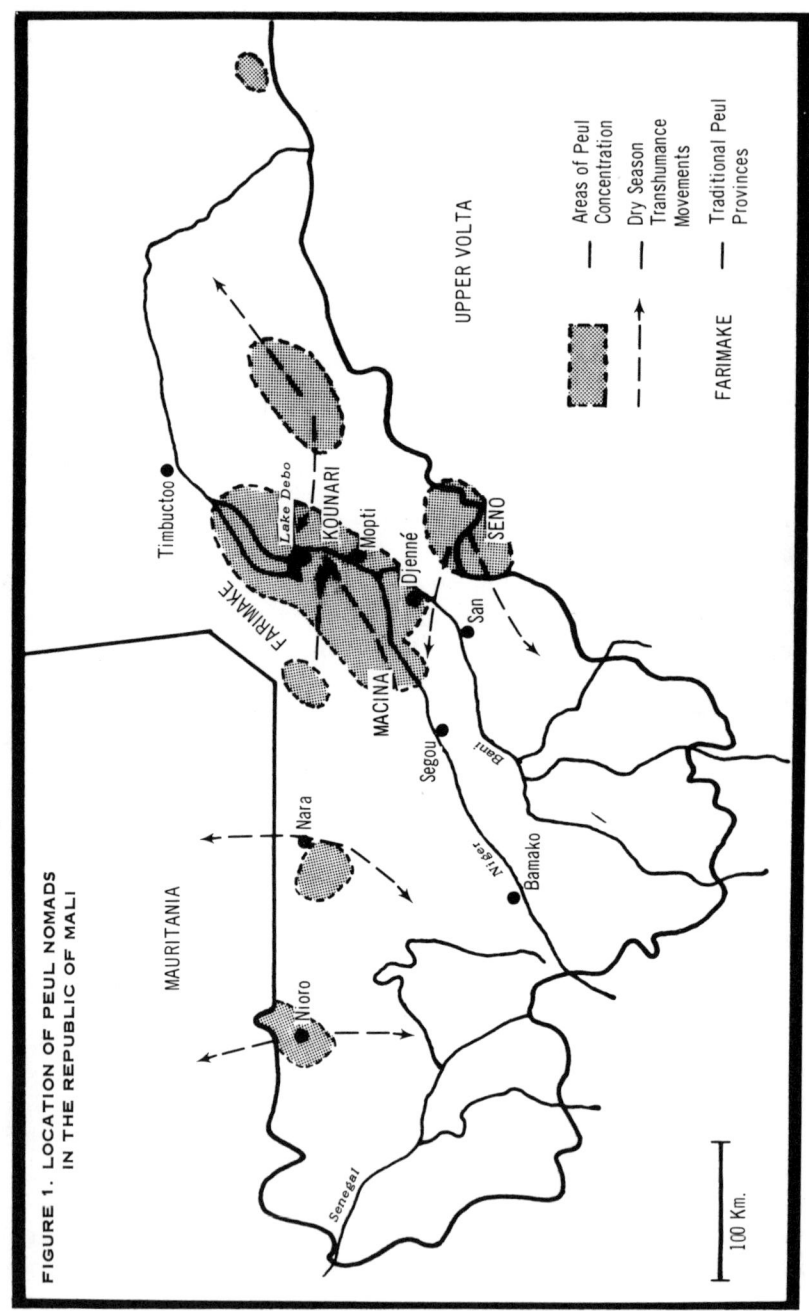

FIGURE 1. LOCATION OF PEUL NOMADS IN THE REPUBLIC OF MALI

point and the final dry season camp which is either on the banks of the Niger or on the shores of one of the great lakes of the inland delta. By common agreement between the herdsmen and the farmers, the herds pass over the fields after the harvest is in. The cattle graze on the fields and the farmers pay the herdsmen for this fertilization with millet or corn. Temporary nomad camps are established year after year on virtually the same fields and there is established an intimate economic and social relationship between families of nomads and sedentary farmers. In some areas, the farmers can predict with considerable accuracy the approximate time that "their nomads" will arrive. Troubles arise when for one reason or another the march has to begin before the harvest is finished. Such was the case when I was with Alfarou Diallo and his convoy and so the passage was one of continuous disagreeable relations between the Peul and the farmers.

As the herds get closer to the edge of the flood plain, they tend to move in a more compact group until they pass through one of the traditional gateways into the plains. There are seventeen such passage points called *gué*, each of them under the control of a village which lays claim to the pastureland surrounding it. Each *gué* is governed by a chief of the pasture, *dioro*, who imposes a tax on each head of cattle passing through. Once the cattle enter, they move through those areas of the plains which have been set aside for them by traditional convention with other clans. Conventions of this kind are sometimes not respected, either through malice, necessity or ignorance and the end result is a physical confrontation between the clans. The flood plains themselves are divided into districts, known as *leydi*, which are the recognized communal property of given clans of Peul. Pasturing in them is governed by a complex weave of traditional verbal agreements in which there is always a wide latitude for differing interpretations. Some areas of the flood plain have been disputed among the Peul for over a century and each year witnesses a new series of disputes. Since independence the situation has been complicated by the fact that the government has said that the plains belong to everyone, including the Tuareg nomads who traditionally never entered them. The yearly disputes are especially common at the end of the dry season when most of the herds are bunched together in a desperate struggle for survival around the few areas where there is still water and grass. Temporary conventions tend to be put aside under such stressful circumstances and the instincts inherent to self-preservation assume control. Physical combat is as much a part of the character of the Peul as herding cattle. Their misunderstandings are never bluffy exchanges of words and insults, but emotion charged encounters of knives, swords, clubs and muskets which often end up with people being killed. "Banging their heads in," as the Peul describe it, occurs almost every year around the shores of Lake Debo where in the scorching heat of June some ten thousand nomads and a half million cattle and sheep fight one another for the few remaining elements the depleted ecology has to offer.

In 1968, when we were camped on the shores of Lake Debo, there was a nasty collision between two fractions of the Dialloubé clan on the southern shores of the lake. The precipitating cause was the usual alleged infringement of grazing rights by one group. It happened that year that there was plenty of water and grass at Lake Debo because of the heavy rains of the previous season. So there was little reason for the wronged group to have been moved to violence. But the Peul view such matters gravely because they never abandon that stirring sense of pride and sacred view of honor which are seriously desecrated by a violation of rights. As usual, the offenders refused to admit wrong and the wronged were frustrated and furious at not being able to regain their honor. Of course the guilty group could not admit their wrong for to have done so would have tainted their own honor. Once this impasse was reached, matters degenerated terribly and there was great temerity on either side when it came to unleashing insults. As so often happens in the hard true life of Africa, the original misunderstanding became a lost shadow in a swelling storm of injured pride and revenge. For the African is deeply in love with his own pride and despises the pride of others and in the defense of the one and the destruction of the other there is no limit to his dedication. The longer the discussion continues, the worse the situation becomes because it only unearths a score of latent resentments and jealousies and sets the disputing parties off on a course of inevitable collision. When the point of no-return is reached, only violence and death can set things right again, for the time being at any rate.

When the fight was finally over, twenty four men lay dead and an unknown number injured. It was only then that things were calm again because death had come in and overwhelmed men with reason and prudence. The Peul say that death and pride cannot live in the same house because death is against man's nature, which for them is to be proud. Death humiliates pride and humbles pretenses, but it resolves the differences between those who remain alive. The nomads hold the death shows men how much they are alike, that there are no

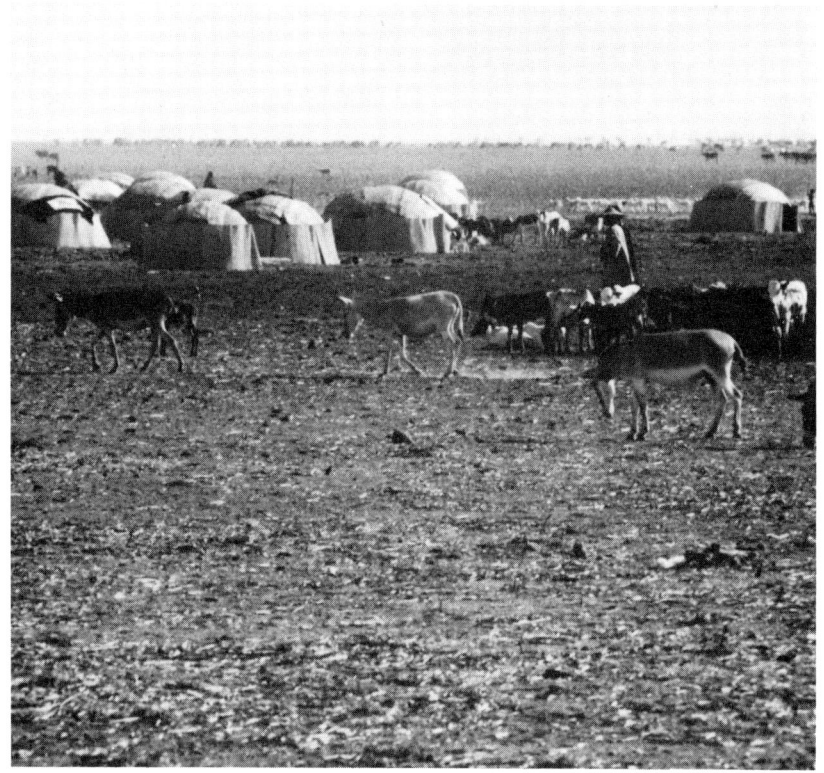

FIGURE 14. A portion of a Peul nomad camp near the shores of Lake Debo.

winners in its unhappiness and discomfort, no pride in sorrow, nor arrogance and vanity in men's hearts when they bury their dead. Death, then, is the final arbitrator in their disputes. But the wisdom gained from the lesson death teaches is quickly lost and has to be obtained again by a people whose failure to learn from the past dooms them to repeat it.

News of this kind travels fast in Africa and within a few days the administrative authorities in the town of Mopti, a hundred miles away, were aware of what had happened. It might have been better in the end had they left things as they were for as it was the matter was closed, a finished affair in the context of traditional Peul law. The disputing parties had paid one another compensations for those who had been killed and had gone their separate ways. They had no desire to take the dispute before the authorities in Mopti because they neither understood nor could accept the peculiar justice handed down by the Bambaras who came from Bamako wearing the same red robes and white hair pieces the French used to wear. The administrators saw things differently. They wanted to show the Peul that the modern administrative machinery which ruled this country was not simply nominal, that Mali's laws and justice had to be respected. How did the Peul view them? Not very well I'm afraid. The Peul saw them as the agents of an outside tyrant, Modibo Keita, as the strong arm of another El Hadj Omar, a king of Segou, the armed force of an unwanted conqueror rather than as a respected ruler. The Peul saw the taxes demanded by these officials as tribute, the same paid by their ancestors to the Bambara kings and the Moroccans. Government was an outside and unwanted force which had no place in the daily lives of the Peul. Government officials were all familiar with the handbook, *La Justice En Republique du Mali,* and tried to apply this offspring of the Napoleonic Code to situations and circumstances not found on any of its pages.

When a contingent of gendarmes arrived at Lake Debo they arrested some fifty men, put them in handcuffs and carried them back to Mopti by truck. Those who were injured were put into the Mopti Hospital where they were patched up by a team of Russian surgeons and the remaining eighteen were sealed up in a small isolation cell which had no windows and an airtight steel door. It is doubtful that the police intended serious harm when they put all of the prisoners into the same small cell. They had never heard of oxygen and so it didn't cross their minds that there wouldn't be enough air for all those men to breathe. They were accustomed to locking up one, two and three men in that room for days on end and saw no reason why eighteen couldn't be locked up just as well. The Peul pounded on the door all night long, crying out that they couldn't breathe. The prison guards as usual turned a deaf ear. When the door was open in the morning four of the nomads were dead and the rest half alive. The town physician examined the bodies, performed autopsies and concluded that death had been caused by suffocation.

The Peul of the delta do not rely on the radio and newspaper for news. It travels by word of mouth, by canoe, horse, donkey, on foot and on trucks with unbelievale speed and accuracy. They weren't shocked by what had happened in the jail in Mopti. Worse things had happened before, all carefully kept secret while the national paper's editorials and Radio Mali accused the countries of the western world of injustice and repression. For the Peul, the suzerain could be unjust, arbitrary and cruel because he was stronger than those he had conquered. And it was as such that the Peul viewed the smotherings in the Mopti jail. Four men had lost their lives, not in a struggle to assert hereditary rights, nor to defend their herds, but through the cruelty of the conqueror. The administrators in Mopti were aware that this is how it would all be viewed by the Peul and foresaw the day when they would dare reprisal against the government. The thought of an armed revolt of the Peul was as terrifying as that of the Tuaregs had already been a few years earlier. The fabric of nationhood was fragile and the necessary repairs had to be made. The government moved with speed, force and directness. The police were arrested and jailed in a military camp several miles from Mopti. The government admitted to having been responsible for a grievous wrong, paid indemnities and released the remaining prisoners. In doing this, they averted a larger catastrophe. But the whole sorry affair only cast them in the light of evil overlords and in the end forced them to settle the account according to the terms of traditional Peul law.

When we arrived with the herds at the edge of the flood plains, it was remarkable to see how abrupt the transition was. The plateau was gray, full of waterless stretches, a hard wild country of fossilized lava flows and thorn trees. But the flood plain was cool and moist, full of pleasant smells and restful green views which stretched long and splendidly into the blue horizon. You could almost draw a line on the ground and in doing so separate the two ecologies. It was as if we were moving from one world into another and entering into harmony with a whole new set of forces and elements which did not exist on the plateau. If you keep company with nomads and their cattle, you have to accept flies as a fact of life and when you enter the flood plains at the end of the rainy season, mosquitoes must be viewed as inevitable nuisances. The flies travel around in great swarms which, when disturbed, make a loud rushing sound. But the mosquitoes are solitary, each one out on his own, each one striving for self-survival. Peul shepherds are well equipped to deal with mosquitoes in the flood plains. They wear thick wool togas, sinyaré, which look terribly uncomfortable on a hot day, but they are the only form of clothing which mosquitoes cannot penetrate. They also wear woolen hockey caps which were introduced into the inland delta many years ago by an enterprising merchant who saw a sizeable profit in protecting the shaven heads of the Peul from the mosquitoes.

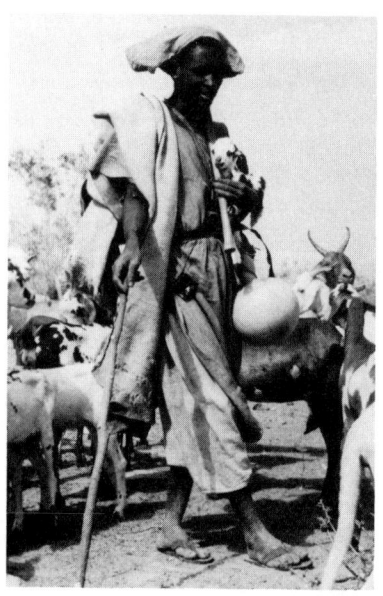

FIGURE 15. A Peul herdsman from Korientze with a herd of sheep and goats.

When it came time to leave Alfarou Diallo's camp it was like moving out of one of those concentrated life experiences which are contemplated many times over in the future. What I had been seeking was simply some basic knowledge about how the Peul moved into the flood plains of the Niger River. And although I found this when I wandered into their lives, I also found something unexpected, a whole new world I never thought existed. It wasn't a world of yesterdays, todays and tomorrows, of hygiene, mechanization and luxury, but one in which life was a procession of todays where hindsight and foresight were submerged by the immediate, by what took place between sunrise and sunset. People worried less in this world because they only confronted the problems of today. They didn't think about what would happen after the next sunrise because that was in God's hands and beyond alteration. There were wishes and hopes, but no long-term goals. This put less stress on everyone, made them unhurried and created an atmosphere where one could get lost in the comfort of deep inner thoughts and enjoy the immediate happiness of today. The Peul had seen the so-called better life pass by them once in a while in the form of a fancy automobile or fine clothes. But for the present, the better life had no place in their world of cattle, water, grass, God,

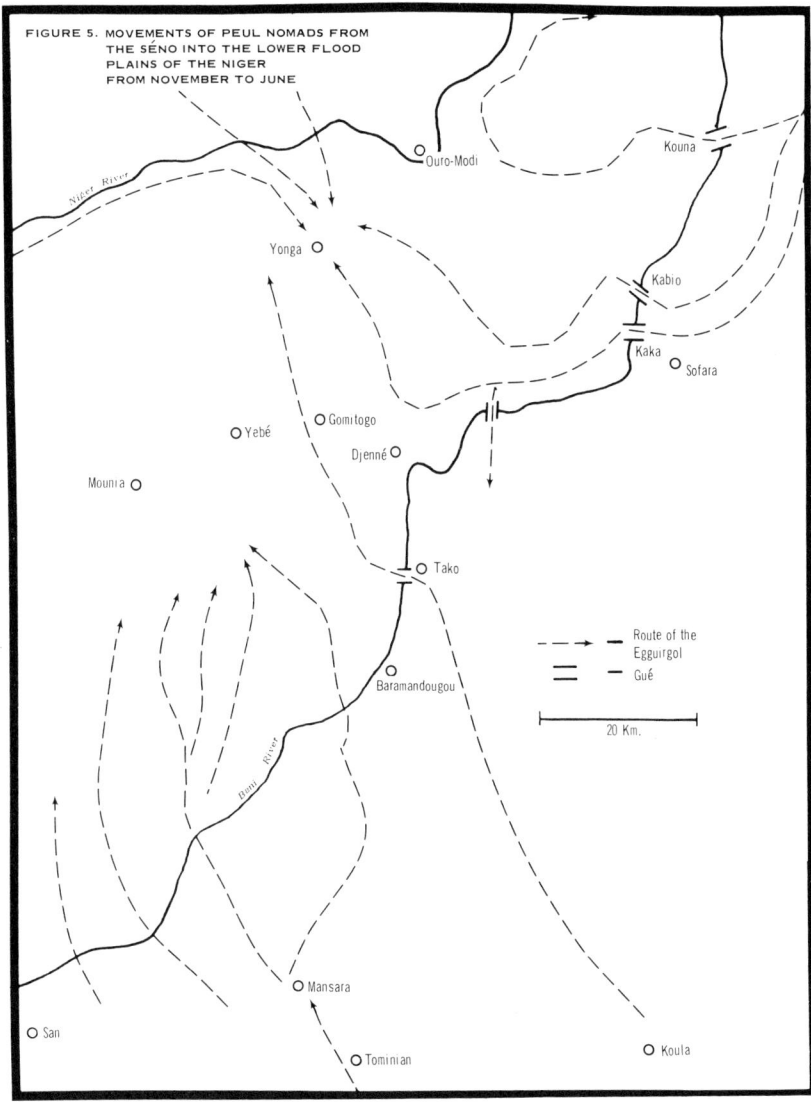

FIGURE 5. MOVEMENTS OF PEUL NOMADS FROM THE SÉNO INTO THE LOWER FLOOD PLAINS OF THE NIGER FROM NOVEMBER TO JUNE

fatalism and unchanging cycles and so it didn't concern them. Although times had not yet changed for the Peul, time was running out for their way of life. From their limited perspective of today, they couldn't see the inevitable and perhaps it was just as well.

We traveled up north to the town of Mopti, arriving there at the height of the "tourist season," when most of the then available accommodations had already been taken up. This didn't really bother us since we had been living in the bush for several weeks, sleeping on cots, taking bucket showers and eating local food. But a comfortable bed in the *campement* and a real shower seemed to me something to look forward to. At that time, it took only a total of eighteen tourists to exhaust all of the available rooms at the government run *campement* and the privately owned Bar du Mali. Unlike most Malians of the era, the gerant of the *campement,* whose name was Badjai, was accommodating and kind and given to quick friendships. He was a very short man whose broad mouth and enormous eyes expressed with a direct eloquence what others would have taken many sentences to say. He was intrinsically a very kind man who often put out extra beds and matresses on the veranda to accommodate those for whom there was no room in the run-down building. It was very late in the evening when we walked in on his experiment in integrated communal living and found men, women and children, both black and white, sleeping all over the veranda with their host running back and forth like a dedicated house mother between the beds and matresses and the rooms and the bar. Although this little haven of shelter had little to recommend it, Badjai tried his best to make it comfortable. He filtered the drinking water, made meals palatable, put up insolvent customers free of charge and kept the linen as clean as the muddy Bani River permitted. Through no fault of his, the rooms had no toilets, only showers, and people succumbed to doing in the showers what should have been done down the hall in the only toilet. The drainage system in the entire place was poor so the showers got blocked up and in the end it was pleasanter to sleep out on the veranda. Badjai patiently put up with the complaints with a smile, accepted blame for the dirty looking linen he had just washed in the river, for the stopped up showers, the roaches, the rats and even the mosquitoes which were worse there than at any other place in the town. One of the first things he told me was that he was going to quit-*demissioner* as he put it because there were too many *emerdements* in the job. He thought that the direction in Bamako was stupid because tourists would never come back to Mopti after having weathered one experience in the campement.

Like many campements in Mali, the one in Mopti not only hosted tourists, but also served as the town hangout. As such, it attracted the dredges of the town, the drinkers, the gamblers, the pimps and prostitutes, children selling black market cigarettes and their mothers' services and the agents of the secret police. It was a sub-world all its own, diverse in its inner structure, but yet all the same on the surface, different and opposite from that of the old men and marabouts which lay across the shallow lagoon in the shadow of the mosque. The bizarre was not out of the ordinary at the Mopti campement and when we walked in we found an exceptionally obese Swedish woman sitting up in a large wrought iron bed which had been put in the middle of the dining room. The bed had been placed directly beneath one of the buzzing fluorescent ceiling lights and neither the pulsating cloud of insects around the light nor the constant shower of cinged corpses falling onto the sheets seemed to bother the woman.

"C'est quelque chose, ah m'sieu!" exclaimed Badjai. "Elle est folle." Then he told me she was an anthropologist, out to study the native tribes. The gerant was not the only one to doubt her professional credentials and it became quickly obvious that her main interest was men, any kind, black or white. He was relieved that she was leaving the next day with a group of Russian mining engineers going overland to Gao. She got out of her bed and after tangling with the noisy steel door, came out sideways with her squat form draped in a silk négligé. She demanded something to drink, but everything else pointed to flirtation. Boundiar had obviously never met the kind before and shifted nervously from one foot to another. He mumbled something about not being in the mood to meet an anthropologist after traveling several thousand kilometers through the bush. Badjai had lots of *bon volonté* but no place to put us and so we decided to go and see the governor of Mopti for a place to stay. Boundiar said he wanted to see the governor alone because they were old school friends and had some private matters to discuss with him. One never knew with Boundiar and so I let him go off alone to see the governor. When Madame anthropologist returned from the bar with a bottle of orange *crush* she said she wanted her bed moved back out to the veranda.

"But I just pushed your bed in there," protested Badjai. "Look at my head!" he exclaimed pointing to a small abrasion in the middle of his bald spot. "I got that carrying matresses today."

"Tant pis pour toi," replied Madame anthropologist in a pitiless voice.

The gerant emitted one of his automatic smiles which never expressed mirth but which successfully enabled him to protect his dignity. "Very well," he sighed. "I'll move it, but this is the last time, madame."

Madame anthropologist guzzled down the rest of her soft drink as the large dilapidated bed screeched its way across the floor to the veranda. Badjai arrived behind the bed, panting, smiling and cursing under his breath in Bambara. The bed had no sooner come to its final resting place than Boundiar returned, strutting like some arrogant and contented tom cat. I hadn't seen him so happy in months, so I suspected that he had been successful in finding a place for us to stay. In all of his successes he had a way about announcing what everyone was anxious to hear at the last possible moment. You knew that in time the news was going to come out and that it would be good. But Boundiar would haul you through years of autobiography, deliver a treatise on his exploits and try to convince you that the benefactor owed his health, wealth and life success to him. When the favor was finally announced, it emerged as the pallid and feeble gesture of an infinitely grateful soul. When Boundiar finally finished telling everyone why the governor owed him so much he produced a handful of keys.

"The governor has given us permission to sleep in the Chinese motel in Sevaré."

"It isn't possible," protested Badjai. "The Chinese are still working on it and the rooms aren't finished yet."

"Chèr ami," interrupted Boundiar, "the governor says that there are finished rooms there and we are going to use them."

"Well the governor is the governor," replied Badjai. "But you had better not spend the night in that motel. The Chinese won't like it. It is still theirs you know. They haven't given it to Mali yet."

Boundiar's response to the gerant's warning was less than polite and carried us into the complicated topic of Mali's sovereignty and independence. According to Boundiar everything which stood on Malian soil was Malian, both animate and inanimate. That argument didn't win the gerant over, but it made it very clear that we were going to spend the night in the Chinese motel.

"Oh, oh, oh!" exclaimed Badjai just as we were getting ready to leave, "If those Chinese find an American in their motel, oh what a calamity." With his hand over his toothless mouth, he backed away from me and reflected for a moment and then seemed ignited by some brilliant idea.

"Maybe you can pass for a Frenchman." I didn't think the idea was an especially good one myself especially when he made the rest of it known. "Park the truck off in the bushes so they won't see that big American insignia and then if they catch you, just say you are French."

"Why doesn't he simply say he is Albanian," said Madame anthropologist.

"Albanian!" cried the gerant. "Why Albanian?"

"Of course Albanian," she said. "Don't you know they get on famously together."

By this time, the other guests who had been eavesdropping on the conversation began to offer advice. Boundiar would have none of it and declared in a loud voice that not only was he going to sleep in the motel but that he was also going to walk into all the rooms, use all the showers and for good measure take a walk on the roof.

"You had better be careful my friend," warned Badjai. "Those Chinese always travel around in groups and if they catch you on the roof of their motel you might meet with an accident and fall off."

When we finally arrived at the motel in Sevaré there was no one there except the old Malian watchman who was equipped with three Mao buttons, a club, a feeble flashlight and a copy of *The Thoughts of Mao* which he couldn't read because he was illiterate. "Where are the Chinese?" asked Boundiar nervously.

The Chinese had gone to their quarters and weren't expected back until six in the morning. But Boundiar was looking for some reassurance that they wouldn't come back during the night. The building was almost completed, extremely attractive and well built. There was a great deal of Chinese building equipment lying about and the walls were pasted up with giant red lettered slogans from Mao's thoughts. The interior was like a transported portion of China, the woods, plaster, terra cotta floors, steel, fixtures, curtains and furniture, all forming part of an inseparable essence which was not African but Chinese. In the face of all of this, Boundiar retreated into his own peculiar form of modesty which insecurity always forced on him.

The rooms weren't numbered yet and the tags on Boundiar's keys were printed with Chinese characters so it took us almost an hour to find out which keys belonged to the doors of the finished rooms. There was a relative luxuriousness about the motel, the slender ceiling fans, screened windows, satin curtains, heavy blonde furniture, flush toilets, night lights, roomy wardrobes and the plaster walls covered with glossy paint. It was certainly the most comfortable accommodation in Mail at that time, but in some ways it seemed an anachronism to find it out in the middle of the Mopti bush. One would have thought it better suited for Bamako where at that time there was a distinct need.

When the Motel de Mopti finally opened, it became very much of a seasonal affair, crowded in the cold months of December and January with quiet groups of elderly tourists from Europe and the States out to see Timbuctoo and the Dogon cliffs. In the beginning, there was never any predictable business routine in its running and one was always sure of the companionship of the unexpected and permitted to experience either frustration or adventure depending on one's outlook on things. During the first two years of operation, five Malian managers tried their luck at running the motel and all were unsuccessful except for one old man who had a small hotel for Africans in Paris. Everyone except the old man had gone to a hotel training school and managed the motel from behind a desk in suit, white shirt and tie. Although they ran things in a self-assured fashion, they were really quite bewildered by it all. Guests complained that they were in a state of perfect immunity to even the smallest requests, but in reality they simply didn't know what was expected of them. Only the old man stayed on his feet, limped around in an open shirt and was inquisitive about people's comfort. He served meals on time, had the linen changed and betrayed his twenty years in France by doing a very non-African thing. He filled the lobby with potted plants and graced the yard with flowers and shrubs.

The first manager burned out the new Chinese generator by omitting to put oil into it. Although he was somewhat indifferent to the calamity, he was resourceful in meeting it. He put kerosine lamps in the rooms, hired women to draw water up out of a well, gave guests a bucket of water to wash with and asked the Chinese for a new generator. The Chinese were outraged and the Malian government embarrassed, and, in the end, the manager left the country. For the past several years, the motel has been managed by a very capable team headed by Monsieur Keita the manager and Monsieur Cissé the accountant. As a result of their management, the motel rooms are first class accommodations and the meals in the dining room the best served in any restaurant in Mali.

When Boundiar, Djigui and Modibo felt the hard beds, they

pronounced them useless and said they were going to sleep on the cots. Like most Malians, they scorned hardness in a bed. Their logic on the subject was quite correct from their point of view. You spend years sleeping on the hard ground, first as a child and then as an adult. Finally, the day comes when you are rich enough to afford a bed. Such a luxury, the logic goes, should be the direct opposite of what you have been used to. And so Malian beds leave an ineffaceable impression on you for their softness. The springs sag and the mattresses are great amorphous masses of stuffing ready to form an instant mold around your body. The springs bend your body into the shape of a horseshoe so that your vertebrae almost touch the ground and your feet and head stick up into the air. And if that weren't enough, the mattress rolls over on you like a shifting drift of snow. The Malians who own these beds say that they are wonderfully comfortable.

It is doubtful that I merit any special distinction for having been the first foreigner to have slept in the Chinese motel at Sevaré, except that I am an American. When the Chinese met me at the doorway the next morning, it wasn't through intent, but because I had overslept and they on time for work. They had already inspected my truck from top to bottom and were busily chatting among themselves when I came out. Now I don't know what they thought of me when we confronted one another and they watched a troop of Malian workers follow me out single file carrying cots, bedding, food boxes, cooking gear, suitcases and a tent. It must have been what I would have thought had I seen them riding down the road in one of our trucks. At that time, the Chinese spoke to virtually no one, except the Malians, and completely dissociated themselves from westerners. Their position on this was so strong that they even refused to ride in vehicles donated to Mali by UNICEF and WHO. Once a Chinese medical team was sent to the town of Markala in Segou where in addition to modern medicine they practiced acupuncture on a large scale. The Ministry of Health offered them a land rover donated by UNICEF. They said they would take it on the provision that the UNICEF insignia be covered up or taken off. The Ministry of Health refused and so the Chinese acupuncture team went on foot, but never complained.

The Chinese finally greeted Boundiar with a collective, "Eee hon," which was how I learned the expression was a greeting and that it didn't represent a cat call on the part of Malian children who often use it to greet foreigners. In fact many Malians refer to the Chinese as "the Eee hon."

The next day we set out for the area of the Bandiagara cliffs where I had to collect some information on the movements of two Peul clans which was essential to the planning of our mobile health program strategy. The cliffs of Bandiagara are one of the most spectacular formations in West Africa. They begin in the south-west as gentle rolling hills and lonely uplifts of great blocks of pink sandstone. Then come the high mountains with long dipping valleys hanging between the rounded peaks. Finally, the cliffs emerge, a solid vertical wall of pink sandstone soaring up fifteen hundred feet into the sky.

You feel a stirring sense of awe when you see this vast sweep of stone standing against the blue of the sky, stretching from horizon to horizon. The cliffs run for a hundred and fifty miles towards Douentza where they lose their vertical accent and tumble into rounded rocky hills and then they end on the white sands of the Gourma as the magnificent monuments of Hombori, great red and purple mesas rising up over three thousand feet.

The land which rolls away from the base of the cliffs towards the Upper Volta frontier is composed of low sand dunes and gentle plains, covered with thorn trees and graceful acacias and hard tufts of twisted grass. It is a country people by the sedentary Dogon farmers and the nomadic Peul herdsmen. On the top of the cliff is a vast rocky plateau,

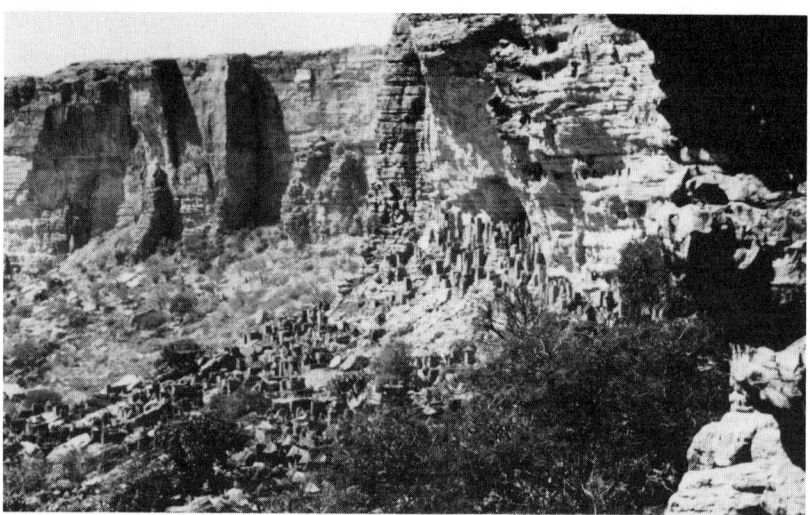

FIGURE 16. A view of the Bandiagara Cliffs showing the village if Irieli. The village's tall cylinder shaped granaries are built up against the base of the cliff.

a landscape of bleak lava flows frozen hard by time, narrow valleys cut with jagged designs into the rock, dolm palms and thorn trees and clusters of baobab monarchs. The sky was clear that day and the land a deep green and the cliffs seemed to draw near in the clear air with oval shadows of gigantic white clouds drifting across their face. Down on the sandy plain and up on the cliffs, the Dogon were in their fields, bringing in the harvest. Off on the cliffs a torrent of rain fell in black vertical rays, but down on the plains it was docile, blowing through the stands of millet like a gentle mist.

Because of the physical isolation inherent to this topography, the Dogon have remained one of the most traditional societies in West Africa and as such they have attracted the attention of scholars and tourists alike. The fact that they are so, meant that when our teams arrived to vaccinate them there would be a great many problems. For societies such as the Dogon, bound as they are to tradition, are often refractory to what is outside of the limits of the traditional. Although my prime interest in entering this area at this time was to study the Peul, I also had to become familiar with the area of the cliffs and the Dogon because they were a crucial link in or fight against smallpox and measles.

The land below the cliffs was either too dry or too wet and now it was too wet. The tracks were soggy and covered with water, the bridges washed out, the mosquitoes unbearable and the only beauty the blue and red mesas and cliffs standing high up in a sea of green millet and corn. The *medécin chef* of the area said that he wanted to accompany us through the area below the cliffs. He was after a manner of speaking a somewhat pitiable sight. He was terribly small and thin and covered his body up with a suit one size too big, wore an enormous hat and large tie and had the shoulders of the jacket padded to make him look bigger. It is often said that such people are at war with the world because fate has dealt them an unfair blow. They fall into the mold of defensiveness and antagonism and never come to live on friendly terms with destiny. I thought myself that he was suffering from an endocrine disorder and felt sorry about the mental state into which it had forced him. He sat in the back of the truck most of the time and for the two weeks he was with us I never saw him without his suit. He also wore a giant sized Mao button and passed the long hours of bush travel reading a pocket edition of *The Thoughts of Mao*. We would have been tolerant of his reading Mao quietly to himself, but he had an annoying habit of reading bold print passages aloud and of then commenting on them. When we made camp for the night he used to pull out the large hard cover edition of Mao he had in his suitcase because he said it was easier to read its bigger print in the light of the kerosine lamp.

I referred to the medécin chef as *Sparky* when speaking to Djigui, Modibo and Boundiar because he reminded me of a character out of the *Our Gang* comedies. Despite the hardships of the trip and the many setbacks in schedules, Sparky's spirits didn't lilt but seemed to grow brighter with every obstacle. He refused to put the seat belt around his almost invisible waist which resulted in his being bounced up and down between the roof and the seat like a Spalding rubber ball. Eventually, I thought he would have to desert his contempt for seat belts, but he didn't even though it meant that he had to cross several hundred miles of bush with one hand on his hat and the other holding the Mao book for dear life. Our first reaction to Sparky was one of comic relief, but as we went along there was a growing awareness that he was dead serious in his reading of Mao. The nomads didn't interest him, neither the Dogon and when I tried discussing medicine he made it known he didn't have time since he was behind in his Mao readings. Some curious nomads thought he was reading the Koran and asked him to read them some passages, but before Sparky had a chance to reply, Boundiar blurted out that the book was written by Mao, the chief of the eee hon people, who didn't believe in God. Certainly Boundiar didn't qualify for canonization as a Moslem saint, but he couldn't resist giving Sparky a hard time. The nomads looked gravely at Sparky and then backed away as if he were some ugly crumbling obscenity. They said that if the eee hon people didn't believe in God then whatever their chief had written was evil and so was anyone who read it.

After several days of fighting mud and water we got through to the administrative center of Koro which stands on a sandy plain, isolated from the rest of Mali by the cliffs and at that time from nearby Upper Volta by political idealogy. By this time, we had all become accustomed to Sparky's high pitched monotone carrying Mao's message into every corner of the cab of my American truck. True, many of the passages were interrupted by the bouncing of the truck and continuity suffered because Sparky always had trouble relocating where he had been cut off, but by the time we reached Koro, Sparky had covered everything from the chapter on the Communist party to the chapter entitled, "Imperialism and All Reactionaries Are Paper Tigers." Sparky found some other Mao fanciers in Koro and fell into an almost immediate idealogical communion with them over Mao's thoughts. Mao seemed to be the

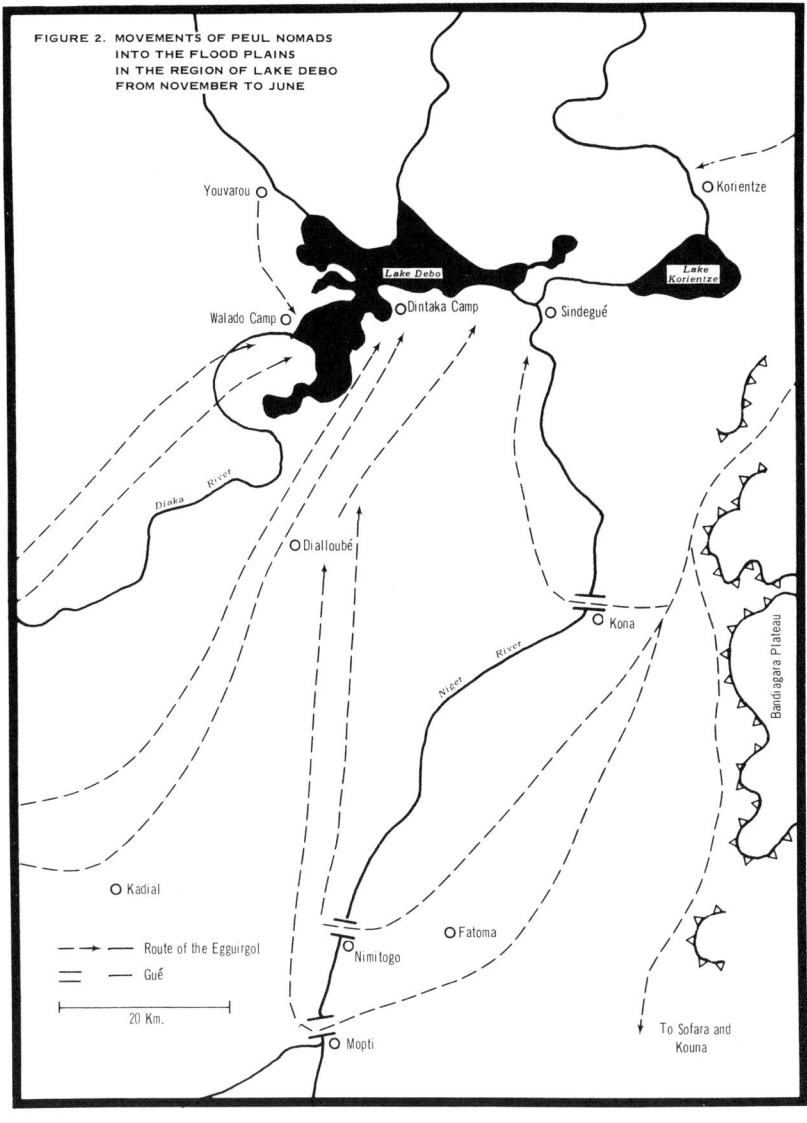

FIGURE 2. MOVEMENTS OF PEUL NOMADS INTO THE FLOOD PLAINS IN THE REGION OF LAKE DEBO FROM NOVEMBER TO JUNE

in thing all over Koro and even the commandant of the cercle had his living room walls covered with messianic color posters of Mao. Mao always stood out four times bigger than any of the other figures in the posters which Sparky said was to emphasize his importance. The commandant had a cheap plaster bust of Lenin on his desk and Sparky spent a lot of time examining it. The commandant remarked that it had been a *cadeau* from some Russians who had passed through Koro.

The presence of so many Mao worshippers in Koro infused Sparky with an expressive boldness which was out of character for him. When he came over to eat supper that night he had the air of someone about to preside over some great triumph. Only his slight neck and small round head surmounted the mountain of rice piled high on his plate. Up until then, I had been caught up in an atmosphere of optimism about Sparky and tried to consider him innocuous, but as he filled his plate for a second time he said with a dry voice that Americans were a dirty race, filthy cowards and an inferior people. In the wake of this explosion of insults, everyone's shock came through as an avalanche of silence, but Sparky beamed with bliss as if he had been the herald of some long awaited joyful news. I held council with myself and decided against doing or saying anything. An awesome silence in the conversation of Africa gives emphasis to what went before, makes good statements better and the bad ones worse, and puts the onus on the speaker. Boundiar had no tolerance for silence and felt compelled to sweep it away with an excited recitation of his own personal feelings. He showed little sense and exercised no emotional control where his own disputes were concerned and would fly into a fearful rage if he thought he was getting the short end of things. When it came to the affairs of others, there was no limit to the punishment he would heap on the adversary, for by punishing the one he complimented the other and in doing so bolstered his own prestige. The storm of insults he unleashed against Sparky began with the Mao book, passed over the ancestors and descended without mercy on Sparky's physical inadequacies. There was always a good deal of humor in whatever Boundiar said and he evolked laughter from the audience when he said that Sparky's basic problem was that his head was too small. Once an idea entered, it filled it up and no new ideas could get in and now his head was full of Mao. He advised Sparky in the next breath to marry a fat woman who could carry him around on her back and for good measure said, "But you had better be careful at night because if she rolls over on you, you will be squashed."

When we took to the road again the next day, Sparky's Mao book was tucked out of sight in his pocket and he himself was a little dark fixture in the back seat held in place by a seat belt. We came to a small Dogon village with the long name of Korporokenie-Na and found an unusual person standing alongside the muddy track. He was dressed in a suit, white shirt and red tie and a new pair of uncreased black pointed shoes and was definitely out of concert with everything else in this bush. He motioned us to stop which we had to do anyway because of the water and then stepped back to avoid getting splashed with mud. When the truck's motor stopped, Boundiar's roaring voice replaced it.

"Just who do you think you are stopping a truck with a red cross on it?" Boundiar was an impressive sight when he was angry. With a fiery tongue he could pour out an avalanche of aggressive rhetoric, accuse, judge and sentence his victim and for good measure call damnation down on everyone. To those who didn't know him, he looked like a mountain of violence, an awesome spectacle of scowled face, clenched fists and masses of tensed up muscles ready to unwind their force on the enemy. Anyone who knew Boundiar saw through the bluff and knew that underneath was a meek coward who would melt into obsequious gestures as soon as the challenge was taken up.

The poor man on the side of the road must have thought he had come up against a lunatic and didn't press a step too far forward. "Don't you know it's against international regulations to stop a truck with a red cross. I'm going to report you to the International Red Cross in Geneva." This time I thought Boundiar had gone too far and told him to shut up. But Boundiar was very magnanimous when it came to handing out prison terms and he had already decided on ten years for the man on the side of the road. When the stranger finally saw me in the truck he smiled and said with a chime of relief in his voice, "Ah, bon, il y a un blanc dans le camion." He then said he had flagged us down on account of the red cross on the truck, but Boundiar told him he was a dirty liar only interested in getting a lift into the next big village, Bankass. "Since when do people go looking for medical help all dressed up in a suit and Bata shoes!" Now there was a lot of truth in what Boundiar said, but I already knew that the man wasn't looking for medical help but for a free ride. The hitchhiker was not a grave citizen and quickly surmised that Boundiar had to be treated as a big joke and so he began to laugh at his insults until finally even Boundiar was laughing. After much discussion the man asked for a lift into Bankass and when I gave my assent he shouted to someone in the bush behind and out came two wives, three children and a ton of baggage inclding a goat. And with all that aboard we started off for Bankass.

In his usual blunt way, Boundiar found out that the man was the local secretary general of the Union Soudanaise-RDA and this was cause for him to rant about one of his favorite topics, the uselessness of politicians. To Boundiar, they were all corrupt thieves and liars seldom interested in anything except lining their own pockets. "Tu n'a pas buffé la caisse encore?" Boundiar demanded. At first, the hitchhiker took it all in good humor, but after several hours his physical and emotional reserve showed signs of depletion and his bouncing between the shift stick and Boundiar's huge hulk didn't help any.

We bumped, swerved, jolted and slid along until the truck became almost hopelessly mired down in a mud trap. "Ce n'est rien," shouted Boundiar to Modibo with optomistic conviciton. He looked out at the back wheels and told Modibo to put the truck in four wheel drive, but that maneuver only got us several more inches into the mud. As the axle descended out of sight I started scanning the bush for available donkeys and horses, but Boundiar scoffed at my suggestion and began digging with a shovel. The deeper Boundiar got into the muddy misery of the trail, the more vehement his criticisms of politicians became. There was a re-kindling of life and courage in Sparky and with discernible discretion and meekness he said he was going to read Mao to himself. Mao had helped surgeons save lives in China and anesthetize people through acupuncture so surely he could help us get the truck out of the mud. On hearing this Boundiar took time out from insulting the hitchhiker to say that there was no longer any doubt in his mind about Sparky's sanity. "Il est fou."

Two hours later Boundiar was a half foot deeper into the mud and so was the truck. Sparky was off on a dry patch of grass, pacing up and down with the solemnity of a priest reading his office. Mao hadn't gotten the truck out of the mud and so Boundiar began denouncing even Mao along with all of the other politicians he knew of and in the most vile language. In a way it was very amusing to hear all of this since Boundiar in the next breath declared that he was a staunch Communist. He looked like a defeated monster standing as he did in a hole covered with mud, sweat and anger. I told the hitchhiker that we had better go and look for help and he agreed. Contemplating Boundiar still shoveling in his hole he said, "Now you big mouth I am going to show you what we politicians can do." And with that he marched off across a soggy millet field. With the politician gone Boundiar started again on Sparky and threatened to rip his Mao book apart. "If I see you reading Mao again, I'll leave you here in the bush all alone and let you see how fast Mao's thoughts will get you rescued." An hour later the politician came back, his suit limpid and muddy and his shoes creased and blunted. But behind him came a line of fifty-three Dogon farmers with their hoes slung over their backs and in five minutes the truck was out and then Boundiar too was silenced.

When we arrived in Bankass the infirmier at the dispensary at the entrance to the village came rushing up to the truck, tremendously excited, and between anxious sighs told us he had a grave emergency on his hands. Only an hour before a Dogon farmer from the cliff village of Gani had been carried into the dispensary on a litter.

"His brains are hanging out!" blurted the infirmier. "And he has been emasculated!"

None of us had even gotten out of the truck yet and our state of exhaustion deadened our immediate reaction to one of complete silence. Not even Boundiar said anything, sitting like an amorphous inert mass covered with dried mud. When I finally regained my physical equilibrium after a few seconds I asked what had happened. Although the infirmier explained everything to me in detail, I didn't grasp much of what he said because I was so exhausted from the trip. It wasn't until later that night and after I had treated the man that he told me the story again in all its detail.

The victim, a middle-aged man named Poundiougou, had gotten into a dispute with some Dogon from another village over the boundary between their fields. At the outset, the dispute was a rhetorical battle but with each passing day tempers became hotter. Finally, relatives and fellow villagers from each side were drawn into the dispute and on the morning of our arrival a physical battle ensued. There were a score of men on either side, using knives, swords and hoes. During the battle, Poundiougou backed his opponent into a thick wall of millet stalks. As he did so he felt a crushing blow on the back of his head. He didn't lose consciousness, but everything went black. Then he felt an arm seizing him around the neck, pulling him down. Two other men pinned his arms against the wet ground and he felt his legs being pulled apart and his trousers being ripped open. Then came the sting of the knife cutting. His fellow villagers finally managed to beat the assailants off.

When we arrived at the dispensary the man was lying on a mat, semicomatose, his head bound up in blood soaked rags. I had him placed on a large wooden table on the open veranda where I examined him in the bright sunlight. He had been struck on the back of the head with a hoe which had inflicted a four inch long laceration through the entire thickness of the scalp. The skull was severely fractured, broken up into tiny sharp fragments which oozed out of the bloody wound with macerated brain tissue. Many of the bone fragments were embedded in the brain.

Poundiougou hadn't been emasculated as the infirmier claimed, but his scrotum had been severely cut. No doubt his assailants would have castrated him had he not been rescued. Our arrival in Bankass was fortuitous for the infirmier since he didn't have any antibiotics and no suture materials. I looked at Boundiar and Djigui and they read my thoughts immediately. Here we were exhausted and covered with mud out in the middle of nowhere, faced with a patient lying on a wooden table who needed a delicate neurosurgical procedure. Even in the finest hospital in the world and in the best hands, the outcome would have been considered dubious at best.

"We will have to treat him," I said. Without further word, Modibo went over to the truck and dragged out the surgical instruments and the large wooden medical box in which we carried everything from antibiotics to snake anti-venom. Boundiar and I went off to wash and then together with Djigui and the local infirmier scrubbed for the procedure. Sparky took care of preparing the instruments and supervised the women as they boiled everything up. The local politician and Modibo served as circulating nurses and the commandant of Bankass kept the crowd of several hundred people away from the veranda. It took two hours of painstaking work to remove the dead tissue and debride the wound and stop the bleeding. After cleaning the wound out I covered the cut surface of the brain with the dura, the thick fibrous envelope which lies on top of the brain. While doing this I sent the politician off to the local blacksmith to obtain a file. The women boiled this and then I used it to file down the jagged edges of bone bordering the hole in the skull. In a modern hospital a plastic plate would have been inserted but that was out of the question here. So I sutured the scalp back into place after irrigating the wound with sterile water and and antibiotic solution.

After finishing this delicate surgical repair, we sutured the wound in his genitals, which was of more concern to his family than the head wound. Poundiougou had been struck on that part of the brain which controls sight. He was completely blind when I treated him, due not only to the destruction of the brain tissue but also to the swelling of the brain caused by the trauma. The following morning Poundiougou was still unconscious and I seriously doubted that he would live.

Many months later when a team of vaccinators arrived in the Dogon village of Gani to vaccinate the population they were greeted with a tremendous reception. The people, seeing the white Dodge truck, thought it was me arriving. The vaccinators found that Poundiougou was alive and well, his sight restored and that the *toubabou ke* (white man) who had saved his life by sewing his head and genitals back together again had become a legend on the cliff.

Chapter VIII
A Beginning

The plan for vaccinating the inland delta of the Niger was submitted and accepted with enthusiasm by the Ministry of Health even though many had doubts we would be successful at such an ambitious undertaking. Unlike any previous health program in Mali, this one was organized not to cover specific administrative areas, but an ecologic zone in such a manner that the greatest number of people would be reached. Success depended on our eight vaccination teams covering 150,000 square miles of mountains, cliffs, sand dunes, plains and swamps, entering over 3,000 villages and a thousand nomad camps, vaccinating a quarter of Mali's population, 1,500,000 people against smallpox, 300,000 children against measles and 600,000 against yellow fever and delivering rudimentary curative medical services to those who were sick, particularly those with river blindness, leprosy and sleeping sickness. All of this had to be done in a period of nine months. The teams were to begin up on the plateau in Koutiala and move along the Mali-Upper Volta frontier towards Douentza, vaccinating the sedentary farmers, seasonal workers in the towns and the merchants in the numerous markets. Then as the waters dried up on the plains, they were to descend towards the Niger and vaccinate the nomads, following the same itineraries as the nomads until they arrived at Lake Debo, the final camping area of the nomads.

In an ordinary year, truck travel across the plains is possible during the months of April, May and June which meant that the teams had to work this area during a limited period of time. That year we had too much rain, more than the old men could remember from any other year. Entire villages were swept away in the swollen currents of the Bani and Niger Rivers whose confluence was ten miles upstream from where it usually was at that time of year. Water on the flood plains was five feet deeper than usual and up in Bamako people living in the riverside quarters of Bozola and Niarela were descending their streets in canoes. By October, it was still raining the way it usually did at the height of the rainy season in August. The water pumping station for Bamako became flooded and only thousands of men and sand bags kept the plant from going under. A city about to have its potable water supply cut off during a flood is charged with an atmosphere of panic and the fatalistic certainty that an epidemic of typhoid fever hovers in the shadows. The river kept rising, its progress faithfully reported by the radio and many fell victim to pessimism. The ministry of health of a country whose capital is hit by the worst flood in its history has to worry on behalf of all the citizenry, calm their fears, make plans for what no one knows will happen and while so besieged undergo a purposeful and conscious self-renewal to meet the disaster. Because the flood was the highest priority for the country as a whole, it was almost impossible to draw anyone's attention to the mass vaccination campaign which was to take place far off in the bush.

It is the comfort of bureaucracies to meet crises by fortifying themselves through enlargement. And so it was that the government formed various commissions, one to study why the river was rising, another to find ways of making it fall, a health commission to prepare for whatever might happen and commissions for food distribution and housing. The hydrologists traveled up into Guinea to find out why the river was rising and came back reporting what everyone already knew, there had been too much rain. Many inundated villages claimed that the river would fall faster if the great dam at Markala were opened. Since the dam was already open, the commission advised that it be better protected against possible sabotage by local peasants who had threatened to blow it up. The task of offering advice to the health authorities suddenly fell to all physicians and we tried as best we could to shine some light into an otherwise dark arena of gloom and come up with some solid suggestions and a reasonable plan of action.

Down river in the town of Koulikoro the river had wrecked havoc, cut the town in two and put the grain barns of the country under water. There were many people homeless there and the Communist Chinese had set up large green tents in which to house them. The Chinese received a lot of propaganda from their tents in Koulikoro and before long all of the diplomats in Bamako were hovering in consultation with their aides about what they should do. It would have been an unwise government which would have followed an optimistic policy about the flood with so much potential aid looming on the horizon and so those charged with studying the rising waters predicted they would continue to rise and those charged with lowering them said they wouldn't fall. The end result was that all sorts of material aid poured into Bamako.

Of all the diplomats in Bamako, the American ambassador, C. Robert Moore, lived closest to the river and although he weathered several anxious days when it seemed he would have to abandon his car for a canoe, he maintained a cool objective view of affairs. Once the river began to fall there was little likelihood that any terrible health crisis would arise and after much discussion and consultation, the American embassy staff decided that no emergency assistance was needed.

However, the Malians' dire predictions and the Chinese tents made the flood problem an arena for international one-upsmanship in microcosmic Bamako. The Russians were determined to outdo the Chinese, the East Germans the West Germans, the Egyptians the Israelis, the French everyone, and the North Vietnamese and North Koreans out to support the Chinese. When all of the medical gifts arrived, I was privileged to see them because they were stored in Lastouillas' warehouse and whenever a new batch came in he would rush into my office with explosive excitement and shout, "Tenez, tenez, venez voir, venez voir." Lastouillas stacked all of the gifts according to the country of origin in an order of precedence which didn't reflect the value of the gift, but his own view of the donor country. The French gave the most, a quarter of a million dollars of very valuable medicines which stood up front in center. The Russian and Chinese gifts were appropriately off to the left, the West German to the right and the Bulgarian and East German far in the back. The French received no public recognition for their generous gift and the Bulgarians who gave the least, five crates of expired samples written in incomprehensible Bulgarian, received the most.

The crisis passed more quickly than the river fell and before long Lastouillas was complaining about the encumbrance posed by the unused emergency aid in his warehouse. It was decided to ship the medicines out as part of the regular supplies given periodically to dispensaries in the bush, but even with this, large quantities remained in Lastouillas' warehouse three years after the flood. Whenever I went into the bush I used to replenish my medical box with these medications and when holding a village clinic would dispense French aspirins, West German bandages, Chinese cotton, East German vitamins, Russian antibiotics,

Czechoslovakian tranquilizers and American anti-malarials. There was a lot of enterprise in Lastouillas' handling of the Bulgarian medicines for he found a Russian woman living ten miles from Bamako in Kati who spoke Bulgarian. His hope was that she would translate all of the writing on the boxes into French, but when she saw the hundreds of samples and calculated the days of tedious work involved, she declined. Lastouillas' contingency plan was more feasible; he shipped all of the five cases out to the only medical post in the country which had a Bulgarian doctor.

Many say that Africa is adverse to precision and makes a fugitive of those who would enslave her unpredictable conduct of affairs to a regular routine. And so it was that they predicted that the plan for the vaccination of the inland delta would be a colossal failure. There is much truth in this point of view of Africa, but it does not mean to say that great undertakings cannot have a successful existence in Africa. You must be very flexible and a very patient person to mastermind a great feat in Africa, someone who views the unexpected as high adventure. The brittle personality finds comfort in routine and is frustrated and driven away by the lack of it and so he doesn't last long in Africa. Because of the wide gap between what he expects and what happens his whole emotional reserve is consumed by anger and frustration which paralyzes him from taking the necessary alternative steps through which success is gained. You must accept that what happens depends to a large extent on you yourself and so you must carry a pocket full of enterprising alternatives to meet every eventuality and be a decisive man who can think up an effective solution to everything. Africa is a very personalized place which feels no need at present for the depersonalized administrative systems of the developed world. Success and failure stem not from the system but from the men who replace their function. If a dynamic man leaves, a ministry collapses, a hospital closes, a program withers away. The bureaucrats of the developed world cannot come to terms with this way of doing things for they are accustomed to working in an organization which moves on independently of those who are in it. People come and others leave, talents are lost or gained and through it all the system goes on. It is as when a president or king dies; the ship of state sails on. Those who approach Africa from this point of view become Africa's greatest failures, but those who accept that all depends on them become her greatest successes.

When we finally sent the eight trucks and thirty-two vaccinators across the savanna to Koutiala the air was warm and dry and the long oval clouds of the rainy season were breaking up into dissipated puffs against a clear sky. We had thought out many devices to insure that this nine month long campaign in the delta would not meet with failure. Because of the flood and the heavy rains, the whole original strategy had to be changed with painstaking care, schedules reset, and new studies made to determine what migratory groups would do in face of the excess water on the plains. The weakest link in the whole operation was our vaccinators and drivers. Although some of them were conscientious, honest and hard working, the majority were young and undisciplined with a strong inclination towards anarchy and sabotage. This was a reflection of their rugged individualism. They were city dwellers and like most such people in Mali were not communally oriented as is the rural villager. They saw no reason why they should sacrifice themselves for nine months on an altar of hard work and self-denial for the same salary they earned when they were in Bamako doing nothing. When I explained that their self-sacrifice would save thousands of lives they replied, "That doesn't matter to us." I carefully analyzed this difference in our points of view and realized that my personal thinking was being determined by a Christian ethic which teaches good works, charity and helping one's fellow man as a virtuous path in life. But their ethic, the Moslem ethic, does not teach this at all. Rather it holds out the promise of paradise to those who believe and who perform the ritual prayers and fastings prescribed in the Koran. Good works and charity are not required, and indeed are not encouraged. So a good Malian Moslem would not readily put anyone before himself nor self-sacrifice for the good of a fellow man. In view of this, I was really wasting my time by trying to appeal to a desire of achieving virtue which did not exist. In the end, it was put to them that their work was a requirement for their salary which if not done would end in their being fired.

My conversations with them on this whole subject always left me depressed and annoyed. They never believed that there was an ounce of self-sacrifice in myself either. Even though I explained to them that I was earning considerably less by working in Mali than I would if I were back in New York they never believed it. They viewed me as they did every foreigner who came to Mali, as someone who was financially profiting from the arrangement. If not, why else would I be there? They would support their argument by saying that I lived in a cement block house and had a truck at my disposition, they presuming that if I were back in New York I would like in a mud and dung building and walk. It was a revealing experience for me to unearth what it was they thought of me, but I realized that they would never feel grateful to me even if I sacrificed the whole of my professional life for the well-being of Mali. As it was, they saw the world through the spectacles of a Moslem ethic and so for them I was an exploiter and profiteer.

There was a striking anachronism about these men because although they occasionally stole medicines, used the trucks for cash paying customers and purposely created false problems out of discontent, they still did their job of vaccinating every village in a meticulous fashion. It was impossible to settle their disputes because they covered everything with a stormy description of irrelevant details and were indignant and obnoxious with anyone who dared question their integrity. The work of these teams had to be continuously assessed to make sure that the vaccines were giving positive results and that an acceptable percentage of the population was being reached. In order to do this, we formed a control team whose job it was to assess ten percent of the vaccinated

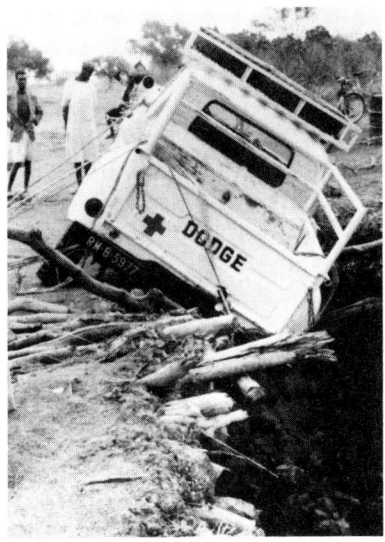

FIGURE 17. A near fatal accident. This vaccination truck almost slipped off the narrow wooden and earthen bridge into a stream fifty feet below. The accident occurred at night after a rain storm had made the earthen surface of the bridge extremely slippery. It took a week and the efforts of hundreds of men to finally get the truck off the edge of the bridge.

population through a method of statistical sampling. In principle this system insured a high standard of work performance from these teams, as long as I myself assessed the work of the control team.

Sending a small army of poorly paid and reluctant men out into the bush to perform an exacting job was no carefree operation. Several days before the list of the team members was posted, most had begun preparing their excuses as to why they couldn't leave. There was a lot of imagination in their excuses and obvious evidence of group coordination since no two were alike. They laid claim to having every possible disease from syphillis to trachoma and to being treated by long drawn out methods which fell into disuse many decades ago. There was a procession of sick brothers, cousins, aunts and uncles, pre-operative mothers and post-operative grandfathers, relatives dying, soon to die or else already dead and awaiting interment, baptisms, court trials, property to be bought or sold, militia duty, marriages and visiting parents. When we told them that only their own personal demise would excuse them from duty, they sunk into sullen contemplation and derogatory murmurings and slid around us like a pack of badgers, reconnoitering, trying to wear us thin to the point of frustration so that we would agree to their demands. If one could weigh up patience and suffering, I would say that my portion of both reached an impressive dimension. The most vexing step was the issuing of their equipment because it represented to them the final act after which there was no possible return. They claimed that the blankets were either too heavy or too light, the cots too firm or too soft, the mosquito nets too big or too small and behind them sauntered in the drivers with delaying tactics of their own. Although all of the trucks had been overhauled by Modibo and Jay and were in excellent shape, they saw reason to delay the departure because of missing reflectors, seat belts which didn't fasten and which they didn't use anyway, upholstery which had holes in it from their cigarettes, year old batteries which worked fine but which didn't suit them because they were a year old and finally ash trays which didn't slide out far enough. One driver made a dramatic last minute stand against leaving because his left directional signal didn't work. When he finally pulled away from the warehouse with his loaded truck it was on a wave of laughter because I had told everyone that the camels and cattle in the bush would be tolerant of a Dodge power wagon which didn't signal its left turns. When I arrived in Koutiala a day after the teams' arrival, the commandant seemed more interested in knowing when the vaccinators would leave his cercle than in when they would start to work.

The logistical problems involved in keeping so many men and all their equipment in the bush were enormous and at times I doubted we would overcome them. Each truck carried its own three hundred pound kerosine operated freezer and artificial ice which when frozen was put into isothermic boxes along with the vaccines. The freezers were set up in a central point out of which the team operated for several days while they were vaccinating the surrounding villages. A vaccinator, called a *frigorist* by Lastouillas kept watch over the freezer and the delicate vaccines. Each team also carried its own supply of medical equipment and a variety of other supplies such as, pens, matches, towels (bought at a sale by Lastouillas), talley sheets, soap, alcohol, jet guns and spare parts, kerosine lamps, bull horns which Jay adapted so that they worked off the batteries of the truck, insect repellant, chairs, tables, cots, cooking stoves, cotton, blankets, mosquito nets, spare parts for the truck, winches, iron sand tracks which we bought in Dakar and which had come down from World War II where they were used as landing strips for planes in North Africa, and water filters. Each team also had a Honda motor bike which was used to transport vaccinators to villages where the truck couldn't travel. In areas where even the Hondas couldn't enter, then they went in on foot or on the backs of donkeys.

The vaccination teams worked according to a master plan drawn up months before by Jay and myself and the Malian administrative and health authorities. Villages in Mali are grouped together into two hundred and seventy eight units known as arrondissements which in turn are grouped into forty-two units known as cercles. The cercles are grouped into six regions. The villages vary in size from two hundred to two thousand inhabitants. The arrondissements are headed by a chief who is responsible for administering all of the villages under him and the cercles are headed by commandants who in turn administer the arrondissements. When we began vaccinating in Koutiala, we sent a team into each of the cercle's eight arrondissements. There they traveled from village to village, according to a daily master schedule previously set up through mutual agreement with the commandant of the cercle, the chiefs of the arrondissements and the village chiefs. Each village had been visited twice before their arrival, once a month before and once a week before, in order to explain to the chiefs and the elders what it was the teams would be doing and on what day they would arrive. This master plan also enabled us to know with a fair degree of certainty the whereabouts of every team each day of the week and to set up the logistical supply system for vaccines and other necessary items. Teams communicated once a week to our headquarters in Koutiala or more frequently if they had problems. Additional supplies and replacement personnel were sent out from Bamako on a regular basis. When Jay and I were in the bush, Lastouillas served as the anchor man in Bamako and would get the needed items to us in a few days time by whatever transport available. We also had to arrange for the vaccination teams to be fed by the local villagers. In addition, we were successful at the outset of this campaign in securing assistance from the World Health Organization in providing the vaccinators with a per diem allowance which amounted to fifty percent of their usual daily wage. The Malian field supervisor who came out with us into the bush acted also as a budget and fiscal officer, arranging for the vaccinators' pay to be sent to their wives or else given to themselves. Most of the vaccinators and drivers had sent their wives to live with their parents. This way the women were safe under the protection of the extended family and the vaccinator also relieved of the burden of supporting his household in his absence.

We also arranged to have the local male nurses of the Grandes Endemies Service accompany the vaccination teams. Since they knew all of the local villages and the topography of the countryside they acted as excellent guides and facilitated acceptance by the villagers of vaccination. They themselves undertook to examine the village populations for evidence of sleeping sickness (trypanosomiasis) which is transmitted by the tsetse fly and for evidence of river blindness (onchocerciasis) transmitted by the simulium fly. They treated patients suffering from these diseases and also those suffering from leprosy and all other major disease problems. Our teams then were not merely vaccination teams, but comprehensive health teams. The area of Koutiala was endemic for sleeping sickness and river blindness, both kinds of flies abounding on the edges of the rivers and streams. The risk to our team personnel was great and so we gave them a protective injection of lomidine against sleeping sickness before they left Bamako. But there was no protective inoculation against river blindness. Many of them contracted this disease, including Djigui, and had to return to Bamako for the long and disabling treatment. Some of the villages in Koutiala were completely disabled by river blindness, over fifty percent of the people being blind. So bad was the situation that often the vaccinators couldn't assemble the population beneath a tree on the village square as was our practice, but had to visit each and every compound. Because people were blind they couldn't make it on their own to the assembly point in the center of the village.

The war against these two scourges has been on for many years.

The French military physicians were the first to uncover the problem and under the guidance of men such at Jamot, Muraz and Richet, established the mobile medical service, the Grandes Endemies, in order to fight these diseases. The battle against sleeping sickness was successful because there are effective and safe drugs for treating the disease and for protecting people exposed to the fly by inoculating them with lomidine. This protects them for six months. However, there is no protective medicine against river blindness, and control of the disease has to be achieved through control of the fly. At the present time, the World Health Organization in conjunction with the European Development Fund and the regional health organization of French speaking African states in West Africa, the OCCGE, are undertaking a massive control program against river blindness. Through aerial spraying and the use of larvicides they are reducing the fly population and opening up the fertile lands along the river valleys which were long ago abandoned by the people because of the ravages of the disease. I myself always thought that there was a great need to develop a new, safe and effective drug for treating the disease, one which would cure it. One of the American ambassadors who came to Mali, Robert O. Blake, beacme very interested in the problem and together we tried to interest drug companies to search for a drug which could relieve the horrible suffering of hundreds of thousands of people. But there was little interest on their part since such a drug would scarcely bring them a great profit on the world market. It would only be in demand by the poor developing countries of Africa and South and Central America who would depend on its being virtually donated free to them, since they can hardly afford to buy medicines.

One of the terrible things about river blindness is that it is a chronic life long disease which begins as generalized body itching. The victims constantly scratch themselves because of the allergic reaction taking place in their skins from the small worms which live there. These small worms or microfilariae as they are scientifically called are produced by an adult female worm which can give birth to about fifty thousand a day. Gradually, the microfilariae move through the skin and into the eyes where they destroy the retina, the lens and the other vital parts, leading to blindness. Victims' skins become severely infected with secondary bacterial infections because of the constant scratching. It is still Ambassador Blake's and my hope that one day we will be successful in interesting someone to search for an effective drug for this terrible scourge of Africa.

Within a week of our starting in Koutiala, a Malian field supervisor was sent down from Bamako by the Director General of Health to take charge of the day-to-day operation of the campaign. Bramane was an *infirmier d'etat*, a young dynamic and efficient organizer, a stalwart of the political party and a declared Marxist. In many ways, he was excellently suited to handle the vaccinators and drivers because he understood their mentality and could deal with them on their terms and so he was a far better choice than Boundiar who by this time had been transferred to another service. Unfortunately, Bramane had an unfounded suspiciousness about Jay and I and the declared conviction that we were not to be trusted since we were Americans. At first, this greatly hindered our working relationship, but with time, the conspiratorial atmosphere disappeared and Bramane found that working with us was a pleasant experience. Even at the outset, Bramane was deferent and polite and eager to please although behind our backs he warned the vaccinators that we were a threat to Mali's security. I always tried to be charitable in summing up Bramane's character, realizing that he had to profess a certain amount of public dislike for us because his closeness to us placed him in outright jeopardy. It was regrettable that Modibo wasn't with us at this time because in him we found loyalty and dependability. We had put him in charge of an old Renault 44 truck which ferried gasoline from our eight thousand gallon stockpile in Koutiala to the teams in the bush. We had all of this gasoline brought up to Koutiala from Bobo-Dioulasso in Upper Volta in tankers. It had been brought to Bobo-Dioulasso from Abidjan on the coast. Because of the thefts of gasoline which had occurred in the past, we decided to put our most trustworthy man in charge.

Because half of the cercle of Koutiala was still inundated with water from the flood, we had to make some last minute changes in the strategy. These areas held one hundred thousand people and we stood little chance of reaching them until March. Several villages on the Bani River had been caught in a flash flood and all of the inhabitants drowned. Several other unexpected problems developed. The Minianka in Koutiala were harvesting their cotton crop and because their fields are far away from their villages, the vaccinators were being greeted by empty villages. The Peul were exceptionally late in making their descent because of the high water, but I wasn't too concerned about them since I knew we would be able to vaccinate them once they got to the flood plain. But the absence of the Minianka from their villages posed a problem which demanded an immediate solution. Finally, after meeting with all of the chiefs, we were able to convince them to keep their people in the villages on the agreed day. Some of the Minianka, however, flatly refused to be seen by the teams, especially those in the arrondissement of Kouniana. They hid their children from the vaccinators and fled into the bush, thinking that the jet guns were real guns and our intention genocide. We were never very successful in talking these villages into cooperating with us.

The town of Koutiala will always be one of my favored spots in Mali. Sitting up in its high valley, the air there is always clear and the sun sets with a fiery trail of red over a winding stream banked with drooping palm trees and enriched with a chorus of doves and crickets. The original Minianka name for this town was Koule Dyakhan, meaning, the village of the blacksmiths. The French found this name too difficult to pronounce and so they changed it to Koutiala which has no meaning in Minianka. The town abounds with blacksmiths, most of them located on the edge of the market place where they present an impressive sight of rows of hand pumped bellows, crashing hammers, red molten iron and roaring furnaces.

We set up our headquarters at the Grandes Endemies Service building on the edge of town. It was a massive fortress like structure with

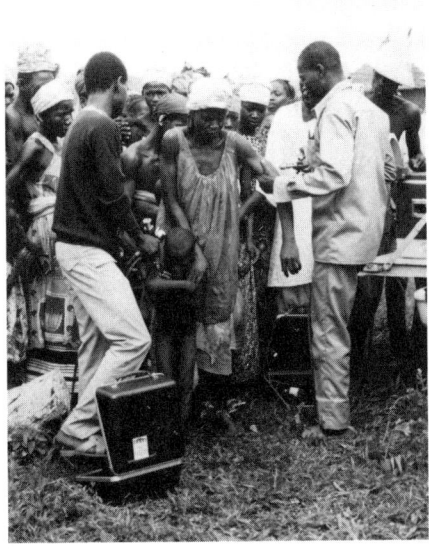

FIGURE 18. A typical village vaccination session. Djigui Diakite *(right)* administers smallpox vaccine while the other vaccinator gives measles vaccine.

an ochre colored patina and broad cool verandas, sitting in the comfortable shade of several massive silk cotton trees. We arranged to take our meals at the Poule Verte campement where Karim the cook kept us well fed with a menue of slightly tough steak and whipped potatoes. The owner of the campement was a Lebanese named George whose brother owned the Auberge campement in Segou. Both George and his brother became quite enthusiastic about the vaccination campaign and hung several of our posters on the walls of their buildings. These posters always disappeared because people found them so attractive that they took them home and hung them on their walls. Bob Baker of the USIS in Bamako had designed the posters before the teams left for Koutiala. It bore the photograph I had taken of a smiling little boy, Mamadou Traoré, being vaccinated with a jet injector. Mamadou's smiling face went all over Mali and looked down from baobab trees, from commandants' bulletin boards, from hotel room walls and from the tents of nomads. It was posted on the interior of the Niger River streamers, in Timbuctoo, in Gao, in Sikasso and in hundreds of other towns and hamlets in Mali. Bob had used blue and white as the colors for the poster because they are the preferred colors among most of Mali's ethnic groups. Little Mamadou, who was the son of the gendarme who worked at the Service d'Hygiene, became so popular that other countries in West Africa asked for permission to post his smiling face in order to attract people to be vaccinated. And so Mamadou's smile went all over West and Central Africa, to Gabon and Nigeria, to Senegal and Mauritania and all the countries in between. Later the Malian Government issued a fifty franc postage stamp depicting the photograph I had taken of Mamadou in order to commemorate the vaccination campaign.

Our vaccination teams moved through Koutiala with astounding speed, through arrondissements whose names sounded like a rhyming litany, Kouniana, M'Pessoba, Consegula, Molobala, Zangasso and Bla. They averaged ten thousand smallpox vaccinations per week and two thousand measles inoculations. In addition, they delivered eight thousand yellow fever inoculations per week and treated thousands of sick villagers. Early on, I had decided upon an operation wherein we could vaccinate the populations of weekly markets, the thought being that at these large gatherings we would reach people who had been missed in the village-to-village campaign. We began with the Koutiala market which was the largest in the area and for this I brought back all of the teams from the bush. We lodged the team members in the unused maternity building, a new structure which had been built by the government, but which was in disuse since the local Minianka women preferred to deliver at home.

Malian markets differ from one another in many ways and their character and purpose is not simply the exchange of goods, but also to provide people with a place to meet and exchange local news. Some markets are held on a fixed day of the week, whereas others are held every five days, meaning that they fall on a different day. In making up a program for markets, we had to study them, find out which ones were on a fixed day of the week and which were "moving markets." Traders come to these markets from far and wide, some traveling for hundreds of miles, on a circuit which takes them to a predetermined number where they habitually sell their wares. These traders travel on large trucks as opposed to local traders who come in small lorries from neighboring towns. The local villagers come on foot or on donkeys in order to sell their agricultural products. Thus it was possible simply by observing people arriving at a market to determine who they were and where they came from. Traders have fixed places in Malian markets, beneath one of a score of straw hangers. The villagers, on the other hand, sit on the periphery of a market, with their backs to the path leading to their village. This custom developed out of the necessity of being close to an exit during the pre-colonial era when markets were subject to physical pillaging and raiding.

Through my studies of the organization of markets, I learned that one had to vaccinate people as they entered a market place. Once inside, it was impossible to reach them because there were too many people milling about and it was impossible to systematically examine everyone for signs of a vaccination scar. This meant that the entrances to the markets had to be blocked and posted with vaccinators before people arrived in the morning. With the help of the militia we were able to do this and to examine everyone for evidence of a smallpox scar. If they had none, they were vaccinated. Because the Koutiala market begins at 6 A.M., Bramane had all of the vaccinators on their feet at 5 A.M., much to their displeasure. Then he had to go over to the militia camp and get them up, which took some doing since the sentry wouldn't let him past the gate. We posted the militiamen and the vaccinators at the six entrances to the market and by 10 A.M. had vaccinated ten thousand people who had not been reached in the village to village campaign. This was the first of the market vaccinations in Mali and over the years we employed the strategy in every market in the country.

The drivers got up much later in the morning and created chaos by driving their trucks all over the little town. It was like watching a bunch of extras in the Keystone Cops. Every time I turned a corner, a white Dodge truck whizzed by in front of me. It took us a few hours to put an end to this because once we stopped one driver and left him in order to go off and chase down another, he in turn would take off again. Bramane performed very well that day and was able to instill a discipline into the operation which I never believed possible.

When I first started traveling with Bramane he spoke and acted as if Marxism were a dynamic and vital force in village life in spite of the fact that most villages in the bush hadn't the faintest idea of what either Marxism or socialism was. One had to admire Bramane's conscientious effort to believe in what obviously was not there, but at the same time accept the fact that the pleasant deception could not go on forever.

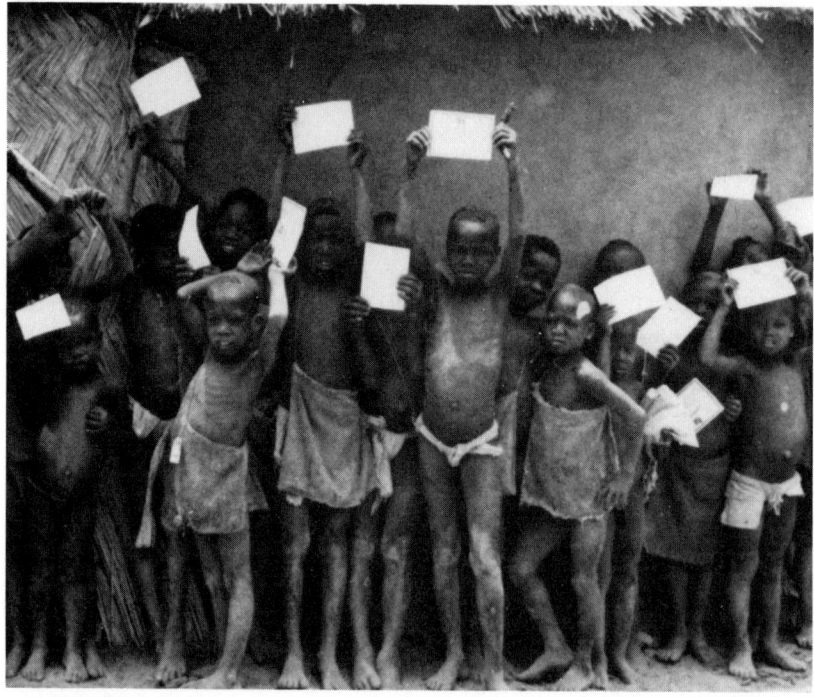

FIGURE 19. Recently vaccinated children in the Region of Sikasso with their vaccination certificates.

Whenever the vaccination results for a given area were not sastisfactory Bramane presented me with reasons which although plausible were simply not true. The Peul nomads often refused to come to the vaccination points in the villages of the sedentary farmers because they had had disputes with the sedentaries, but Bramane maintained that it was because the villages were too far away from their camps. My verbalizing of the truth never intimidated Bramane into compromise and even when we went into nomad camps and the real truth emerged he stuck to his original position. There was a high percentage of villages in Koutiala which were animist and our vaccination campaign coincided with their annual secret society rites. According to Bramane most of the population was Moslem and those who weren't were Catholic, but he was never able to give me a satisfactory reply when I asked why there were so few mosques in the area and no churches. The Mali which Bramane saw in Koutiala was very different from the one he believed to exist, trusting the descriptions of the country's political poets. Like the commandant he found it impossible to come to terms with reality.

One warm sunny afternoon soon after we had vaccinated the market, a vaccination team came back to town and told Bramane in Bambara that six villages refused to be vaccinated because they were in the midst of their most important fetish ceremony. In a way it pleased me to let Bramane think that I didn't understand any Bambara so when I asked him what the trouble was he said that the villagers couldn't be vaccinated because they were too busy harvesting their crops. I don't think I ever saw Bramane as uncomfortable as at the moment I announced my intention of going into the villages myself to see what was going on. He fell naturally to disuading me by saying that the trip was too difficult, the track impassable and the area infested with tsetse flies. Over his loud protests I pulled Modibo off the Renault truck and with Djigui drove into the area the next day, dragging a reluctant Bramane with me. Contrary to what Bramane had said, it was clean rolling country full of hill top vistas and pleasant deep valleys where for as far as you could see everything shimmered in shades of blue and green. The springs of the truck sighed and sang as we inched along the rutted muddy track, crossed creaking log bridges and splashed across the glittering rush of swollen creeks. There were a lot of tsetse flies in the area, especially around the streams where they buzzed around the truck in hoards. Insect repellant is useless in keeping them away because in the heat and dry air it evaporates from the skin in twenty minutes and is no longer effective. If one maintains a speed of forty kilometers per hour the tsetse flies can't keep up with the vehicle and one effectively avoids them. But at slower speeds they descend like vultures onto a vehicle and get inside through every hole and crevice imaginable. I told everyone to close the windows to keep the flies out, especially at the river crossings where our slow speed going through the water and the concentration of flies created ideal conditions for our being bothered by them. Bramane said he wouldn't close his window because there wouldn't be enough air in the truck for him to breathe. I told him that if it were air he wanted he could go out onto the back of the truck and ride there. He finally closed his window. The tsetse fly is as large as a horse fly, but folds its wings over on its back in a scissors like fashion. The female fly is a voracious blood sucker and needs a blood meal every few days. They bite through thick clothing and inflict a sting which is extremely painful. In biting, they transmit a protozoa known as a trypanosome which multiplies at the site of the bite and then invades the blood stream, later lodging in the brain where an encephalitis ensues. At that stage of the disease the victim lapses into a stupor, hence the name "sleeping sickness." Generally, tsetse flies prefer to bite wild animals such as wart hogs and antelope, but in the absence of these or when in contact with man they will bite humans. When they bite an infected animal or human they suck up the trypanosome which after developing in their bodies migrates to the salivary glands, ready to be injected when the fly bites the next victim. So it is that the protozoa is transmitted from one person to another or from animals to man. Tsetse flies do not like direct sunlight and dry heat and for this reason stay close to the river beds where there is plenty of moisture and shade. They usually bite early in the morning and at dusk, the same as does the fly which transmits river blindness, because it is cool and the sun not strong. However, I have known of tsetse flies to bite even at night when there is a full moon and if they are hungry enough they will bite even when there is not a moon, being guided by any light near their intended victim. For this reason, many of the teams encountered difficulties with the flies which were attracted by the strong headlights of the trucks at night.

By six in the evening, we reached a clear hill top from where we saw the sun set into a long bank of tumbling clouds in a splash of red and orange. Down below us in a broad valley was a large Bambara village, a mosaic of clustered conical straw roofs, gardens and cattle pens. There was a continuous chorus of loud drumming, clanging bells and the precise clicking of wooden rattles coming from the center of the village and it meant that the great Komo fetish had been taken out of its sanctuary. I asked Djigui to go down into the village and speak to the old men about allowing the team to enter the village. Neither Modibo nor Bramane belonged to the Komo nor did I, and so only Djigui could get into the village since he was a member of the cult. As he described it later on, he was stopped at the edge of the village by some men who said, "Go away from here. Don't you know that the Komo has come out!" When Djigui replied that he was *Komo dé* (a child of the Komo) and showed the finger signs known only to initiates, they let him pass through to the center of the village where he found a masked dancer and the fetish moving around the village square surrounded by the members of the society.

As soon as the masked dancer saw Djigui he rushed up to him with threatening gestures, circled around him several times and screamed out in anger. Djigui finally did what he knew he had to do; he raised his left hand up and with his fifth and index finger pointed out cried out, "Eeeee, ee, eeeee, ee!" The dancer calmed down and trotted around Djigui with gay steps and once the passwords had been given danced off shouting, "Another of my children is here." People maintain that long ago in this area and not so long ago in other places the masked dancer was obliged to kill any non-initiate on the spot. Even today a non-initiated person does not dare enter a village when the Komo is out of its sanctuary. The women and children of the village are obliged to remain in their houses for the seven days the ceremony takes place and are not permitted out even to urinate or defeacte . They must take care of these needs by using large calabashes kept inside of the houses. The actual fetish in this village was a small round mound of river mud, cotton, bits of wood and bone covered with a sacrificial patina of chicken and sheep blood. The members of the Komo believe that the spirit of the supreme being *Faro,* resides in the fetish. Societies such as the Komo serve as social controls. They punish murderers, thieves and other criminals and maintain a respect for social law and order. They unite the people of different villages on the common ground of religious belief and in so doing foster political alliances and territorial cohesion.

When Djigui finally came back up the hill towards eleven P.M., he was accompanied by the chief of the village who was also the head of the society, the *Komo Tigui.* Judging from his state and also Djigui's it was obvious that there was a good deal of drinking going on in the village. Djigui was livlier than ever, and although not feeling any pain, was able to give me a precise run down on what was going on.

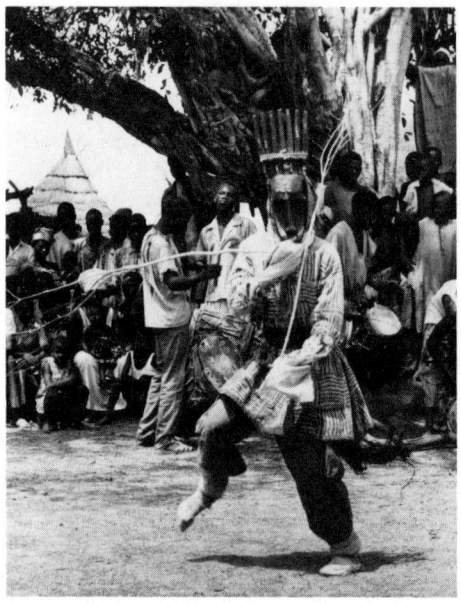

FIGURE 20. A young Bambara man dancing with a seven honored *N'Tomo Society* mask. This society is the first of six into which Bambara males are traditionally initiated. The purpose of the *N'Tomo Society* is to prepare boys for the gradual acquistion of knoweldge about man and the universe. The seven horned mask represents man's masculinity and femininity.

I was surprised also that the old man approached the matter of the Komo in a very direct fashion. Bramane had long since fallen into silence and I didn't worsen matters for him by pulling him into the conversation. The Komo Tigui told me that the six villages which were allied to this Komo held their ceremonies between sunset and sunrise. Contrary to what the vaccinators had told us, he had no objection to our vaccinating the villages during the daylight hours when the fetish was inside of its sanctuary. It seemed that the vaccinators, on hearing that a Komo ceremony was taking place in the area, simply headed in the opposite direction. In talking things over with Modibo and Djigui I came to the conclusion that the best time to vaccinate these people was about noon since before then everyone was too hung over from the night before and by four in the afternoon, the drinking began once again. When we finally settled the affair with the Komo Tigui he agreed to allow the women and children to come out of their houses for the vaccinations and made a parting gesture by offering to initiate me into the Komo. This was Djigui's doing and I was properly initiated. Two days later we sent two teams back into the area to vaccinate the six villages. Because none of the people wash for several weeks before the ceremony and during it, we had to use enormous quantities of alcohol to clean off their arms. The odor coming from this mass of humanity was so offensive that even Djigui and Modibo felt sick to their stomachs.

There was much more frankness in Bramane's character after this experience and it ushered in a better era in our relations. A few days later, when we drove north to San, he was surprisingly more conversant than he had ever been about animism and seemed to be negotiating with his own opinions on many subjects. Bramane's good humor never left his face even when he was immersed in intense concentration, and in spite of his opposite stand on many issues he always echoed a seemingly agreeing refrain of three descending notes, "bon, bon, bon," whenever I spoke. I once told Bramane that were he back in the United States a decade ago he would have qualified for a job as the National Broadcasting Company's station break gong. He didn't catch the meaning of this as first, but when I explained it to him he laughed.

When we got to the village of Kimparana late in the afternoon, an unexpected thunder storm broke on the hills surrounding us and finally swept down into the valley through which the road cut a tortuous course. It all began with the descent of an ominous darkness, threatening gusts of wind, the crackling of leaves and dry sand blowing through the air. At first, the drops fell a few at a time but within a few moments the water crashed down in torrents and turned the road bed into a swollen river. Modibo had to stop the truck for an hour during which time we sat encircled by a dense curtain of water which cut us off from all of our surroundings. Small lakes welled up on ground one would have thought dry enough to soak up the Atlantic and the violent rush of the red muddy water on the roadway rocked the truck from side to side. There is nothing in Africa to challenge the soverignty of a storm and before it everything in the savanna stops. Canoes are anchored, bustling markets disperse, farmers leave their fields and people working in city offices gaze out as if some great drama is being played before them. There is no audible sound other than the rain falling onto the ground, into the grass and the trees and finally onto itself. A profound stillness pervades everything living. Birds stop singing, the cicadas silence their endless drilling sound and men are moved by some strange and unknown feeling into talking in whispers. One doesn't wait with impatience for a storm to end in Mali because it is the only welcomed force which can defeat the crushing heat, clear the air of its thick heat waves and put a pleasing scent into everything which is comforting and cool. We waited out the storm discussing the role which storms might have played in determining the course of Malian history, a subject which Bramane said was as appropriate as any under the circumstances. He finally concluded that storms stopped the march of El Hadj Omar's army, delayed explorers like Mungo Park and Réné Caille and aided socialism and Marxism. With some imagination, it was possible to see some truth in the first part of Bramane's conclusion, but we all failed to see how storms helped socialism and Marxism. Bramane's explanation was more poetic than illuminating, as were many of the things he said, but it seemed a fitting way for the conversation to end as the sun burst through the now misty clouds.

There is always a wonderful feeling of relaxation after a storm which puts you into the best of condition for any new challenge. It is just as well that it is this way because when we arrived in Kimparana and spoke to the chief of the arrondissement we learned that the control team was sorely in need of controlling. In a frank and direct manner, he told me that several days before two men had come through on red Honda motor bikes, the tallest of whom made claim to being the "inspector general." The chief was suspicious enough about this claim to say that it was his understanding that the vaccination campaign was being directed by the Americans and a Malian named Bramane. But they told him that all of that was changed now and that the "inspector general" was running affairs. The chief thought it might be true so he treated the "inspector general" royally and sent word out into the villages that they were to do the same. From his description, the self-proclaimed "inspector general" was Karamoko Sanogo, a burly six foot Bozo whose mind and body of generous proportions moved with a ponderous slowness which didn't reflect any careful pre-mediation, but simply the fact that he was slow. Although Karamoko was by no means the intellectual beacon of the rank and file, I thought him honest and reliable and capable of doing the required assessing. New ideas came slowly to Karamoko and after much suffering, but once they took root he never forgot them. He enjoyed a reputation as an excellent letter writer because he was never without an old French book which Lastouillas had given him entitled, "How To Write Love Letters." Karamoko took great pride in sending letters to me attached to his reports and they showed both a lack of thinking and his arbitrary use of passages from the love letter book. They came as a Christmas card on Easter Sunday and with a sentiment which was inappropriate to the occasion. It took many months before Karamoko got the idea that I and other people were not very flattered by his referring to us as "fragrant morning flower," and "passionately loved one." When I asked Karamoko if he knew what these expressions meant he said, "No, I don't. But they are in the book so they must be good." When we finally found Karamoko and the other controller, he was comfortably seated beneath a huge orange umbrella in the camp of West German road engineers who were building the new road between Segou and San. Karamoko's inspector generalship had given him a passport to the finest German beer and a comfortable bed in an air conditioned room in the camp, but when we arrived he reverted to drinking water and spent the night on a straw mat underneath the orange umbrella.

When the work in Koutiala was finished, the commandant and the local committee for the defense of the revolution gave us a large reception at George's Poule Verte. We had vaccinated 184,654 people against smallpox and 55,610 children against measles. Only Karim the cook was sullen because the women of the town had made chicken, rice and lamb, his only contribution being a soup which no one wanted. We all ate some and finally he beamed. George cranked on the electric generator and three neon lights shone where there was generally only the faint flickering of orange kerosine lamps. The commandant asked me to deliver an address which Bramane helped me to compose by the light of an old kerosine lamp on the back porch. Bramane said it would be a good idea if I ended my speech by shouting, "Long live the revolution, long live international cooperation between all peoples of the world, long live liberty, fraternity and equality, long live good health to everyone." I explained to Bramane that in America we didn't end speeches that way to which he replied, "That is too bad. They are really lacking something then." As lacking as my speech was in Bramane's eyes because I left out all of the "long lives" it conveyed what it was I really felt. I read it beneath the unsteady light of the insect covered neon bulbs and because the bugs kept falling down my back I wiggled quite a bit. I don't remember everything I said to the teams and the local officials, but I did let them know what a fine thing had just been accomplished. In reading the speech my thoughts were not so much about the words written on the paper but about the people in front of me, Bramane, Djigui, Modibo, the commandant, the vaccinators, the drivers and the chiefs. I saw through them the villages being vaccinated, the joy on the faces of thousands of work weary mothers as their children were vaccinated, the squirms and screams of the children and the laughter of the adults. Although most of our vaccinators hadn't undertaken this great effort for the purpose of bettering the lives of their fellow men, in the end this is what they achieved. I thought about them all, the ones who wore Mao buttons and those who wore buttons of Hollywood movie stars of the 1940's. It was not in buttons alone that one saw anachronisms in Mali.

Chapter IX
The Festival of Return

Once a year in December, tens of thousands of Peul nomads converge on an isolated village, Diafarabe, which lies hidden in a quiltwork of swamps and flood plains in the middle of Mali. They come down from the dry sahel in the north in great convoys with their thousands of head of cattle. This great gathering lasts for a day, during which the Peul hold their annual ceremonial crossing of the Diaka River, a branch of the Niger. This festive crossing of the river was instituted by Cheikou Ahmadou in order to commenmorate the passage of the herds from the harsh country of the sahel into the rich grass filled flood plains. The Peul call it the *degal,* the festival of return.

The obvious advantage of such a festival to us was the gathering of so many thousands of nomads in a given spot where we would vaccinate them and take care of their other medical problems. So while Jay and Bramane led six vaccination teams across the plateau into the country of the Bobo and the Dogon, I traveled up the Niger with a convoy of four canoes with two vaccination teams, a staff of infirmiers and Djigui for a distance of a hundred and twenty miles in order to reach Diafarabe. Djigui was in high spirits as we set out from Mopti since he had learned that his wife had just given birth to a son, his first, down in Bamako. Little did we suspect that this joy would soon be turned into terrible sorrow when the baby died of neonatal tetanus seven days after birth.

The Niger was tremendously swollen and wide, the shore line invisible beneath water which stood two feet deep on the surrounding plains. This swamp had that power which stems from immensity and silence. It was a world of blues and greens except when the sun gave it a silvery glow. You could see the sun rise here between the reeds, a giant red disc, as lonely and as big as a sun rising over the ocean. There is something very maritime about the inland delta. You feel the openness of the sea all around you, the lack of limit, the absence of difference. The wind moves the same, tossing the tops of the borgus grass into gentle waves. Even the storks and herons seem to be the same one finds legging their way along a deserted ocean beach. The amiable sound of wood and water dominate, the splash of the oars, the thumping of bare feet on the gunnels, the rubbing of the soft bow on the tops of the white caps. The two have a real affection for one another. There was little boat traffic on this stretch of the Niger, just long canvas covered canoes submerged deep into the water with orderly rows of crowded passengers and heterogeneous heaps of baggage and goods. They disappeared in a flash from the main channel, off onto the narrow arms of the river which snake their way through the tall borgus grass to hidden island villages. We passed the villages of the Bozo fishermen where their long nets hung from tired kapoc trees like delicate lace in a fancy shop window. Their villages are always inviting, a pleasant place to stay with warm and friendly people. The river ahead always looked like a dead end and it was hard to tell where the true channel was with a score of ragged peninsulas jutting out as limiting black lines. The lonely palm trees danced on them in the mirage a few feet off the ground.

When I was young I used to read books like *Sanders of the River* and dream that one day in the romantic future I would be sailing down some thrilling African waterway. Were youth to realize its dreams when romanticism and sentimentality are still very much alive what wonderful experiences would be had. But maturity and age tarnish the glow of youth romanticism and the experiences come during the pragmatic era of our lives.

After two days of tedious paddling we rowed into Diafarabe where the river widened into a calm glassy surface and moved off to the southwest with ease and unlimited freedom into one of those great landscapes and splendid views which are the essence of Africa. Along the river the air was cool and charged with the noise of a drama being played out by thousands of screaming nomads and their excited herds of cattle. It was a menacing mass of men and animals, spilling all over the orange colored terraces of the river's steep bank, flying off into the skyline like an enormous bellowing dragon. Never before in my life had I seen such a sight. The smoke and booming of nineteenth cenutry flint lock muskets filled the air and from the opposite shore there came the hypnotic and enchanting din of flutes and drums playing the same short tune over and over again. All of the Peul from northern Mali were there, herdsmen, warriors, chiefs and nobles, waiting on the opposite bank for the signal to cross the river. For over a hundred years the Peul have patiently waited for that signal to cross the river. The herdsmen were young and in spite of being staunch Moslems had been drinking locally brewed *dolo* earlier in the morning. The assortment of clothes they wore was reminiscent of paintings depicting life in the middle ages. Some wore red hats which stood up like toppling chimney stacks and some wore broad straw platters which looked like left overs from a consistory in Rome.

They ran and shouted with great agitation between the frightened cattle, thrusting their broad spears and clubs high into the air. Even from where we sat in our canoes, we could hear the distinct note of the chanting. Djigui and the vaccinators took in a deep breath and with a quick look told me they were a bit frightened by it all.

"Don't worry," said Djigui to the others with his usual air of confidence. "Dr. Imperato will know exactly what to do." Little did he realize at that point that I didn't have the faintest idea as to how we were going to vaccinate this enormous band of half-tamed nomads.

The old men and the chiefs sat placidly in a dignified flotilla of canoes, their consumptive chests wrapped up in yards of silk and cotton. These herds were theirs, the investment of a lifetime and the living symbol of their prestige and affluence and certainly there was no greater pleasure for these old men than to look at their wealth and to parade it before the entire establishment. One saw satisfaction and pride radiating beneath their wrinkled bark-like faces. It was a pride not only of their herds, but also of themselves, a pride of status, importance and greatness. For in that composite mass of cattle, dust and noise lay embodied the earthly strivings, the goal of decades of hard work, the spiritual and the emotional whole of many men. In a strange way, difficult for us to understand, those cattle stood for success and goodness, for a greatness among peers born of devoted effort and submission to the will of God. They were the reward of obedience to God's will, to the teachings of the prophet. So it wasn't then just a matter of wealth, but equally one of the holiness and Koranic obedience of those whose reward this cattle wealth was.

The old men engaged in streams of quiet conversation and perhaps some of them thought about the days when they were young and swimming the river in the *degal* next to their fathers' herds. As they talked the herds were driven into the water with a great splash according to an order of precedence. The herds from Djenne went first, followed by those from Sossobe, Soufroulaye, Pondori, Sebera and a score of other traditional chiefdoms. Each herd was led into the water by gaily decorated bulls which had ribbons attached to their horns and tails. The crossing took four hours and when the last of the herds reached the opposite shore pandemonium broke loose.

The date for this great event in the moving lives of the Peul is not fixed. It depends on the level of the river and on previous events in the Peul calendar. Day after day the herds had come down from the sahel and browsed along the river bank while the oracles were consulted and a day for the crossing set. In order to be prepared for this day, I had previously arranged with the chief medical officer of the cercle of Tenenkou in which Diafarabe is located to telegraph to our base in Bamako as soon as he received word that the Peul were crossing the river. When his telegram arrived in Bamako, Jay and I were in the bush in Koutiala and so Lastouillas called me by telephone and over the static filled line shouted, "The Peul cross on the fourth of December." Lastoillas didn't think we would be able to get to Diafarabe in time to be there for the crossing.

"It is only four days off," he said. "You will never make it." But I was determined to. In an ordinary year one can get into Diabarabe over the dike road which runs along the left bank of the Niger from Markala to Macina. But that road was now flooded and so there was no other way into Diafarabe other than by boat. The logistics of handling the Diafarabe program were complex. I needed to have a freezer and vaccine shipped into Diafarabe from Bamako by boat along with additional vaccinators to help with the campaign.

"There's a river boat leaving tomorrow night from Koulikoro," shouted Lastouillas. "I'll put the freezer and the vaccine on it." To fulfill that order was no easy task, and the rest of that day was hectic for Lastouillas. First he had to arrange to ship the material and the vaccines on the train from Bamako to Koulikoro and secure passage for the vaccinators on the same train. Then he had to arrange to have the material and the vaccines transferred from the train to the river steamer, *General Soumare* and secure passage on it for the vaccinators. The train was to leave Bamako at 7 P.M. for the hour trip to Koulikoro and the boat at 9 P.M. In an Africa noted for its delayed train schedules, this was tempting disaster, but Lastouillas went ahead anyway.

The following afternoon, Lastouillas and the vaccination team and their mountain of equipment stood on the rickety Bamako station. Lastouillas noticed that they had large quantities of food with them.

"Why are you bringing all that food? " he asked. "They'll feed you up there."

The boys laughed. "And if they don't." They weren't taking any chances. None of them had ever been on a train before nor on a boat so they were both apprehensive and excited. When the train pulled out on time Lastouillas breathed a sigh of relief.

While Lastouillas was getting the vaccinators off on the train for Koulikoro, Djigui and I and the rest of our party were somewhere on the Niger in our canoes. We spent two nights along the river bank, the last in the Bozo village of Dia-Bozo where a week before a terrible tragedy had occurred. On a Thursday afternoon seventy villagers were in a long canoe on the Niger returning from the weekly fair at Mopti. About two miles from the village, the canoe broke in two, spilling the passengers and tons of baggage into the deep and swift current. Only six people managed to swim to shore, the remaining being carried off by the swift current or sinking under around the broken canoe. Because the survivors didn't remember all of those who had been in the canoe, it wasn't until several days passed that families presumed their loved ones lost since they didn't return on the other canoes and couldn't be found in Mopti. Dia-Bozo was a very sad place and most of the time the old men were praying in one of the two great mud mosques.

We got up at 5 A.M. after a restful night just as the sun rose out of the grass along the river bank. The old chief of Dia-Bozo walked down to the river bank with me, silent, pensive and sad. He didn't say anything as we shook hands and parted, nor did I. Our communication was through touch and sight and conveyed what we both felt. I will always remember Dia-Bozo with its two beautiful mosques and their elaborate minarets and turrets, standing high up on the *toggue,* presiding with benign passivity over tragedy and sorrow.

After several cool hours on the river, we sailed into the waters of the Diaka which were placid. The Diaka is a small river which swings off gently to the left of the Niger in a great arching curve. Its banks are sandy and flat, unlike the tall precipitous walls which confine the Niger. Diafarabe stands up on a cliff-like peninsula between the two rivers. As we sailed past the village, scores of little kids ran down the sandy embankments towards the river edge shouting, *"toubabou, toubabou"* (white man). We went on to the house of the chief which stood on a small hill behind the village. Like so many of the houses of the arrondissement chiefs this one was the usual stereotyped cement box with a verenda in the front and back and a tin roof. A Malian tri-color, green, orange and red, fluttered from an improvised pole, but because the orange had long since faded to white it looked like the Italian flag. The commandant of the cercle of Tenenkou was there, having come down in his long canoe. We tied our canoes to posts and then went up the steep shore.

The chief's veranda was a shocking array of flowing white and red *bou bous,* marabouts in indigo turbans and Peul chiefs in broad straw hats. They were warm and friendly and pleased about our plan to vaccinate the herdsmen as they crossed the river. The chief of the arrondissement, however, was visibly tense and unpleasant which Djigui said was due to his being investigated for corrupt practices by the local committee for the defense of the revolution. Before I had a chance to say very much, the chief blurted out of context that I was not to take any photographs for security reasons. This attempt to visibly and dramatically demonstrate his revolutionary fervor was foiled by the commandant who said I could take all the photographs I desired. And to the painful embarrassment of the chief, he asked that Djigui take a photograph of himself with the chiefs and I.

After much palavering, we got back into the canoes and headed for the far side of the peninsula where all of the nomads were gathered. The program called for an inspection of the herds by the commandant before the elders gave the signal to begin the crossing. Our smaller canoes moved more quickly than the commandant's long boat and we arrived on the far side of the Diaka well ahead of him. When his canoe came into sight, it was a wonder to me that it was still capable of floating. "You know," Djigui exclaimed, "there are about two centimeters between the top of the water and the edge of that canoe." One more passenger and the commandant's canoe would have been at the bottom. We beached our canoes on the wet sand where we found the vaccinators who had come down from Bamako. They were busy talking to some old men about their train and boat trip from Bamako. Until I overheard them talking, I never realized what a big event this trip was in their lives. They said they didn't have to eat the rice they had brought along because the people who ran the boat fed them and even gave them a room to sleep in. They went on to say that there had been a delay in Segou because some white people were coming from

Bamako by road to catch the boat and the boat couldn't leave without them. "The white people are important," one of them added to emphasize the statement. Djigui jumped into the conversation at this point and told them in very direct terms that they were all wrong. "That boat never waits for anyone, white or black!" And Djigui was right.

Finally, the signal was given to cross and amid great fanfare the herds from Djenne were driven into the river. They were accompanied by a flotilla of canoes, swimming herdsmen, some with their tall sheep's skin hats still in place and small boats carrying calves and sheep to the opposite shore. We paddled across the river between hundreds of horned heads bobbing up and down in the water. In many ways, I felt very insignificant and non-essential to this great African festival. It was not that I was unwelcomed, but rather that I saw myself out of place with no definite role to play. For in spite of their confused look, such festivals are well organized events in which everyone knows his part and in which there are no real spectators. In the degal, the young men and the cattle had the stage, charging across the river like an enormous tidal wave of motion and noise, cheered on by regiments of young girls dressed in their finest clothes and jewels.

The alien shadow of government, although non-essential in the Peul's

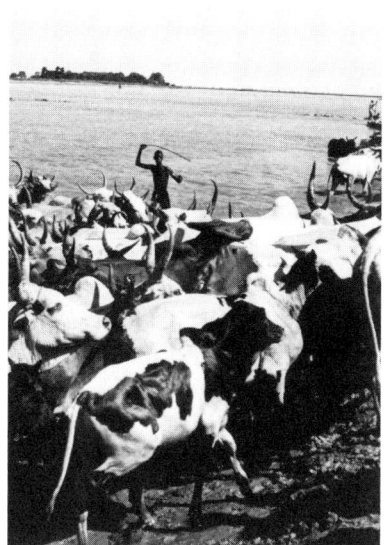

FIGURE 21. Peul cattle emerging from the Diaka River during the *Degal* at Diafarabe.

eyes, had long ago moved into this festival in the hope of exercising its authority and implementing its social and economic reforms. But against the calm self-confident traditionalism of the Peul, it stood like a pallid sapling trying to self-propagate itself through the Sahara. The chief of the arrondissement and the local militia had constructed a wooden stand from which to view the traditional tournaments and contests. The commandant invited me to sit under it, which I did uncomfortably with Djigui and the rest of my staff. The militia kept eyeing us as if we were about to commit some outrageous and threatening act. They were all armed with two foot long pieces of rubber hosing which they later tried to use on the nomads.

The highlight of the celebration was an African version of an American rodeo show in which herdsmen demonstrated their prowess by driving unruly herds of bulls into an arena formed by walls of participants. They drove the herds headlong into the crowd, turning them away at the last possible second to the cheers and applause of the women. The militia had their hands full trying to prevent the herdsmen from driving their herds into the reviewing stand. I felt that the shepherds made a purposeful effort to charge their herds into the reviewing stand, knowing that with a movement of their clubs they could turn the animals around in perfect coordination. There were bareback contests and cattle wrestling tournaments and through it all the women and children never lost their enthusiasm for cheering and clapping. Finally, a bull was ceremoniously killed, his throat being slit, after which the shepherds danced around the body shouting and singing.

The commandant and the other officials gave a series of dull speeches exhorting the nomads to become good socialists, but the Peul could not have cared less about socialism and deadened most of what they said with musket blasts and inattention. I don't think that those who gave the speeches really believed in what they said, but they had to say it. They tried to force their way into the lives of the Peul with threats and intimidation, into that world which consists of deliberate and quiet action, of independence and self-reliance and which makes no accommodation for the outsider. The Peul have an inborn ability to meet threats with politeness and evasion. They see themselves as a separate and independent polity conducting relations with whatever government which happens to be in power in the spirit of an equal.

The Peul nomads at the degal cooperated in being vaccinated. The chiefs and the marabouts led the way, sinewy old men with beards as white as their robes. The women followed them, a gentle queue of striking elegance, in gold and silks. Earlier in the day, I had seen these same women washing clothes in sudsy patches of water at the riverside. But even while doing something as mundane as washing clothes, Peul women maintain their noble elegance. The children and the herdsmen were last, rushing on me with a loud chorus of *toubabou*. It wasn't an insult in any sense, but more of a bantering reminder I was a stranger, not one of them . By the end of the day we had vaccinated thirty thousand nomads and treated hundreds of them for a variety of illnesses. The following day Diafarabe was dramatically quiet, the nomads and their herds having dispersed into the plains in a dozen directions.

Chapter X

The Wind Illness

After many weeks, during which we moved across eight thousand square miles of rolling hills and wooded valleys and vaccinated a quarter of a million people, we came to a fertile strip of country which lies along the banks of the Bani River. It was an enormous expanse of land full of smooth grasslands where the grass was taller than the tops of our trucks, but in other areas the land was planted with millet, corn and checkerboard squares of rice. It was a crossroads of the races where the Dogon, Peul, Bambara, Bobo-Oulé, Marka and Bozo all came together, where herdsmen mixed with farmers and Moslems with animists and in some mysterious and bewildering way got on well together. It was a great and adventurous challenge to come to know all of these diverse peoples, to unravel their view of life and to see the world through their eyes. In doing so you gained a new perspective of things, learned of beings who live in the sky and under the earth and off in the four directions and came to see that what is so clearly obvious to them is not so to you and vice versa. One had to learn where the gods and spirits lived, how they worked and moved in the world, and accept that they played an important role in determining events and setting the direction of men's lives. Although many people were Moslem, no more of the old animist cult had been abandoned than was absolutely necessary and what was compatible with the new from the old remained. In some places the old animist gods had become Moslem genies who lived in rivers and on the tops of hills, in the trunks of great baobab trees and at the bottom of wells. It was God and this great pantheon of spirits and mortal beings who could manipulate their power who caused disease, unleashed epidemics and in the end healed the sick.

It would have been senseless to have tried to put people into concert with our beliefs and with what science held to be the only believable truth. Rather, success lay in presenting what we were offering in terms which they could understand. Vaccines then had to be seen not as antigens which stimulated the production of antibodies which protected against virus-caused diseases, but as talismans and amulets which infused health and protected against the spiritual causes of disease. It shocked many that we should have established our relationship with people on their own terms and in doing so have mocked the solemnity with which scientific truth is usually held. Had we done otherwise I don't think we would have been successful.

Bramane thought himself lucky in being able to set up a temporary headquarters in an old building opposite the jail in the town of San. Personally, I thought the arrangement a painful one since sunrise coincided with the exit of prison work gangs, lunchtime with their re-entry into the prison and sunset with a chorus of their complaints. Bramane, however, was happy with the location and said that it gave him better leverage over the vaccinators and in the course of time he instilled some discipline by threatening to move some of them across the street into the jail. Bramane's threats and the presence of the jail never quite delivered the desired result and we found it necessary to send some of our team members back to Bamako. Although Bramane's expressions of exasperation became chronic he had impressive powers of self-renewal and was able to carry the heavy burden of our vaccinators' antics with admirable patience. Their game was to tire him out until he sunk out of sight and left them a clear field to do as they pleased. They usually had the advantage over him because it was he who visited them in the bush and in doing so suffered the heat, dust and exhaustion. When he eventually found them, rested and refreshed in the shade of a cool mango tree they bombarded him with a final cop de grace of complaints, insults and annoyances until he retreated back into the heat and dust of the trail he had come in on. There was much bias in their own reasoning, but joined as they were by common bonds of discontent, they could not see it. There was no end to the schemes they invented, but when they were caught their excuses were like remembered verses of poetry which we listened to with unimaginative indifference and the conviction that we would never accept them. In spite of this, there was always the paradox that they would throw themselves on our mercy whenever they got into real difficulty and depended on us for their every need.

One would have thought that our constant presence was assurance enough that their fate and well-being weighed heavily on our minds, but such was not the case at all. In the comfort of one another's company, they reached the conclusion that we cared nothing for them and so resolved to make the best of things through their own devices. Their major complaint was that they were being slowly starved to death in spite of the fact that most of them were gaining weight from the generous free meals they were getting in the villages. I was never able to reach an understanding with them on this issue through reason because Malians hold that there is no relationship between a man's weight and the quantity and quality of the food he eats. People who don't worry get fat and those who do worry become thin. The vaccinators held many discussions over my ignorance of this obvious fact of their lives and never came to believe that weight had anything to do with one's food intake. As a result, I never got anywhere with them when I pointed out the scientific inconsistency of their weight gain and their claims of starvation. They saw themselves as the victims of an injustice and decided to take matters into their own hands by eating sumptuous meals in restaurants whenever they came into the town of San to report. There was nothing objectionable about their eating in San's "restaurants," provided they paid for it, but Bramane had to brave the enemy again when the bills for these meals were sent to him. There was no modesty in what they ordered, eggs, coffee and bread with butter for breakfast, steak, potatoes and salad for lunch and three courses along with desert for supper, all of which represented a tremendous change from their Bamako diet of *bouille,* millet cakes and rice. Bramane tried to find a solution to the problem by telling all of the restaurant owners in San that he wouldn't pay any of the vaccinators' bills and by arranging for the teams to eat their meals in San in one restaurant. He paid the owner a certain amount out of the vaccinators' per diem allowance and assured me that everyone was getting three good meals per day. It wasn't long before the vaccinators began complaining about the quality of the food in the restaurant and finally we were forced to go down and have a meal with them in order to validate what they had said. Unfortunately for the vaccinators, the cook carried in a steaming basin of aromatic rice and chicken. There was an uproar of indignation from the vaccinators and shouts of "That isn't what he has been feeding us all along," but the cook maintained that this was one of the average meals he had been serving them. When Bramane and I finally sided with the cook against the vaccinators, it was on the grounds of their increasing weight gain.

Our vaccinators had no sympathy for recalcitrant populations and lacked the patience necessary to explain to frightened people what it was we were offering. This proved to be a serious disadvantage in this part of Mali because many were unfamiliar with vaccination and thought that the jet guns were real revolvers and our intention genocide. Others viewed us as tax collectors or government agents out to confiscate their grain and so it wasn't rare in certain areas for entire villages to flee into the bush as our teams approached or to hide themselves in their grain storage barns. Whenever people fled or hid, our vaccinators packed up and left and came back reporting that they were too stupid to be vaccinated. It was a curious thing that our vaccinators should have thought intelligence a pre-requisite for being vaccinated and Bramane pointed out to them that if such were so then none of them should have ever been vaccinated. As it was, this pattern of friendly disengagement between our vaccinators and the villagers was mutually agreeable to the principles, the one being glad to be left alone and the other delighted to be relieved of work. It seemed to us that a free union between the two was absolutely necessary if we were going to accomplish anything and Bramane thought up many plans to get the population to cooperate. The first of Bramane's plans was one of those creations which you know from the outset is doomed to failure, but which you can nonetheless watch being executed from a detached perspective with relative calm. He decided to provide the chiefs of the teams with old account ledgers borrowed from the SOMIEX grocery warehouse in San. According to Bramane's plan, the ledgers were to be opened in front of those few villagers who had remained behind in the village as decoys as the others fled and it be announced that the names of all the villagers were recorded in the book. The next step called for the team leader to say that all those who didn't come out to be vaccinated would have a check mark put next to their names and be subsequently fined. Bramane might have been able to have squeezed some success out of this plan were it not for the fact that the first few decoys he came up against were *anciens combattants* who made a proclamation of their literacy only after they had read down the lines of the ledger from *alumettes* to *savon*. Bramane had an ample gift for moral indignation and an exceedingly dramatic reaction whenever his ingeniousness went aground. His sympathy was not with people's ignorance of what it was he wanted them to do but with his own damaged pride and so it was natural for his next plan of action to have had a taint of vengeance in it. Fortunately for Bramane, he had a chronic nagging conscience which made him feel uncomfortable whenever he thought out this new plan down to the last detail and so it was only half-heartedly executed.

The teams were to be accompanied by members of the popular militia who through a display of uniforms and unloaded rifles were supposed to induce people to the receiving end of the jet guns. Although some villages honored the militia's presence with attention, in most, they were greeted with the mockery that a deserted village renders to unwanted visitors.

I, myself, thought that the militia had undertaken this exercise not so much as some great enterprise, but as a light hearted diversion from their usual tedious routine. I was never able to follow the logic of their tactics and in most instances they didn't have any strategy for trapping fleeing villagers even in circumstances where it seemed obvious to me what should have been done. Their greatest defeat came in the area of the Dogon cliffs where after scaling mesas and cliffs a thousand feet high they edged up over the top, panting, and dehydrated just in time to see the head of the last villager disappearing down the other side. None of Bramane's plans ever solved the problem and it was only after measles swept through the unvaccinated populations and took its mortality toll of fifty percent and higher that people saw the value of vaccination. It was regrettable that these villages had to pay so high a price in order to sweep away innocent ignorance and we all wished that it could have been otherwise. The spectre of measles unleashing devastation only among those children who had been hidden from the vaccination teams altered traditional ideas centuries old and transformed what seemed like eternal recalcitrance into a model of cooperation and understanding.

While we were working along the banks of the Bani River, a severe outbreak of measles occurred in several villages which had hidden from the vaccination teams. The chief of one of these villages sent a message to us saying that many of the children were dying from *fingnabana*, "wind illness," which we know to be measles, and asked that we come and stop the epidemic with our guns. We already knew that in the village in question, Sossobee, people had been hidden from the vaccination teams two months earlier and that a request for us to come now and with our guns meant that a great change of attitude had occurred. The village was not an easy one to reach at that time of year because it stood on an island in the middle of the flood plains where the water was still five deep and so one had to go in by canoe.

It has never been my good fortune to sail on a river in Mali in either a large or sturdy boat and I always arrive on the shore and with painful certainty know that it will be a leaky canoe, a listing barge

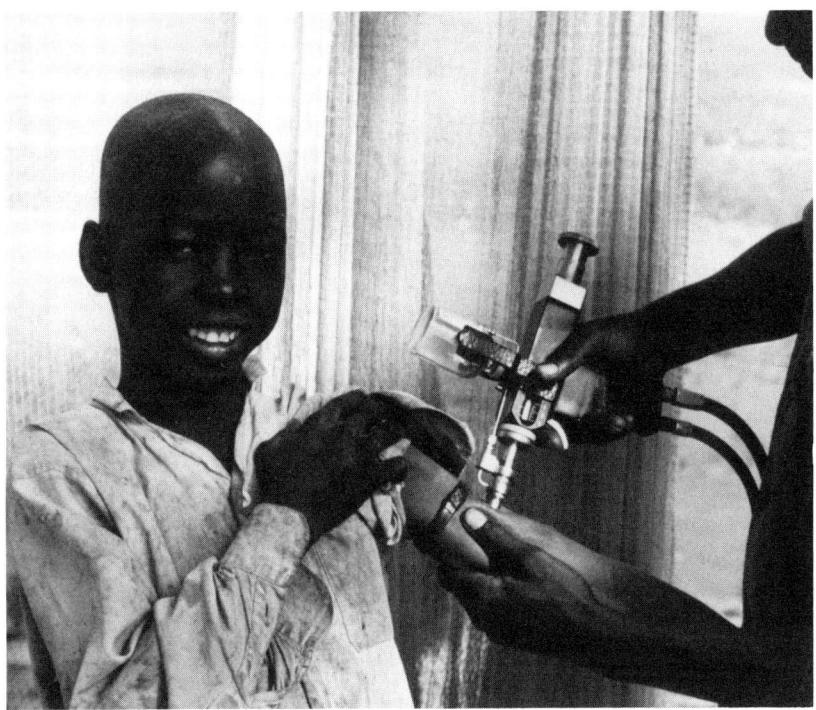

FIGURE 22. A young Bozo boy being vaccinated on the flood plains near San.

and if I am very lucky a motor boat whose motor is always breaking down. I begin these ordeals by saying to myself "No I won't enter that canoe" and finish the day murmuring "Never again, never again." Long hours are spent bailing out water and praying that the obese man or woman in the back won't stand up. Invariably they do, provoking an alarm of protests and screams from everyone else. Most Malian canoes are no match for a river when it is in a disagreeable mood. They take on water, lose their balance and rapidly give up the fight. Those who ride them know nothing of the center of gravity theory and if a canoe capsizes it is attributed to water genies, witches or to God, but never to the person who stood up in it. The Bani and Niger can be friends or foes the same day. They can throw up sand bars, dead end channels and adverse currents if they have a mind to or carry you swiftly and safely on the crest of their rushing backs and deliver you to your destination hours before you are expected. That day the Bani was our foe and we fought it for three hours on its own terms.

It was late in the afternoon when we turned into a quiet narrow channel where only the oars made a pleasant and soothing sound in the quiet water. The mosquitoes were intolerable, flying out in hoards from the walls of moist grass. Sossobee came on us all at once, a cluster of gray mud and straw clinging to a hillock above a sea of brilliant green. It was an island haven, a patch of dry land cut off from the outside world by water and swamp, but custom and by time. Whenever you arrive in a Malian village, you are met by a wave of noisy and happy children, by their lively outpouring of generous curiosity which knows no bounds. The boys come first, in clusters of giggles, whispers and smiles, prankishly testing each other's bravery by pushing one another forward. You hear the soft shuffle of bashful feet and children's whispered conversations coming from behind the trees and fences. But in Sossobee all these sounds of normalcy had been silenced and in their place was an abnormal stillness, a disquieting calm which in this part of Africa meant that some great catastrophe had rushed in on their lives and left behind an enormous disaster. The shadow of suffering and death hung over the place and filled it with an uncomfortable quiet, altered the usual noisy and lively pattern of things and driven people into that remote solitude and isolation which are their refuge when life and well-being are threatened.

We walked up a narrow winding path which cut through the tall grass and led to the cool shadow of a mango tree. There is always much enjoyment in Mali whenever you move out of the hot sun and into the shade and you feel the infusion of a new vitality which renders you capable of doing what you had despaired of out in the sun. Normally, the old men would have been seated beneath the tree, on straw mats, logs and stones, deliberating over the happenings of the past with a pattern and speech accented by the chewing of kola nuts and the brushing of teeth with the wooden sticks of the *gwossay* tree. They would have greeted us with an excited chorus of "Ani oula" and then have moved up the ladder of politeness until they had inquired about the health and welfare of all our relations and friends. There would have been smiles and laughs and exclamations and surprise when I answered in Bambara and then one of them would have dared to say, "Is it possible that this white man speaks Bambara?" and the others would have said, "Of course he does. Didn't you hear him?" They would have launched into excited conversations to test both my knowledge and vocabulary and then when the novelty had worn off gotten involved in the business of my visit. But the shade of Sossobee had been emptied of human sounds, deprived of the joy and the warmth of smiles and laughs and glistening eyes and had become not a desired and pleasant relief from the sun, but an uncomfortable chilly place. We stood underneath the tree for what seemed like a very long time until one very forlorn old man came out from behind a mud wall and stood before us, sullen and motionless as if he had lost the power of speech. Under the circumstances, his manner was appropriate for this was not the time for the usual effusive and lengthy joyful greetings delivered when men met. We of the developed world meet grief by expressing our distress. We console the sorrowing with words and gestures, with letters and telephone calls and try to divert their attention from what they have lost to what is still there. The Bambara's reaction to sorrow and disaster is not as ours guided and governed by convention and formality, but is rather instinctual and natural, an affair of emotion and not of procedure and so they fall into silence and retreat away from social interaction into the comfort of solitude.

When the men of the village finally came out into the square they had the appearance of a senate of Venetian doges in turbans, mufflers and flowing robes, presiding over some grave affair of state. The women came behind them as a gentle queue of submissive suffering and the fact that very few of them had children on their backs in itself announced that something terrible had happened. Under normal circumstances the initiative for launching a conversation would have been theirs but now it fell to us to begin by saying why we had come, that we knew about the measles epidemic and all the children who had died. The chief who sat next to me on a straw mat said that one hundred and twenty eight children had died in a month's time, almost half of those who had contracted measles. The epidemic began several weeks after a small girl from a neighboring village arrived in Sossobee with measles, but the chief and the elders did not draw any connection between the first case and the subsequent epidemic. For them the epidemic was a manifestation of God's will, the result of an evil wind which had blown in from the swamps and plains of the delta and penetrated the skins of their children. It wasn't long before scores of children were ill with coughs, running eyes and fever and shortly thereafter rashes came out. The people of Sossobee like all the Bambara attempted to bring out the rash as quickly as possible in their children because they have over the years made the empirical observation that once the rash appears the prodromal symptoms disappear. The children were given honey by mouth and had their skins rubbed with honey, monkey feces and dirt from termite hills so that the rash would come out. Because of the tremendous concern for the rash to appear, children were not washed with water and were kept in the dark interior of their huts until the illness was over. The children were given purges of tamarind juice in order to drive the illness out of the interior of the body and into the skin.

Although the sick children were dehydrated from their high fevers and from being kept in the hot unventilated huts, their parents refused to give them anything to drink for fear of impeding the development of the rash. They diminished their food intake, prohibited them from eating meat and put honey, goat's milk, tamarind juice and peanut flour solution in their eyes in the hope of preventing blinding corneal ulcers. Parents abstained from sexual relations because they believed that it worsens measles in their children. The people of Sossobee firmly believed that all of the practices and treaments they employed were for the benefit of their sick children and could not understand that sick children with high fevers needed protein and fluids, that serious eye infections with permanent damage resulted from the ophthalmic preparations they used, that purges were nefarious and solutions rubbed on the skin the cause of serious dermatitis. What was undertaken with the finest of intentions was in reality a major cause of the high morbidity and mortality associated with the epidemic.

The old men were surprisingly forward in admitting that they had observed that those children who had been vaccinated did not contract the wind illness and it was for this reason that they had asked us to come. I knew it would create a great stir the moment I asked why the children had not been vaccinated and when I put the question to them there was a short pause, a silent but meaningful communication between eyes. The chief was not entirely without self-consciousness when he finally spoke and said that all of the unvaccinated children had been away traveling when the vaccination team visited Sossobee. I didn't reply right away, but let silence tell him my thoughts, that what he had said was not believed. When I finally spoke he received my words with impressive dignity. I said they were all good and holy Moslems anxious to please God, men of truth who viewed lies as a defilement of their souls. I then asked the chief to repeat what he had said because I had not fully understood it since my knowledge of Bambara was limited.

No one looked ashamed when the truth finally came out because the lie had not been heard.

They had heard for several months that there were large white trucks going from village to village with guns which put some kind of medicine into people's skin. They didn't think this could be true because in their view guns had only one purpose — to kill. After much discussion among themselves, they came to the conclusion that the guns were instruments of genocide, the medicine a slow acting poison which eventually killed because it was a *koroti*. A koroti is a particle of millet, a piece of wood or drop of liquid which an enemy injects into the skin of his victim with the intent of doing harm or causing death. A koroti can travel long distances, over land and water and through the air and enter the victim's skin when he least expects it. Modibo and Ahmadou were firm believers in koroti and took pains to protect themselves from them even though I often proclaimed my disbelief in them. They would spend as much as a week's wage for talismans to make their skins impenetrable to koroti which in itself testified to the seriousness of their belief.

Many of the old men in Sossobee had been convinced that the koroti coming out of our jet guns were capable of traveling from Mopti and San and entering their skins. Some of them had gone to distant villages to witness the vaccinations and reported that they had seen the guns being fired up into the air in the direction of other villages. This interpretation of our vaccinators cleaning their guns with distilled water drove them to implement every available measure to protect themselves from what was so obvious, our shooting of koroti up into the air. Talismans were hung in the trees and bushes around the village to intercept the koroti as they fell from the air, heads of families went to the marabouts to buy koranic charms and sacrifices of chicken blood were made to the old fetish statues which the men still guarded in a sacred grove on the edge of the village. The final eventuality was the arrival of the team in the village and they rehearsed for weeks in advance what they would do when that day arrived. The women and children were to be hidden in the grain barns along with some of the men and the rest of the male population was to take up positions of defense in the interior of the village. Bramane, trying to be funny, interjected that the operation in Sossobee had started off with anti-aircraft activity and ended with everyone taking shelter in bunkers.

Early one afternoon, word reached Sossobee with some Bozo fishermen that a vaccination team was coming up the river with their jet guns. Wild pandemonium broke out; the women and children were rushed up into the grain barns and the men prepared their muskets. Down on the river the vaccination team was sitting on the bottom of a leaky canoe fighting the heat, the mosquitoes and a swollen current. Things had gotten off to a bad start that day because they had been charged by a hippo within the first half hour they were on the river. Progress up the river was slow because of the current and the oarsmen's preoccupation with recounting gory tales of how their friends and relatives had been charged by hippos, their canoes smashed and they themselves dragged down to the bottom. When the vaccinators tried to find solace by eliciting assurances that there would be no more hippos in their future they were told that the river was teeming with them. Had they known at the time that as they approached Sossobee a dozen Bambara muskets were pointed in their direction they would have turned around in an instant and braved all the hippos in the Bani. The vaccinators deliberated over their self-defense and decided that their only weapon against the hippos was a transistor radio which they began playing, the thought being that the noise would frighten the hippos off. By the time their canoe slid ashore at Sossobee with the transistor radio blaring in the center, the population was well concealed and the defenders at their command posts. No one greeted them on the river bank and with much disgust they carried their equipment up to the village square. As the vaccinators sat down beneath the mango tree, close to seven hundred frightened souls were hiding in the grain barns, convinced that their very lives were hanging in the balance. Several men came out to talk to the team and in a premeditated and non-cooperative manner told them that the villagers had gone off to attend a market upstream. The team leader was a battle-scarred veteran of such tactics and said with unhurried firmness that the team would simply wait for them to come back. Unfortunately for the vaccination team, they had no food with them. When the sun began to set that evening they were not offered anything to eat and were told there was plenty of water to drink in the muddy river. From the outset, the men of Sossobee had the upper hand and by early evening they had forced the team into the decision of leaving and spending the night on the opposite bank. There was a rejoicing as the small canoe disappeared into the dark shadows of the river and the grain barns were opened to let out the women and children who had been locked up in them for over five hours. They had no way of knowing that in a cold box in that canoe lay their only hope against a disaster which loomed ahead in their future and that they would be shortly asking the vaccination team to return with their jet guns.

The Bambara of Sossobee were good hearted people who understood things well on their terms, as part of their world. We were invaders in their lives and it was very natural for them to have thought of us in terms of themselves, of what we were giving in terms of what they knew. Had they known that what we had would benefit them they would have been eager to cooperate and accept. As it was, they didn't see things this way until a measles epidemic showed them what they had not known. Ideas changed, attitudes were reversed, but there was no admission of error or remorse, for what had been done was the product of firm conviction and a desire to preserve the common good. When measles came to Sossobee it struck fear into the heart of every mother because it is known to be an indiscriminate killer which passes through villages and kills most of the children below four years of age. It leaves some of its survivors premanently blind and malnourished and others mentally retarded. It usually comes in March and April when the dry season is at its peak, when the sun rolls high up and bakes the earth dry and changes the grass into ugly tufts of brown straw. It comes when the rushing brooks have turned into stagnant wallows, when stiffling dust fill the air and the lungs which breathe it, when the grain barns are low, when the heat has driven all of the strength and resistance out of the human body. It strikes when man and nature are at their lowest ebb. And then when the rains come in June and the air clears up and becomes cool, the millet stalks shoot up out of the soggy ground, rivers swell, the grain barns fill up, grass turns a velvety green and measles disappears, like a phantom out of Islamic mythology. Some say that it hides on the top of the Manding Hills, at the bottom of the Niger River with the water genies, in the heart of the monkey bread tree. They see it lurking on sand dunes and at the bottom of wells, in the swirling dust of a whirlwind, in fetish houses and in the branches of sacred trees. The Moslems say it comes from God, but the animists aren't always sure.

There was a time when no mother in this part of Africa counted on her children surviving to adulthood until they had had measles and over the years they made up proverbs to underscore this belief. The Dogon say, "If your child has not yet had measles you do not have a child," and the Peul say, "Never be proud of the beauty of your children until they have had measles." The old women maintain that measles comes with the Harmattan, that dry wind which blows heat and dust off the Sahara from January to June, blanketing most of West Africa with a sand fog. Although old women know nothing about the germ theory of diease, it may be that measles is transmitted more efficiently when there is a lot of dust in the air. Old Malian women are not epidemiologists, but they know that measles does not come to the same village every year, but that it runs cycles of two to three years. When measles came to Sossobee it was at a time of year when it was not expected and so people were taken by surprise. In recent years, we have learned in sophisticated epidemiological terms what the old women have known for centuries about measles. Measles epidemics occur at the peak of the dry season primarily because children are in closer contact with one another and transmission is rendered easier. When the rains begin, children are sent off into their family fields where they live in temporary houses and have little or no contact with other children. When a measles epidemic strikes ,it usually touches every child and the survivors are permanently immunized. It requires from two to three years for enough children to be born into this population to support another epidemic.

We visited all of the houses where the surviving children were being kept and found them in the final stages of disease. Almost none of the children in the village had escaped the disease and so it was futile to vaccinate. Rather we spent our time taking care of the sick, treating their complications and giving instructions to the mothers for improving the children's diets. Some of the children had developed corneal cataracts as a result of measles. These opaque white scars covered the pupils of their eyes and made them blind for life. Their mothers believed that we could dissolve the scars with medicines. But when I told them that we could do nothing for them, they accepted it with fatalistic resignation and said that it was God's will that their children were blind. The people of Sossobee were very grateful for everything we did for the children and demonstrated their appreciation with gifts of chickens, calabashes of milk and bunches of mangoes. I saw in these gestures of thanks more than just appreciation. I saw that the people of this village had come to see things on our terms and that an important break with the traditions of the past had occurred.

Chapter XI
Land of the Cliff Dwellers

It was an interesting drive to Bandiagara in the center of the Dogon country, the red laterite road twisting and turning around great uplifts of gray boulders and jagged mesas, giving us a splendid view of the ever fading flood plains which lay behind around Mopti. During the previous weeks, we had spent a good deal of time in canoes, gliding through lakes of weeds and lotuses, crocodiles and egrets in order to vaccinate the Bozo fishermen who live on the southern periphery of the flood plains. Their misty green world grew dimmer as we climbed up higher into the dry hot escarpment. There is nothing very inviting about the landscape of the Bandiagara Plateau. It is a harsh and rocky country scarred by great ravines and deep gorges, redeemed in the name of comfort only by clusters of shady acacia trees and courts of baobab monarchs. Soil is scarce in this sea of rocks and the Dogon who live here cultivate their crops of millet and onions on table cloth sized patches of ground around the stream beds. The soil which is brought from great distances is carefully laid out a foot deep on the surface of the hot black rocks and held in place by a low wall of gravel and more rocks. Crops are planted, grown and harvested in this artificially created farm land which has to be watered from the nearby streams several times a day for anything to survive. There is no other agricultural group in Mali which expends so much physical effort and tenacity in farming as do the Dogon.

The plateau is an arid ecology which is gradually becoming drier for reasons which are not fully understood, except by the Dogon who say that it is due to the displeasure of the ancestors. Over the forty years since the French began measuring rainfall on the plateau, the amount of rain has decreased by fifty percent. The Yame River, the largest on the plateau, once flowed the year round. But now it is a vast bed of sand for most of the year reflecting the hot glare of the sun from the bottom of a deep canyon. Only the rib-like markings on the sand speak for water which passed before. Around its banks are clusters of hot gray-green thornbush where goats nibble on the tiny leaves. The crocodiles which once lived in the river, long ago migrated to the Bani into which the Yame flows. The Dogon honor the crocodile as a sacred animal for according to a legend, Nangabounou, the founder of the town of Bandiagara was led to the Yame by a crocodile.

There are two hundred and fifty thousand Dogon living in an area of fifteen thousand square miles. Until rather recently, the majority lived on the plateau and in villages along the edge of the massive Bandiagara Cliff. Their villages were built as fortresses, high up out of sight on top of the mesas or in the face of the cliff which is fifteen hundred feet tall and a hundred and fifty miles long. They were a society which lived on a constant war footing, struggling for survival against the harsh elements of the environment and competing among themselves for the meager resources of the land. Although the Dogon fought many battles with the Moslem Peul and their other enemies, more often than not they fought among themselves, village against village, clan against clan. These were not massive pitched battles, but rather small chronic internecine struggles, fought over land and water, between which reigned an uneasy calm. For untold generations, life was a predictable procession of births and deaths, drought and famine, rituals and sacrifices and the never-ending struggle against the Peul and other Dogon villages. Then the Europeans came.

In 1893, the French general, Archinard, marched on Bandiagara on his way down the Niger valley and then across the plateau to the edge of the cliff at Sanga where the *hogon* (the spiritual and temporal chief) capitulated after three days of fighting. The Bandiagara Plateau was claimed for France and the Dogons' impregnable tower of solitude opened to the outside world. Then in 1905, Lieutenant Louis Desplagnes led an archeological and ethnographic expedition into the plateau and cliff, conducting the first detailed study of the Dogon which was later published in his book, *Le Plateau Central Nigerien,* now almost forgotten as is the author himself. But it took many years to pacify the country, until 1920 in fact, when the last battle took place between the village of Tabi and the French Colonel Mangeot. It required eight days of fighting before the village capitulated.

Gradually, and in degrees, the outside world drifted across the hot gray rocks into the lives of the Dogon. Administrators came with the apparatus of modern government, schools were opened and mission stations established, bringing the Dogon into contact for the first time with new European values and goals. They slowly came down from their rocky citadels, traveled to Mopti and Bamako and entered the cash economy and tasted modern city life. It was as if some great cloisture had been opened and all allowed to come and go as they pleased. Some chose to remain with the traditions and the security of the past and thus the process of change is never the same in either degree or kind in every village. It is least evident in the more isolated villages situated on the edge of the cliff. But slowly people are leaving their mountain top fortresses and building new villages out on the open plains below the cliffs or at the bases of the rocky mesas. The Dogon animist religion, perhaps the most complex in this part of Africa, stood for centuries as a placid island, unchallenged and undisturbed on top of a roof of the world, surrounded by a turbulent sea of Islam. But today Islam and Christianity are gently replacing animism, pushing all of the gods and ancestors further back into the historical past.

In 1930, an American missionary, The Reverend Francis J. McKinney and his wife Laura traveled on horseback across the sea of frozen lava flows to Sanga where they set up a mission station in a mud house with a thatched roof. During the forty-two years they were to remain at Sanga, they saw it transformed from a remote administrative outpost to a thriving and picturesque village with a church and a mosque, schools and a dispensary and a tourist rest house catering to the two thousand tourists who come each year to see the Dogon, their masked dances and the cliffs. But it wasn't this sort of village when they first arrived. They studied the Dogon language of which there are twelve dialects and Mrs. McKinney translated the Bible into Dogon. They traveled on foot over the rocky plateau and on horseback across the plains, established outstations and gave the Dogon a modern medical dispensary. When they retired in 1972, they left the Sanga mission in the hands of their eldest son John who was born in Mopti and raised by the Dogon.

A year after the McKinneys' arrival in Sanga, a French anthropologist from the Sorbonne in Paris, Marcel Griaule, led an ethnographic expedition across Africa from Dakar to Djibouti. In the course of this journey, he was taken to Sanga where he was to declare that he had never seen a people in Africa so remarkable as the Dogon. It is difficult to put into words what Griaule felt, but virtually all who have ever traveled through the Dogon country have come away with the same reaction. One is awed and amazed by the landscape, overwhelmed by the massive purple and pink sandstone cliffs which stand taller than the new trade towers in New York City. The villages are an architectural conformity of soaring cylindrical granaries and rectangular mud houses, built up against the base of the cliff or tottering on its edge. A thousand feet up in the face of the cliff are grottoes in which the Dogon bury their dead, hoisting the bodies up by ropes. In other areas, there are large caves in the face of the cliff, five hundred feet above the ground in which the ruins of small villages stand, built the Dogon say by a race of pygmies called the *Tellem* who inhabited the country centuries ago. Who were the *Tellem* and where did they go. Did they really build the miniature villages in the caves high up in the cliffs, caves which even the Dogon have never been able to get up into. And if they did, how did they ever ascend the sheer vertical wall of stone to get to their villages. There are still no final answers to these questions.

It was not simply the topography which impressed Griaule, but more the culture it had preserved. For twenty-five years he and his colleagues intermittently studied most aspects of Dogon life, from their complex cosmological concepts and religious beliefs to their fantastic masks and sculpture. They published an enormous corpus of ethnographical data. To some, these studies do not appear wholly convincing because they are the result of intensive and prolonged research carried out in the small area of Sanga using a limited number of selected intelligent informants. Pervading the results, so the criticism goes, is a deterministic European logic and a discernible theoretical framework which over the years may have been absorbed by their informants, quite unconsciously and unknown to the investigators.

The Dogon medical assistants who were to work with us in Bandiagara often remarked, "The Dogon told Griaule what they thought he wanted to hear." I personally do not believe that the Griaule expeditions fell victim to the calamity this summary judgement implies. But Yambo Ouloguem, Mali's most celebrated writer and himself a Dogon of the family of paramount chiefs of Bandiagara, upholds this view in his famous book, *Bound to Violence*. I always thought myself that it was as one old Dogon chief told me . "In every dish," he said, "there is the food and there is the sauce. They were given dishes with more than the usual share of sauce."

When Professor Griaule died in 1956, the Dogon held a *Dama* ceremony in his honor. This is a traditional death anniversary ceremony in which the mask society, the *Awa,* dances for several days with some or all of the seventy eight masks the Dogon possess. The purpose of the *Dama* is to transfer the soul of the decreased to the world of the ancestors. This event was much publicized at the time, described as the worshipful last gesture of a grateful African people toward a European god. But the Dogon who were there will now tell you that the idea was not theirs but one developed by the French administration and presented to them as something they had to do. As a result of a variety of intended and unintended circumstances, Professor Griaule and his colleagues enjoyed an academic monopoly of the Dogon for many decades. Consequently, their studies have never been corroborated by outside anthropologists. The chances for such corroboration being per-

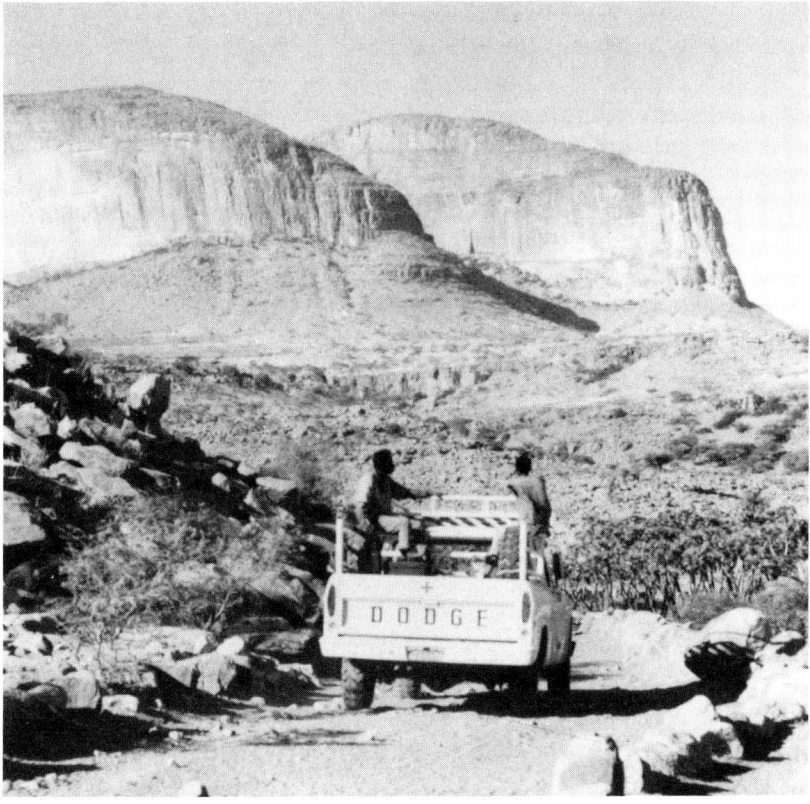

FIGURE 23. Dr. Imperato's truck making its way through the mountains of Hombori. In the background are the peaks of Hombori Tondo.

formed become less with each passing year as Dogon traditional beliefs are dying with the passing older generations. It is certain then that the studies of Marcel Griaule and his colleagues will be much discussed and debated in the years to come.

We discussed the Dogon in a lively manner as we rode over the corrugated road at the head of our convoy of eight trucks. Bramane's attitude was one of discernible antipathy, perhaps because he was an intellectual and a Moslem; Modibo was neutral and Djigui distinctly sympathetic, they having an appeal to those inner remnants of animism still present in his heart. We had anticipated many problems in working on the cliffs and I personally felt less up to the challenge since only a few weeks before I had returned from a military hospital in Germany where I had been hospitalized with infectious hepatitis. I was still not fully recovered and certainly never suspected that very shortly I would be going back into a hospital again with an even more serious illness.

Most of the Dogon country lies in the modern administrative cercles of Bandiagara and Douentza which have a combined population of 300,000 distributed in twelve arrondissements and 483 villages. We had already been to Bandiagara and Douentza to prepare the campaign with the commandants and the arrondissement chiefs. Large sections of several arrondissements were inaccessible by truck and the vaccinators would have to go in on foot. Bramane and I had made arrangements for local Dogon guides to take them along the cliffs and down into the valleys. In addition, we assigned infirmiers of the Grandes Endemies sector at Bandiagara to each of the teams. All of them were Dogon with many years of itinerant medical experience in this region. They were in a sense the barefoot doctors of Mali. The medecin-chef of Bandiagara, Mabo Kassambara, was a Dogon from the remote mountainous arrondissement of Kendie. His home village of Borko lay hidden deep in the back of a cavernous valley below a two thousand foot high escarpment next to permanent springs which made the valley a garden the year round. Mabo was an extremely bright infirmier who had received a year's training in East Germany. He was a very influential person not only in his arrondissement but throughout the plateau and had a seemingly unlimited number of friends wherever he went. People came to him not only to seek his medical assistance but also his advice and opinions which they valued greatly. He had traveled into every nook and cranny on the Bandiagara Plateau as chief medical officer of the region except one remote zone not far from his home village where it is said that there is a human form mumified into stone in a cave. Mabo and I often planned to visit this region and the cave where the mummy supposedly rests but these plans never materialized. His knowledge of Dogon history and customs was encyclopedic and what he did not know someone he knew surely did. He traveled regularly with Djigui and I, and had someone taped our conversations over the churning of the wheels of the truck, the playback would have sounded like an ethnographic conference. I often remarked that our trips together were traveling seminars on Dogon culture woven in while riding in the truck and after the day's work had been done.

Our headquarters in Bandiagara was at the modest dispensary where on the night of our arrival a cobra slithered up out of the sink drain and almost bit a curious vaccinator who was bending down to look at whatever might be inside. The vaccinators and drivers saw this as a bad omen and it demoralized them considerably. As it was, most of them were unhappy about working with the Dogon because they had heard all sorts of erroneous tales about human sacrifices and cannibalism and feared they would end up in some communal pot. Bramane was less than successful in reassuring them because he himself wasn't all that sure that the stories were untrue. Supporting their fear was the fact that the Dogon were beginning to celebrate the Sigui Festival that year. This festival is held very sixty years and lasts for five years, successively moving down the cliff through all of the important villages. The Sigui marks the replacement of the ruling elders by the next generation and provides for the transfer of all sacred and secret religious knowledge from the retiring elders to their younger successors. During the ceremonies, the incoming group learns the secret language of the Sigui through which this knowledge is communicated and through which the Dogon speak with the ancestors. The Dogon replace all of their masks at the time of the Sigui and carve a Great Mask measuring some fifty feet long which is used for the next sixty years during funeral ceremonies.

The vaccination teams were convinced that so important a ceremony couldn't take place without humans being sacrificed. It was only after we had seen some of the rituals of the Sigui that their fears of being sacrificed were dispelled. Now we were all anxious to see the Sigui and so while Jay and Modibo went up to Douentza, Djigui, Mabo, Bramane and I drove across the plateau in a truck with a very inexperienced driver by the name of Mamadou. We arrived in Sanga just as some of the commercial masked dances were being performed for a group of Russian and Czechoslovakian newsmen. The Malian Tourist Office landover was also there with a handful of stout hearted tourists, including a strange bearded boy from Brooklyn who later told me he had come to Africa "to study the primitive tribtes." Whenever Modibo passed this landrover on the roads in Bandiagara it was always with great trepidation because the brakes didn't work, it had only one headlight and no spare tires, not to mention the deficiencies of the driver which were many and varied.

The masked dances in Sanga had by that time become available for hire to visting tourists who paid the equivalent of fifty cents a dancer for a twenty minute session. In later years, the price rose considerably as the area was opened to increasing numbers of tourists. Organizing these dances and serving as the chief guide in Sanga was a remarkable man by the name of Ogobara Dolo. In the days before independence, Ogobra had been appointed the paramount chief of the Sanga district by the French, a powerful position of great prestige in the Dogon country. But in the traditional scheme of things, Ogobara's power was quite limited. Although a practicing Moslem, he retained, I think, some of the mystical traditions of his forefathers in ways which were not so easily discerned. Recent years had seen him take on the job of chief guide for tourists in Sanga for the Malian Tourist Office. It was his responsibility to provide the guides who took tourists on one of two walks, Le Grand Tour and Le Petit Tour, and for certain people he himself would lead the party down and up the cliffs. All of this brought Ogobara into contact with many types of people from all over the world thereby making of him a shrewd judge of character. Visitors were always trying to seduce him into selling ancestral statuary and masks or into leading them to some dark hidden corner where they might buy them from someone else. The Malian government considers this art its national patrimony and consequently has forbidden its being taken out of the country. Others came probing with an obsessive mania for finding a metaphysical meaning to everything from the way the Dogon sat on a worn out log to the way they ate. To soften these assaults, Ogobara was always benign and vague rather than personal and intense in his feelings towards visitors. He dealt with them I thought in an extremely practical way, giving as little as possible while obtaining the most from the relationship.

Our relationship with Ogobara was on completely different terms and over the years we worked with him we found him to be a kind and sincere man, keenly conscious of his historical past, fiercely partisan to his own people and willing to move all in order to help them. By the time I had gotten to know him, he had already traveled all over the world with the masked dancers, to Paris and New York and even to Alaska. But in spite of these frequent and long associations with the outside world he never lost his inner spirituality and those fine and recognizable subtleties of his race. Although a man of great property he led an austere life devoid of pretense and nascent arrogance. He rarely spoke of his foreign travels and then mostly when asked and always in a way which was arid of great display.

Ogobara confided to Mabo that although the Sigui Festival had been officially scheduled to being the next day in the village of Youga, the foxy old elders had actually started the ceremonies two days before. The ceremony had been launched on time according to the Dogons' calculations of stellar and lunar movements. But they had purposely given the government officials an inaccurate date in order to avoid the foreseen invasion of outsiders from Bamako and Europe. The Malian Tourist Office was scarcely capable of handling any great influx of visitors to the cliffs because they lacked accommodations, transport facilities, personnel, and had an extremely weak administrative and organizational structure. Ignoring all of these inadequacies, they launched a massive publicity campaign about the Sigui Festival, passing out mimeo-

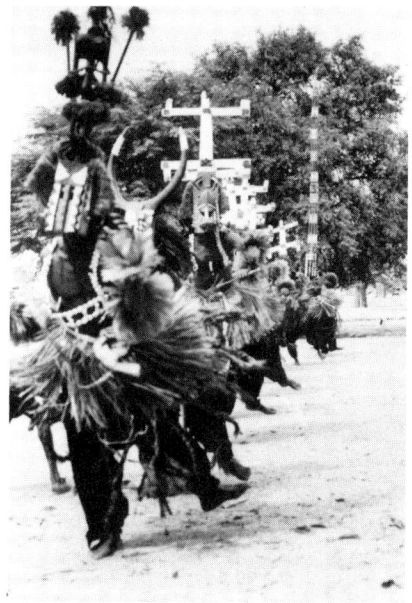

FIGURE 24. Masked dancers of the Dogon *Awa Society* performing at Sanga.

graphed sheets all over Bamako and abroad. Foreigners living in Mali were fully aware of the shortcomings of the tourist office and among them the response was predictably bland. Those of them who did go to the cliffs went in with their own vehicles and life supports. But people living abroad were easily seduced and came out on an expensive tour package, interpreting such items as accommodations to mean a room with a bed, not a veranda floor with a mat. While some of them may have disbelieved what Griaule had written, they certainly could not ignore it. He had given birth to a tempting legend, stirred up men's imaginations and by doing so beckoned them to discover it all for themselves. In his own way, Griaule had brought the long Dogon sleep to an end and prepared the way for the great disruption.

The tourist office's program was a hastily-conceived project spawned on the belief that the Dogon would do as the government wished. It was clear now that they would not and this was the message which Ogobara was asked to convey to the twenty people who had come from Europe for the festival. The tourist office had also presented the festival as a singularly impressive dramatic event which in fact it was not and disappointment was bound to be the result among those who came with this soporific view. Under the circumstances, the guilty officials chose the easiest way out. They remained obscure under the falcon eye of the anticipating crowd. It fell to Ogobara to tell the visitors the news and certainly he reasoned that their reaction would be violent which it was. In a few short well-worded sentences, the delusion was smashed and forebearance and patience disappeared, unleashing a repressed verbal tidal wave of criticisms about incompetency, treachery and misrepresentation. Matters went from bad to worse after that as the ranks of the disgruntled were swelled by a dozen West Germans and twenty Russians from Bamako. Eighty people were crowded in and around the campement which had four rooms, one toilet, two refrigerators and an obliging but nervous French manager by the name of Monsieur Molinari. The eighty welded themselves around a common cause which was their determination to see the Sigui, Germans, East and West, Russians, Frenchmen, Britons, Swiss, Americans and a Brazilian who practiced yoga.

Sundown and the relaxing cool air and Monsieur Molinari's house mother conversation and good meal didn't bring any solace to the visitors who then decided they would go to Youga themselves to see the festival without the tourist office staff. The imbroglio became worse when the gendarmes came and the governor of Mopti and a host of officials from Bamako. They decided that no one was to go to Youga, fearing that the presence of the tourists would generate a terrible fracas. But Ogobara was a schooled diplomat and eventually his persuasive advice overruled the governor's imprudent high handedness and so the following morning before sunrise the army of ethnographic pilgrims, tourists, newsmen and officials set off across the cliff for Youga with Ogobara in the lead. We were among them.

Somewhere on the ten mile trail they overtook Madame Germaine Dieterlen, Professor Griaule's chief collaborator, who had spent the night several miles from Sanga. With her was Jean Rouch, a well known ethnographer and cameraman and his crew as well as interpreters and servants. The effect of her presence on the trail to Youga was therapeutic for the crowd's morale because they reasoned that if she were going to Youga then something must be taking place. Madame Dieterlen, a serious scholar, was scarcely overjoyed by this massive invasion into a once in a lifetime ethnographic event. The two groups observed one another at close range for a few moments, the one boisterous and excited, treating Madame Dieterlen herself as an object of curiosity, the other reserved and polite and much relieved when Ogobara moved his charges on.

The already irate people of Youga were not very willing hosts and tried to confine the crowd by declaring most of the village off limits for religious reasons. Such a declaration had absolutely no effect and tourists pounced headlong into every nook and cranny of the village trying to ferret out the material fragments of metaphysical thought and religious symbolism everywhere they turned. It was like a pack of hungry children being let loose in a candy factory. The Dogon were quite unprepared for this shock wave of curious visitors and had no prepared defense. The women shrieked, the children wailed and the men made threats in baratone voices, but eventually all of the villagers retreated behind closed doors. An uneasy silence reigned and only the high wind blew its howl across the boulders.

The gendarmes rounded the tourists up and got them all back to a central location, except for a few newsmen who managed to hide behind some boulders. Ogobara knew that the crowd was clamoring for an ethnographic circus and would settle for nothing less. He and the elders came to an agreement. The villagers would perform some of the ceremonies of the Sigui on the provision that no photographs be taken. Everyone agreed to this, except the newsmen who were safely perched out of sight. But at the first sight of the dancers dressed in their white bonnets, trotting forward in single file, shutters clicked from the waistlines while contented faces look straight ahead as if their fingers had done nothing. Ogobara neither liked nor approved this tactic and sounded a warning but it fell on ears deadened by awe and excitement and a self-generated sense of responsibility. It was their duty to preserve this for posterity, or so they said. Posterity was of no concern to the dancers; a bargain was a bargain and it had been broken so they withdrew in anger. Then the governor ordered everyone's film confiscated on the spot, an act which didn't have the intended effect of endearing him to the Dogon because they too thought it summary and severe. The group met this tyranny with ingenuity and gave the gendarmes rolls of unexposed film, but lamented the seizure just the same for whatever dramatic effect it was worth. Madame Dieterlen had her exposed film confiscated but it was later returned in Bamako through the intercession of the French Ambassador.

By early afternoon, the heat had driven whatever enthusiasm remained out of the army of zealots and like a great carpet being rolled up they retreated to Sanga. There morale rose to a new height when an old Dogon died and a massive funeral ceremony got underway.

When I left Sanga a few days later I thought to myself that this was probably the last Sigui Festival and perhaps the most unique one because of what happened. We drove back to Bandiagara over an extremely difficult track and hadn't traveled for more than an hour when the truck came to a stuttering halt and bellows of black smoke rose up from beneath the hood. On looking we found a hole in the radiator large enough to accommodate several fingers. It was then that Mamadou announced with pride that he had already discovered the hole in Sanga and had plugged it up with mud and soap while we were in Youga! Mamadou's inventive response to necessity was admirable, but that didn't stop me from giving him hell until I had physically exhausted myself. Some returning German tourists took us into Bandiagara and two days later Modibo went up to install a new radiator. When the truck was repaired, Mamadou set off again, but five miles down the road ran into a cow, overturned the truck and demolished it in a ravine. The announcement of this disaster was made by Mamadou himself, remarkably safe and sound without as much as a scratch. He came into my room and in almost poetic language said, "An act of God has occurred," to which my initial reaction was, "He's drunk!" Then he told me that God had put a cow on the track in his way and forced him to drive into it. I didn't refute what he said but I did fill out the insurance report myself since acts of God were not covered.

In modern times there had never been a campaign in the Dogon country like the one we launched. It was an enormous and fearsome undertaking; for the country had never been systematically combed from village to village and the savage nature of the terrain alone was enough to promise failure. There were all sorts of dangers for the men and ourselves; we were again exposed to river blindness along the banks of the Yame and to guinea worms in the village wells; puff adders and cobras got into the blankets, they abounded on the plateau and at night the roar of lions shattered our sleep.

Djigui was exquisitely sensitive to lions because he came from an area of Mali where there are still large numbers of them which terrify villages in the bush. It was always his custom to ask about lions wherever we camped for the night, in a discreet way which didn't betray his cowardice in the affair. During one of these routine inquiries, the chief of a village said, "There are no lions here."

"No lions?" exclaimed Djigui. "Impossible!"

The chief grew somewhat irritated at his word being doubted and said abruptly, "I guarantee that you can sleep on the outskirts of this village every night of the year and never see or hear a lion." Djigui nodded his head in amazement. "But," the chief added, "you had better be careful because there are a lot of lionesses," and with that he marched off leaving Djigui open-mouthed.

We had of course wisely decided that if we were to go into this venture and be successful everything would have to be planned and executed with impeccable thoroughness. Communications and logistical support were the principal problems for there were no bridges, roads nor decent tracks. We went about organizing the campaign in the most sensible way we could think of based on the intelligence we had gathered from many sources and the first hand experience of Mabo and his infirmiers. Four sub-headquarters were established in the arrondissements where the freezers, vaccines and supplies were kept, hauled in through backbreaking work with donkeys and porters. The central headquarters maintained communication with Lastouillas in Bamako and stayed in close contact with the four sub-headquarters. I did not keep this headquarters stationary, but moved it geographically so that it was always in the center of activity. In some ways the logistical problems were less as we moved towards the cliff since the trucks could not be used. A distance of ten miles per day had been set as the maximum for the vaccinators to walk. While this is far less than what most Malians are accustomed to we had to calculate the vertical ascents required, especially the scaling of mesas. Each team moved out of its sub-headquarters according to an itinerary which brought them back again in three days, their path being in the shape of a swooping arch. Itineraries of five or even seven days would have been possible had it not been for the fact that the ice chests couldn't keep the vaccine cold for more than three days. Returning to sub-headquarters, the teams took on new vaccine and artificial ice and set off again.

I often remarked to Bramane that this was a most unusual medical campaign, more of a struggle against the topography of the country than a campaign against disease, an exercise in logistics and strategy rather than a healing mission and I thought that no good military man could ever fail to approve of the precision and professionalism with which the whole complicated operation was put into motion. Inevitably we all began to show signs of fatigue, especially the vaccinators who were being pushed as far as anyone had ever dared. While they and the infirmiers had a skilled experience in dealing with villagers, convincing them to be vaccinated, they were often defeated by interminable palavering and ouright refusal in some places. They often came back reporting that villagers perched high up on the mesas looked down on their slowly moving columns, making no attempt to help them haul up the heavy baggage. Then as they lifted themselves higher and higher up on the face of the mesa or cliff, the villagers scattered, running away over the rocks with sure footed swiftness. I had instructed the teams to wait in the villages until someone came, which invariably happened and then began the long drawn out ritual of palavering. The villagers usually sent initial reconnaissance men who were very young and devoid of decision making powers. Once everything was explained to them they would disappear into the rocks and return after a while with some older men and the cycle was repeated several times until the chief appeared. Even though these chiefs and elders had assented to being vaccinated when our initial preparatory teams went through the region, once the vaccination teams arrived negotiations had to re-open and start from the beginning. It reminded me very much of the bargaining techniques of Malian merchants. You could bargain with them one day for an item and succeed in reducing their asking price by fifty percent, or even more. If you were not in agreement with the merchant for even that price you would leave and perhaps return the next day expecting to start the bargaining again where you had left it off the day before. But the merchants invariably started at the same original asking price, nullifying all of the bargaining efforts of the previous day. A similar phenomenon was operative among the Dogon when it came to accepting health services. The actual moment of acceptance was the climax to the whole affair and the vaccination operation somewhat of an anti-climax. I had greatly underestimated the amount of time this palavering required and after a while had to reset the schedules. It bothered Bramane that such palavering had to take place at all, but he should have known, as I often pointed out to him that things did not move very quickly in the Dogon country. Bewildering though it seemed, it was the Dogons' way of doing things in cautious considered steps.

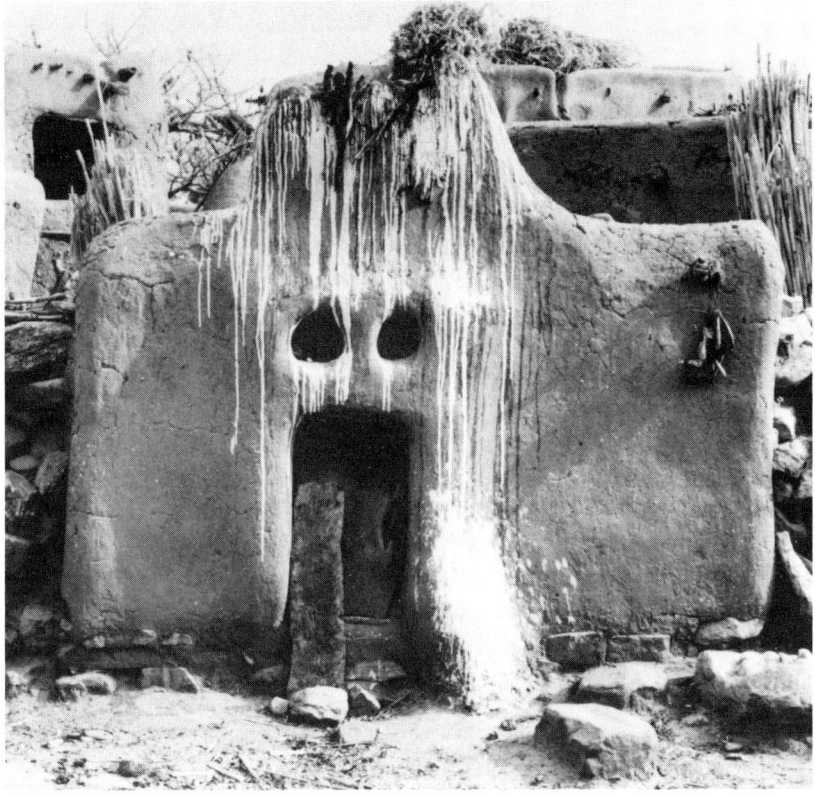

FIGURE 25. A Dogon village shrine. Within such shrines are kept statues representing ancestral spirits. The white material is a sacrificial liqud composed of millet porridge and milk which is poured on the shrine periodically. On right, in front, are herbal offerings.

While we were in the remote arrondissement of Oua, a telegraphic message arrived in the embassy in Bamako from Washington announcing that the Surgeon General of the United States Public Health Service, Dr. William Stewart, planned to visit Mali in order to examine our campaign. The message stated that he had heard of the campaign's success and wanted to see it first hand. This news arrived shortly before Bramane and Mabo returned from a cliff village where the people had not only fled but also rolled boulders off the cliff onto the vaccinators and fired at them with their muskets. It had taken Mabo three days of palavering to finally get the village elders to agree to accepting vaccination. But he had to bring in another team to give the inoculations since the original team refused with good reason to go near the village.

Jay and I finally had to leave the Dogon country in order to go down to Bamako where we put the ponderous machinery of two government bureaucracies into motion. First we had to inform the Malian government of the Surgeon General's desire to visit Mali and hope that they would extend an invitation. The Minister of Health was delighted by the prospect of the visit and readily invited the Surgeon General. Once this formality was concluded we set out to work with the Malians in arranging the details of the trip. I proposed to them that we take the Surgeon General and his party to the Dogon country where the teams were working, and specifically to Sanga which was the Minister of Health's home village. Once this was agreed upon scores of details had to be attended to, the itinerary planned, logistics established for feeding and housing the party and meetings held with all of the local officials in order to explain to them the purpose of the visit.

Dr. Stewart planned to fly into Mali aboard the plane of the military attaché from Dakar and this necessitated obtaining a clearance from the Malian Ministry of Defense for it to land and travel in the interior of the country. Obtaining this clearance in the past had always been an impossible task, but Ambassador Moore was optimistic and made the diplomatic request through regular channels. The pilot of the plane, Colonel Shanks, requested we arrange for fuel in both Bamako and Mopti but when Jay contacted the Bureau of Civil Aviation they politely said they could do nothing until they received clearance from the Ministry of Defense.

In the midst of all these uncertainties, the Minister of Health went off to Mopti and Sanga to prepare the reception ceremonies. The day after he left and two days before the expected arrival of the Surgeon General, a telegram arrived from Washington from the Secretary of

Health, Education and Welfare, instructing Dr. Stewart to return to Washington immediately. At the embassy, panic broke out. The Minister of Health was in Mopti organizing the reception, the protocol office had sent us their final resumé of official functions and receptions and now the visit was being called off. The fact of course that the Ministry of Defense hadn't as yet given their permission for the plane to land did not obviously dampen the energetic arrangements of either the Ministry of Health or of the Malian protocol office. Using beautiful syntax, Ambassador Moore sent a cable back to Washington indicating that a cancellation of the trip at ths point would be a diplomatic calamity. We all breathed a sigh of relief when a cable came in from the Surgeon General himself stating that the trip was still on.

There still remained the all important problem of the plane's landing in Bamako. The plane was scheduled to arrive on a Wednesday at 9:00 A.M. By Noon on Tuesday we had still not received official word as to whether it would be permitted to land. Stanley Clark, the director of the United States Agency for International Development in Mali made a discreet inquiry by phone at the Ministry of Defense. He was told that a decision would be handed down at 3:00 P.M. I sat in Stan's office until the messenger arrived from the defense ministry, counting the minutes off on my wrist watch. Finally, the phone rang. It was Dao the receptionist in the embassy lobby. "There is a letter here from the Ministry of Defense," he said in a calm voice which reflected his unawareness of what was transpiring.

When Stan opened the envelope, he looked gravely at the letter for a second and then exclaimed, "Impossible! They have refused permission for the plane to land." We were all struck dumb.

Ambassador Moore was a veteran of such crises and took this one in stride. In less than ten minutes he had the strategy for dealing with the problem clearly laid out. Stan and I were to go immediately to the Ministry of Health and see the *directeur du cabinet,* explain the problem to him and ask that he have the decision changed by the Ministry of Defense. If for any reason this failed, then the ambassador would go to see the foreign minister. The Surgeon General and his party were in Sierra Leone, completely unaware that all of this was going on and in the midst of our ten minute conference on diplomatic strategy a cable arrived from Colonel Shanks in Freetown reminding us about arranging for gasoline for the plane.

By 3:30 P.M., Stan Clark and I were at the Ministry of Health after having raced up the hair pin curves of Koulouba at breakneck speed. The directeur du cabinet wasn't in his office but down in town teaching a course in pharmacology at the secondary school of health. So down the hill we raced toward the school, arriving at the directeur's classroom at 3:45 P.M. We barged into the classroom much to his shock and that of the students, but once we explained the dilemma he dismissed the class and raced back up to his office where he made a series of telephone calls which culminated in Stan's being received by the Ministry of Defense at 5:00 P.M. The minister was quite taken aback by the whole turn of events, or so he pretended to be and said that he hadn't signed the refusal note, which we doubted. In dissecting the course of events much later we came to the conclusion that he had signed refusal not realizing that the plane was carrying in an important diplomatic delegation. He apologized to Stan for the inconvenience, affirmed that he would investigate the matter of the request being denied and then gave his assent to the plane landing in Bamako and elsewhere in Mali. At 5:40 P.M. Jay was at the Bureau of Civil Aviation arranging the gasoline needs and by 6:00 P.M. a cable went off to Freetown informing Colonel Shanks that all was well and that the party was anxiously being awaited in the Malian capital. Then we all went off to Stan's garden for a good stiff drink!

Bamako's airport is a very somnolent place, its big red terminal building standing out on the edge of town like a giant albatross. This day seemed an exception because there was a Caravelle leaving for Paris and a DC 3 flying up to Mauritania. Paris-cut business suits brushed shoulders with *bou bous* and camel saddles were thrown onto piles of sleek luggage. The lounge was choked with people, including thirty Chinese sporting buttons and books. The military attaché plane circled overhead and finally came down on the tarmac. Directions from the tower must have been confusing because the plane taxied toward the terminal building just as the big Caravelle moved to go out. Obviously, size was destined to win out. The Malian portocol officer gave us the signal to walk out onto the tarmac which we did just in time to get blasted with the sand filled exhaust wind of the Caravelle and see the Surgeon General's plane turn around and taxi away. It was futile to clean off the dust from our white shirts or to straighten our hair which felt as if it had been tied up in knots overnight.

The Surgeon General finally stepped from his plane, a big softspoken man who put everyone at ease within a matter of seconds with his gentle manner and unpretentious casual bearing. There was no false grand air about him and the Malians succumbed to his sincerity, warm charm and air of quiet authority. He was whisked up to the VIP lounge where Rudy Ellert-Beck, the USAID operations officer translated his speech for Radio Mali into French and then there followed a day full of official meetings and receptions crowned with a stag dinner at the ambassador's residence where Stan Clark and I set the place cards incorrectly, putting everyone who was supposed to be on the ambassador's right on his left and vice versa. Under the strain of the circumstances it was an admissable error about which we often joked.

The following morning we flew up to Mopti where the Minister of Health, Doctor Somine Dolo, was at the air strip with a delegation of two hundred people including two dance troupes, an honor guard of Bambara hunters in traditional dress and an orchestra of drums and xylophones. The Surgeon General was swallowed up in a tidal wave of white bou bous led by the Minister and carried off to meet a line of dignitaries. Bramane managed to get me off to the side after I got out of the plane and told me that the three trucks we had instructed him to put aside for the delegation were all washed and shining as brightly as the day they came off the assembly line. He had taken them to the hospital in Mopti the night before where there was the one and only water hose in town and had hired an army of children to scrub them down.

The procession of trucks and cars finally left the air strip and rolled over the long dike into the town of Mopti. The flood plains on either side were full of Peul herdsmen, moving with their herds towards the river. It was one great panorama of blue sky, cool breeze and green turf and they didn't have to do much more than ride over the dike to see what it was all about, the Peul, the inland delta and nomadism. The Mopti gendarmes were out in force, directing traffic from perches which on a score of my previous visits to the town had always been empty. Bramane had covered the town with posters, with so many in fact that enough of them survived the nocturnal raids of the Moptians to make an impressive if not artificial sight. Bramane and Djigui were vocal about so many of the posters having been taken down by the townspeople who then hung them in their houses.

"But don't worry," said Bramane, "we put a couple of hundred on the road to Sanga."

"You did what?" I gasped. Bramane who had become the self-appointed Potemkin of this trip didn't perceive my alarm.

After a fish brunch at the governor's house in Mopti, the caravan of three Dodge trucks and thirteen landrovers rolled out over the dike and on up into the rocky hills of Bandiagara. It wasn't too long before some of Bramane's posters became embarrassingly obvious, plastered onto any and everything which in the least looked stationary. Dr. David Sencer, the Director of the Center for Disease Control, who was riding in my truck along with Bramane and Djigui commented about all the posters.

"It's strange," he said, "that all of them are facing towards us."

It wasn't strange to me at all because Bramane and Djigui told me they had put all of the posters up so that they faced the road as one rode into Sanga.

"Is he happy to see all of these posters?" asked Bramane overhearing Dr. Sencer's remarks. I told Bramane that his posters were perplexing to Dr. Sencer who wanted to know why it was that they were all facing the same way.

"So that they can see them," said Bramane quite honestly.

The last straw with Bramane's posters came when we passed a group of nomads standing on the edge of the road holding one up towards us. "I had to pay them a hundred francs," said Bramane seriously." and that was after a lost of bargaining." Dr. Sencer smiled. Bramane had not made a very good Potemkin.

We twisted our way through the rocks to Sanga and a mile outside of the village heard the deep drums and the high pitched chanting rumbling across the valley. Five thousand people were chanting and swaying in rhythm when the caravan negotiated the last rise and descended onto the flat plain before the village. It was according to Ogobara the greatest assemblage which the village of Sanga had ever witnessed with everyone present from the ancient *hogons* to newborn youngsters. Mr. and Mrs. McKinney were there with their granddaughter, standing beneath the cool shade of several ancient silk cotton trees with Ogobara and the commandant.

Dr. Stewart gave a speech which Jay translated into French and which Ogobara then translated into Dogon. Then the people were vaccinated, the long lines spilling up over the rocks and across the narrow canyons. Dr. Dolo then hosted a lunch prepared by Mr. Molinari who was less nervous than anyone had expected because I had given him a tranquilizer. There then followed a walking tour of the cliff and a performance of masked dances which was the best I had ever seen in Sanga. Toward evening there was a *mechoui* (roast lamb) beneath the stars and a serenade with flutes and guitars. The McKinneys very graciously gave us their guest house which enabled us to house most of the visitors comfortably. Jay and I slept on a veranda with Bramane and Djigui. It fell to 45 degree Farenheit that night and a cold wind howled over the cliff and down through the deep canyons. But it was a beautiful night with a full moon beating down with a clear yellow light through the cold air. I pulled up my blankets and fell asleep.

Chapter XII
The Venice of Mali

Shortly after the Surgeon General left we moved the teams up into the rocky hills of Douentza and out into the bleak wilderness of Hombori. By the end of April all of the villages on the Bandiagara Plateau were finished and I re-grouped the vaccination teams in the town of Mopti for the launching of the final phase of the campaign in the flood plains around Lake Debo. I drove down to Mopti with Bramane and Modibo, battered for most of the way by one of those suffocating wind storms which blow heat and sand across the inland delta with great velocity in the months of March and April.

The town of Mopti is young by historical standards, having been developed by the French from a small Bozo fishing village into the thriving administrative and commercial capital of the delta. Its present day population of fifty thousand is crowded onto three small islands which stand at the confluence of the Bani and Niger Rivers. The islands are connected to one another by dikes and to the higher ground of the mainland by a causeway thirteen kilometers long. The causeway is banked with stunted sycamores and fig trees planted by the French to keep its sides from washing away. The air is cooler as one rides out towards Mopti and the presence of thousands of water fowl gliding over the broad puddles on the plains and flying into the infinite view in ordered flocks makes you feel as if the ocean were but a few miles away. The town itself is laced with canals and lagoons on which the Bozo fishermen pole their gondola-like canoes and it is thus that the town has the aspect of Venice. During the rains Mopti stands surrounded by water, an island in the sea, but in the dry season the green strips on either side of the rivers' banks grow ever narrower and beyond is a vast dry plain accented by mirages quivering in the mid-day heat.

Most of the population lives on the island of Kommugel, a crowded mass of two and three storied mud brick houses banking narrow tortuous streets. The buildings are gray in color, decorated with intricate geometric designs, terraces, turrets, parapets and narrow outdoor staircases winding their way up above the roofs of the city. The great mosque which was built in 1935 by a French administrator towers above the city as an imposing array of mud columns, minarets and broad gray walls studded with projecting wooden poles. The protruding wooden poles have no structural purpose, but serve as scaffolding for the masons who re-surface the building after the rains.

Mopti is the great crossroads of the middle Niger, a distinction

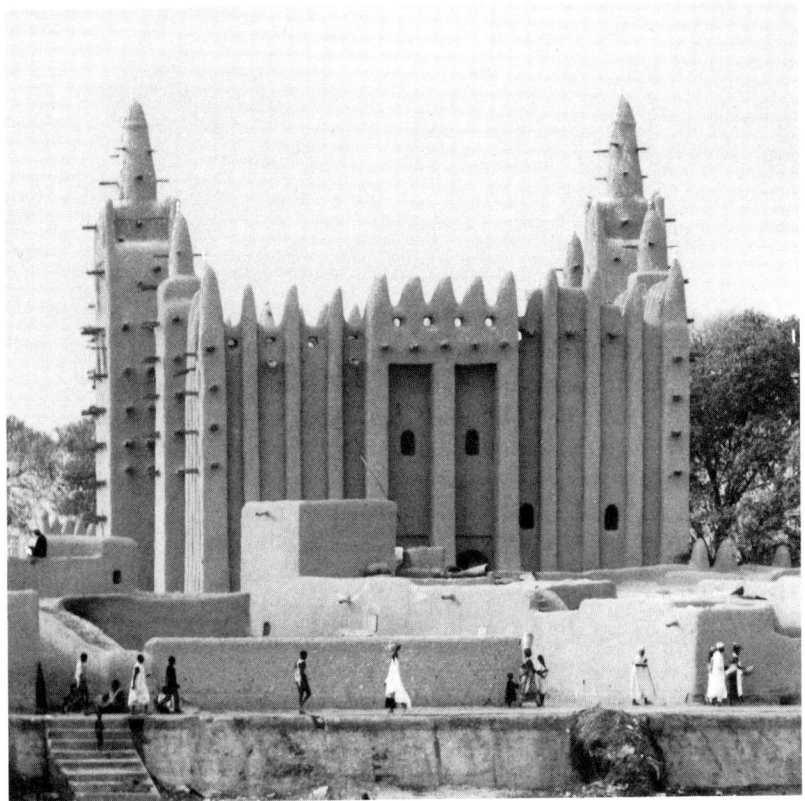

FIGURE 26. The great mosque at Mopti. This was built entirely of wooden poles and mud brick by masons from Djenne under the direction of a French administrator in 1935.

it gradually took away from Timbuctoo and Djenne during the past fifty years. Here commerce is the very life of the city and existence animated by the ever present sense of arriving and departing. Its markets are a fabulous hotch-potch of the races of West Africa from the fairest Arabs to the blackest Africans. On Thursdays when the weekly fair is held, traders and buyers from hundreds of miles around are present, from Timbuctoo and Gao, from Mauritania and Senegal, from Nigeria and Ghana and from North Africa. It is full of heaps of spices, salt from the Sahara, leather goods and saddles, beautifully painted pottery, firearms and swords, piles of silver coins and Maria Teresa Dollars, cotton, wool, cloth, foodstuffs of every sort, mounds of Peul blankets decorated with colorful geometric designs and mountains of dried fish. The stalls and shops are packed with a department store variety of goods, hidden away under patinated wooden counters, up on rickety shelves and suspended from the ceilings. The aroma of the merchandise rushes in on you at the doorways, telling you beforehand what lies ahead in the cool darkness of the shops. Merchants and buyers lead a quiet life, squatting in the alleys and in front of the stalls in the heat and dust, bargaining from early morning until the swallows and bats fly out over the river at dusk.

It always seemed an extraordinary thing to me that Mopti being so much in contact with the outside world was still so much cut off from it. It was as if western culture had scarcely sent a ripple down the river for the inhabitants still followed that way of life worked out centuries ago by the ancestors. It is a life and a culture which depend on canoes and the river and the camel and the caravan, a genuine capsule of the past to which paved roads and trucks are but non-essential additives. The touchstone of this life is that traditional commerce which once belonged to Timbuctoo and Djenne. It is permeated with a traditional consciousness stretching back over the centuries to another era and yet it reflects in a revealing way the present day life of the inland delta.

Even if Mopti is picturesque it is also drastically crude and unhealthful, a city where contagious diseases such as typhoid fever and malaria are endemic. Because the water table beneath the islands is so high, cesspools cannot be dug and so they are built as small rooms on the ground floor of the houses with the toilets above them on the second floor. Seepage occurs and often the walls break, flooding the streets with the contents. Special urinals are also built on the second floors with drain pipes which stick out over the gutter below. Unknowing visitors have often been the victims of unpleasant accidents by walking beneath the pipes. Many people though urinate and defecate in the lagoons and in the river, facilitating the transmission of disease. The town's water supply comes from the rivers and from wells all of which are heavily contaminated. The Bani River at this point makes its closest approach to becoming a sewer and several bacteriologic surveys have confirmed this impression. In the absence of a palpable aspect of even rudimentary hygiene, it is not surprising that gastrointestinal disease is rife in the town.

One would think that there would not have been much inducement for Europeans to have settled in Mopti and view it as being pathetically reckless if they did. Clearly there are special reasons why some Europeans chose to live in this unhealthful place. This micro-world of Europeans was not so obviously visible to visitors unless they spent some time in the town. In their own peculiar way the settlers all seemed happy and adjusted, but somehow I detected that all was not well with them. In recent years their ranks had been swollen by technical advisors who had come to Mopti for varying reasons and short periods of time. One might suppose that all of these people formed a closely knit community, clinging to one another in such a remote place. But this was very far from being the case. The permanent settlers were a strange cast of characters, spun off from the periphery of European society into these far off surroundings. They did not really mesh into the local African society nor were they any longer a part of Europe. Rather, they floated in a social limbo between the two, pitied by other Europeans and inscrutable to the Africans.

The dean of the settlers was a Monsieur Bignat who lived on the opposite bank of the Niger in his own small settlement appropriately named Bignatville. When I first met him, he had been in Mopti for thirty-two years. He had married a Peul woman and had had several children, most of whom had been sent to school in Bamako and Paris. Bignat's children had the option of living in one of three worlds, the African, the European or their father's limbo and that they chose to live as Europeans in Bamako and France did not surprise me. Bignat rarely crossed the river to Mopti, but stayed most of the time in his own settlement whose architecture was a peculiar synthesis of European and African styles. Like Bignat himself it was neither one nor the other, but nonetheless distinctive.

Unlike some of the other settlers, Bignat was not a piece of wrecked timber washed up on this far off shore. Through him ran the strong feelings of the non-conformist; his was an odyssey of the defiance of the rigid rules of European society, of success in defeating the norm. While crossing the river to meet him I had anticipated coming upon a recluse shut off from the whole world, a lonely figure all unto himself, bent over his own misery. What a surprise it was then to find a hospitable and friendly old man, radiating poise and courtesy, conversant on music and art, history and politics and full of general human conversation. He was placid and well balanced, I thought, a man who enjoyed the horizons of the modern world from the comfort of another century. He thought very highly of what I was doing and conversed in great detail about the terrible epidemics of yellow fever and bubonic plague he had seen in Saint Lous in Senegal many decades ago. Bignat supported himself by manufacturing soft drinks in a small building behind the house. He made *limonade, crush d'orange* and *eau gaseuze* which were sold up and down the river in opaque green bottles. Over in Mopti he sold it to an agent, a Frenchman by the name of Monsieur Roque.

Monsieur Roque had been in Mopti for thirty years and in addition to selling Bignat's soft drinks from beneath a dilapidated straw awning also operated the only movie house in town. This tumble down open air affair did a good business and ran without much overhead. Monsieur Roque operated the projector himself which was set out on a rickety wooden table in the center of the middle aisle. As the theater filled up with several hundred spectators he sat enthroned on a chair in the middle aisle next to the projector with one finger on the switch. This gave the performances the dramatic effect which the films often lacked. Monsieur Roque kept the audience waiting in anticipation for the second the switch would be thrown. For those few moments every evening he was the celebrity of Mopti. All of this came to a crashing end when the government nationalized Monsieur Roque's movie theater.

Monsieur Roque had two cousins, the Simone brothers, who were the oldest European inhabitants of Mopti, they having been born there. Back in the 1890's their parents wandered down the Niger in search of egret feathers and crocodile skins and finding both in the vicinity of Mopti settled there. Both of the Simone brothers had melancholic morbid personalities and a gift of bringing themselves into trouble with relative ease. They were a very sad sight to see, dressed in their tattered khaki shorts, sandals and frayed polo shirts, shut up from the whole world in their dilapidated mud brick house where rats, flies and roaches paraded with the arrogance of ownership. The furnishings were bare, and decrepit, reflecting the spirit of those whose home this was. Henry, the oldest of the two owned a pre-World War II vintage radio which was his chief contact with the outside world. Some decades ago he had subscribed to *Paris Match* magazine and still read the patinated dusty numbers which stood in heaps all over the main room. The house was rarely cleaned and was cluttered up with dust and several generations of spider webs.

The Simone brothers squeezed out a living in Mopti from the meager rents they collected on the houses their parents had owned. Occasionally, they helped Roque selling Bignat's soft drinks, but when I met them there had been a falling out over issues which were clearly undefined. A great crisis entered their lives one day when the second floor of their house collapsed down into the ground floor which had by necessity been recently rented out to the SOMIEX for use as a grocery store. With the floor went the radio and the issues of *Paris Match* and a kerosene operated refrigerator which miraculously landed right side up in a heap of pulverized mud brick.

"I am going back to France," declared Henri Simone in response to this disaster and although these words were not said with any great conviction he did manage to get the French embassy to repatriate him as an indigent. In France, he found people who were understanding of his life tragedy, but all this understanding and public assistance could not dispel the misery of a misfit. So he returned to Mopti, to the dust and grime and an endless procession of days filled with a quiet narcotizing routine.

Jean Durmant had been in Mopti for fifteen years, gainfully employed as a building contractor. Although he built fine edifices, like many building contractors I have known he himself lived in a run down building. His home was the second floor of a mud brick house which tilted sharply to one side and in later years it finally fell over and collapsed. The floor of the living roo mwas so slanted that one had to push the dinner plate up on the table if one sat on the low side of the incline. Eating soup was always an enormous problem but one never felt embarrassed in the presence of Durmant who was an outgoing man full of good humor. The doorway to this house lay on the other side of an open gutter which was always full of greenish looking stagnant water. Once on the other side of the immense door you had to climb up a large and rickety wooden staircase whose steps were unevenly spaced. Underneath this staircase the landlord kept two large pigs which were well hidden from the eyes of the fanatical Moslem population.

Durmant eventually left Mopti and returned to France. "If I remain any longer, I'll be trapped like the others," he said and in doing so summed up the unpleasantness of their tragedy.

Onto this stage there fell a cast of lesser characters who made up for the brevity of their stay with especially bizzare performances. A Turkish physician came to work in the dispensary, but it soon became clear that he was not a real medical doctor. So lacking was he in medical knowledge that he went out to investigate an outbreak of smallpox without ever having been vaccinated himself in recent years. He contracted the disease and almost died. Afterwards he left Mopti quite suddenly and went to work in Senegal and then in Morocco where the news of his lack of credentials finally caught up with him. He was replaced by a French physician who had spent many years working in a remote Sahara outpost in Algeria which should have evoked suspicions about his ability to get along in society. He soon declared himself a Marxist and took delight in carrying a large sign in Mopti's May Day parade which read, "Down With The Imperialists."

There also came an American male teacher who fathered a child with one of the town's leading prostitutes. The boy was four years old when I first saw him pimping for his mother at the campement. He was a beautiful child with fair smooth skin and sandy colored hair. She had taught him to tell people that he was an American and to spot Amercans among the tourists. This routine never brought home the customers she had hoped for; it only corrupted the morals of a small child who grew up knowing no other way of life.

So many of these foreigners had like fallen timbers drifted into the still waters of Mopti, rotated and turned until they were either washed out again or else sank into the unseen mire of the place. They had all drifted out of the complexities of the modern world into the intoxicating calm of this far off place. But strangely they sought contact with those who were still part of the complex world. Perhaps it was to hear their own conviction repeated, that the modern world was a fatiguing place from which it was better to flee.

The pillars of normalcy in Mopti were a Lebanese merchant family, the Jajas and André and Rosey Szabo who worked for the Food and Agriculture Organization of the United Nations. Jaja was a fattish man with a red puffed face accented by spectacles which were as thick as Coke bottle bottoms. He and his sons ran a lucrative chain of gasoline stations, hardware stores and a grocery. They traveled every year to France, entertained lavishly with twelve course dinners and could maintain a persistent conversation on world affairs with relative ease. Like so many fat people, Jaja was affable and kind, but he had a shrewd business head. It was always possible to have faith in his hospitality and hearty manner, but when it came to business he was hard and unyielding, all of which made him a great success on every count. Jaja's kindly interest in me was not so much medical but rather as Bramane observed, matrimonial since he had some very eligible daughters.

André Szabo was an Israeli fisheries expert who ran his home like a Communist establishment, taking in wanderers, diplomats, friends and ordinary vagabonds. He was a rousing man, full of a vigorous readiness to do anything for anyone. He had been flung out into West Africa like some burning stone out of an erupting volcano, full of zeal to do and create, to change and improve everything with which he had contact. As he worked, he generated newer and bigger ideas such as motorized convoys of fishing canoes, refrigeration equipment for the fishing boats, a fish canning factory and finally an export trade for Mali in fresh fish via air to Paris. I never saw him sitting peacefully still for even a short while. He was always on the run, even while eating dinner, driving at a terrific speed towards new creations with an untamed imagination and a lion's roar. He was enormously enterprising and having no sympathy with exasperation and frustration, achieved the impossible through dramatic and joyful adventure. In a compulsive way he was always engaged in some great and noble conspiracy, to improve the lot of the fishermen and to modernize one of Mali's few resources. The Malians never appreciated his worth, until he left, and then they did it indirectly according to their manner by moaning his loss.

Rosey was by contrast an impressive figure of benevolent placidity, content in being an inspiring quality for André. There was no trait of drudgery in her character and in a quiet and almost imperceptible way she could redirect and harness much of André's eruptive energy. She spoke French with an accent which Jewish mothers in Brooklyn used to embellish English and was endowed with Jewish motherliness. She took an interest in all of the small details whenever I left their home to go out into the bush again. From the balcony above she would send down a chime of last minute concern about water and food, handkerchiefs and blankets. Even as the truck pulled away along the dike beneath the shade of the sycamores Rosey would remain on her perch until we were out of sight in the horizon.

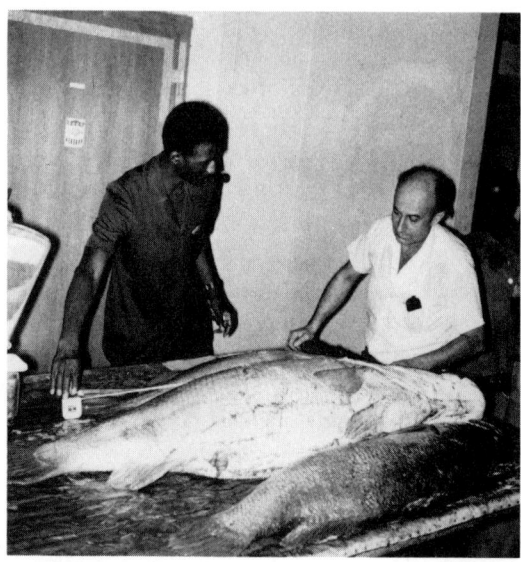

FIGURE 27. Dr. Konare *(left)* of the Water and Forests Service and Andre Szabo examine fish brought in by the members of the Mopti fishing cooperative.

The Szabos lived on the second floor of the Water and Forests building. It was in comparison to even Bamako a pioneer's existence. But the home had a special charm and warmth which compensated for the lack of comforts. It was in many ways a delightful apartment, encircled by a spacious veranda on three sides and which overlooked the dike and the Bani River beyond. From the back room where I usually stayed the flood plain spread out towards the horizon and throbbed at night with a symphony of bird calls and insect noises. The sound of the river lapping at the sides of the dike played as a delightful background throughout the night, broken only by the splash of the oars and muffled conversations of fishermen heading downstream. The Bani and Niger met at their doorstep and in the morning as we ate breakfast in the high airy dining room I could look down onto the river, see the breeze dancing over the white caps and inflating the sails of the long canoes. It was a thrill to see and hear the big white hulk of the *General Soumare* pushing her way through the turquoise water on the Niger, effusing a great eruption of white foam as she swerved in a wide arch onto the Bani. As the boat passed beneath the Szabo's veranda on her way to the port her decks were full of waving passengers and there was the first of a series of long loud whistles from her tall stack. This beautiful and exciting vision came in through the wide open doors of the veranda as I sipped my coffee and planned my day.

The day after we arrived in Mopti the *General Soumare* sailed into port on her way down the river to Timbuctoo and Gao. Four of our teams were to sail with her at dusk, going on to Niafunke where they would vaccinate the nomads north of Lake Debo. Four days afterwards we placed four of the trucks on two barges along with the drivers and Modibo and arranged for them to be pulled to Niafunke by a tug boat. What was supposed to be a three day journey turned into a twelve day nightmare because the tug boat captain didn't know the channels well enough and became mired in the marshes on the far side of Lake Debo. After fighting sand bars and scraping the bottom of the river they arrived at Niafunke where a woman passenger fell into the river and drowned leaving behind three small children. It was a portent of difficult times ahead. The remaining teams descended into the flood plains at Djenne and Tenenkou and then went on to the shores of Lake Debo. Because the teams were scattered in four widely separated areas logistics became an enormous problem and communications were virtually non-existant. A deluge of problems arose, dead batteries, broken axles, burned out motors and refrigerators which heated up like ovens instead of freezing. But in spite of all this the teams maintained a quick pace and moved through the nomad camps towards the great lake. As the teams converged on the lake, Bramane and I went about planning the strategy for reaching the thousands of fishermen and nomads camped on the shores. In order to reach the fishermen, the governor of Mopti suggested I speak to the president of the Bozo fishing cooperative in Mopti. And so one morning Bramane and I made our way through the noisy tangle of the Mopti market to his office.

It was the day of the weekly fair and the river was lined with a solid bank of beached canoes and long boats with swollen sails. The market itself teemed with waves of Bobo women in indigo boubous, balancing aromatic wicker baskets of dried fish on their heads and young men dumping out mountains of fresh fish from the waists of their boats. It was the height of the dry season and the river lay thirty feet below the top of the dike whose sloping sides were covered with thousands of people. The piles of dried fish were bundled into straw mats shaped like rectangular boxes and thrown up onto the waiting lorries for transport to Ghana and the Ivory Coast. Higher and higher they would go until the truck would almost reach the height of a second story building. These trucks were a familiar sight on the roads in central Mali, swaying back and forth from side to side around a center of gravity which was five feet higher than the roof of the cab.

We climbed up on the top of the bank and edged our way through a group of straw shelters shared by the indigo dyers and the wizened old men whose patinated hammers shaped long narrow canoes from hard teak wood. Bramane conversed about indigo, saying it was made from a certain tree which grew on the Bandiagara Plateau. I said it came in cans from England which Bramane discovered was the case. "Then it isn't real indigo," he said.

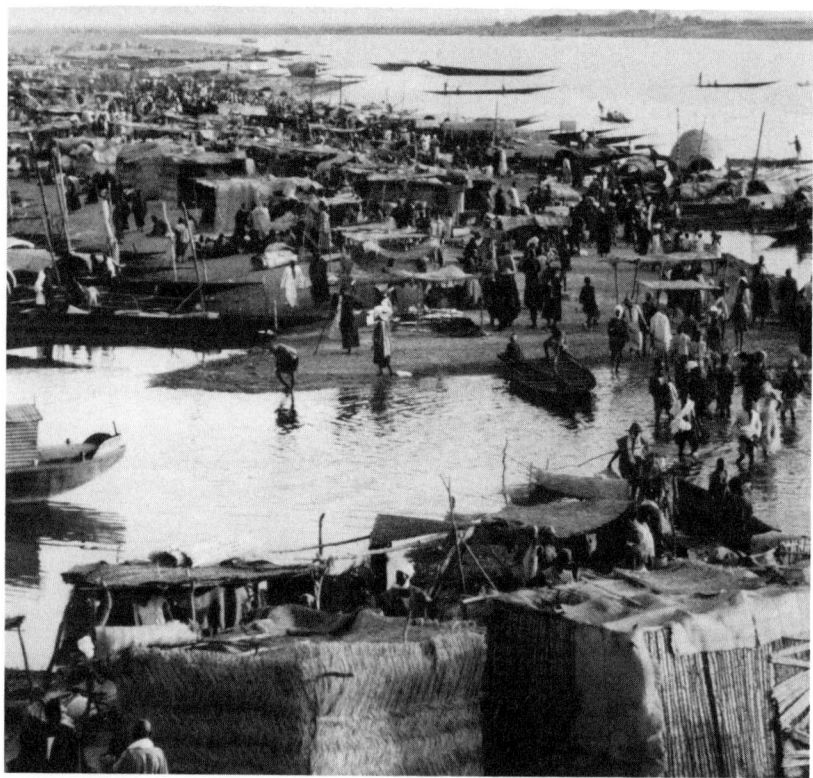

FIGURE 28. The port of Mopti. The numerous straw mat sheds house vendors and artisans. During the high water period the entire area depicted here lies under ten feet of water.

"Why not?" I answered.

"Because it is imported." Bramane's logic was unclear to me and I didn't reply but the indigo women started up a cyclone of discussion with him which ended in their telling him to mind his own business.

We got to the small cement building which housed the fishing cooperative offices. It was like the canoes below, packed with people, noise and straw mats which hung by ropes from the ceiling. The straw mats separated the building into separate "offices." The office of the president of the cooperative was two straw mats away from where we entered, but those who knew the lay of the land could walk directly into this office by coming through a back door. It didn't strike me that the clatter of noise and the crush of humanity were particularly condusive to efficient office procedures. Bramane said it looked busy which was more important. The president's secretary told us to sit down on a long shiny bench which faced his desk. There we sat looking at him for about ten minutes while he looked at us, neither of us saying a word. He left for a few minutes and came back saying the president was having a conference but would adjourn it since the health profession came first ahead of all other matters. From the loudness of the shouts and the argumentative mood of the participants, it was hard to call the encounter on the other side of the mat a conference.

As I walked over to the other side of the mat, the president told the conference participants to leave because the meeting was very private. They went over to the side of the mat where Bramane and I had just been and could naturally hear everything which was being said. In spite of this, the president opened our talk by saying that he preferred to discuss health matters in private which made everyone on the other side of the mat strain all the more to hear what was being said. Bramane changed the course of the conversation by asking why the Bozo had a president. "You are supposed to have kings and chiefs," he said.

"C'est plus moderne," answered the president. Bramane and the chief got involved in a lengthy discussion of the advantages and disadvantages of kings and presidents, Bramane expressing monarchical sentiments which were obviously at variance with his Marxist political beliefs. Once this thoroughly inconclusive discussion was through, we got into the business of our meeting.

The president of the cooperative was an enormous man who like all Bozo people was very black. The Bozo are reputed to be the blackest people in Mali, a fact which the president later spoke about, telling us that Bozo were the original inhabitants of the Niger Valley. The president used to travel around Mopti on a chauffered motor bike.

When I explained to the president that we wanted to vaccinate all of the fishermen grouped around Lake Debo he replied that he would do everything possible to help us. The cooperative had a fleet of long canoes with Johnson outboards stationed up and down the river and along the shores of the lake. To vaccinate the fishermen was simply a matter of getting into several motorized canoes and riding down the river and around Lake Debo, or so the president said. That of course was easier said than done. The president didn't know the exact location of the fishing camps, but he was willing to give us the canoes. All that we had to tell him was where and when we wanted them, something I couldn't do because I didn't know where the camps were nor the canoes for that matter. The president was full of good intentions but devoid of hard facts and a comprehension of what it was we wanted from him. So I politely told him that now that our "prise de contact" had been made I would work with his subordinates in setting up a program for the fishermen. He agreed to this and then sputtered off on his chauffeured motor bike which was parked behind the back door.

André Szabo finally came to my rescue and put me in touch with a man who was the liaison officer for the Ministry of Water and Forests for the fishing cooperative. Mama Tangara knew all of the Bozo chiefs; he knew where all of the camps *(daga)* were located between Mopti and Lake Debo. And so two days later I went off with him and Bramane to the shores of Lake Debo to set up the day-to-day schedule and to coordinate the use of the cooperative's canoes. After two weeks of exhausting work, we came up with a master plan designed to reach all of the one hundred and fifty one camps in two weeks time. It only remained now to put this plan into operation.

Chapter XIII

Illness

Naturally there were delays in the teams getting over to Lake Debo and quite a bit of normal apathy which sets in towards the end of a long hard campaign. The men's health had begun to fail, a combination of their being physically run down and their moving through a malaria and typhoid fever endemic zone. It was certainly with a compassionate heart that I tried to infuse a blaze of energy into this last effort. That they had stood up so well for this long was nothing less than a mircale. In demanding the achievement of this last worthy objective, Jay and I stood quite alone and never before during the long hard campaign had we felt the heavy burden of solitude which responsibility demands. How acclaimed we would have been if we had announced that we had done enough and could go home.

The plains were a cauldron of heat from which there was no escape. The thermometer in my own truck never fell below 110 degree Farenheit. Except for milk there was little food in the region and the water in the lowered rivers and lakes muddy and contaminated. In each of the teams a vaccinator had to be assigned full time to boiling and filtering the water. We had salt and rice sent in to the teams, but under the heat and hardship of this harsh place their morale only grew all the more wretched. The nomads were not at all hospitable, only permissive at best which increased the uncertainty and suffering of it all. Against such overwhelming hardship the only comfort was a sense of duty and responsibility which the vaccinator's didn't have. So I doubted that they would see it through to the end and expected an open revolt at any moment. Bramane and I went from team to team, bolstering morale as best we could.

Day-by-day the teams pushed themselves along, ignored in many camps, harried in others and thoroughly wretched. Djigui was in the

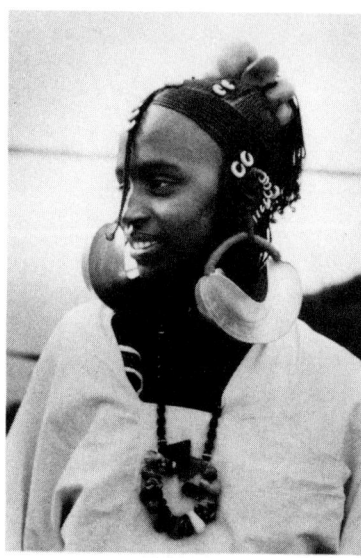

Figure 29. A young Peul woman from the inland delta of the Niger. The large gondola shaped earrings as well as the small rings in her hair are twenty-two karat gold and her tiara composed of amber stones.

south, in Tenekou and Djenne, moving with three teams up the flood plains to the vast plain at Dintaka which lay on the southern shores of the lake and Modibo moved down from the north with four teams through the swamp of the Farimake. The remainder completed the pincer movement, coming in from the east across the Kona plain. Once more I went up to Niafunke and down to Djenne to give them heart if nothing more and then over to Lake Debo. The country around the lake was full of an immemorial stillness, the plains spreading away to the west where the green banks of the Niger are just visible to the practiced eye. To the north are other lakes, Niangaye, Do, Korientze and Agagoungou, great sheets of shallow water covered in the dry season with a veneer of brilliant green algae. Only the thatched huts of the Bozo and the tents of the nomads tamed the landscape which is still one of enormous space and emptiness full of a frightening silence.

Never thinking that my own physical collapse was imminent, I returned to Mopti, feeling tired but well. There had been a report of a suspected case of smallpox in Sanga and I decided to inspect it myself, profiting at the same time to take some friends into the Dogon country. So leaving Bramane, Djigui and Modibo in charge for a few

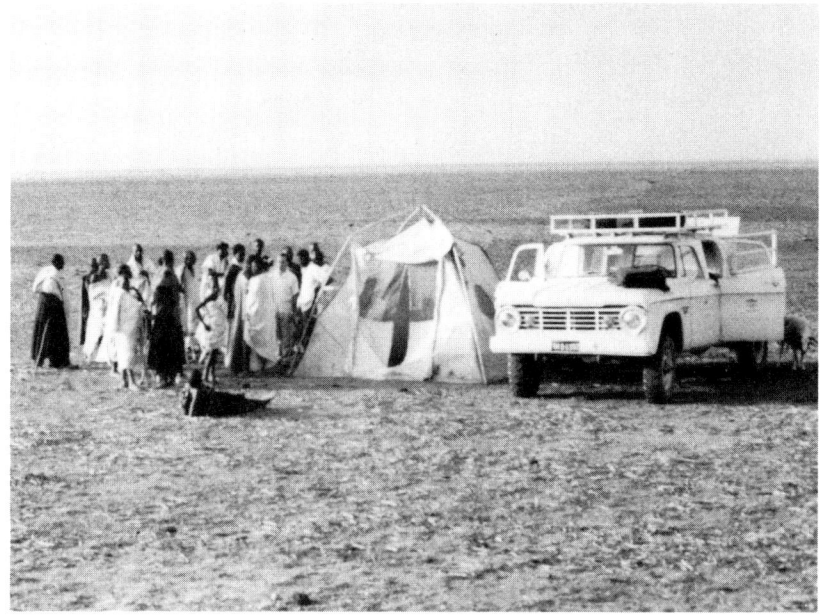

FIGURE 30. Dr. Imperato holding a clinic near the shores of Lake Debo in the arrondissement of Youvarou. In the background on the right attached to the truck is Albert, a ram, presented to Dr. Imperato by the Peul chiefs of the area.

days, I left for Sanga. With me came Ladislas Segy, a world authority on African art and his wife, Helena and Ted Clark, the son of the United States Ambassador to Mali. It was a refreshing change of pace, full of uplifting conversations about art and music, history and philosophy. When we arrived in Sanga I learned that Ogobara was slightly ill, but on examining him found that it was nothing serious. However, it was enough of an illness to prevent him from accompanying us on a tour of cliff down to the village of Irieli. He sent his son in his place and the following morning while the air was still clear and brisk we started off across the high windy plateau, through shaded villages where indigo robed Dogon women pounded millet and filled round earthen jars with cold water from deep wells. We descended the gradual incline onto the lower plateau and then crossed a broad clear stream and then edged our way towards the cliffs along a narrow precipice which overlooked a deep forested canyon.

Before arriving at the edge of the cliff I told Oumar, Ogobara's son, that we would visit one of the accessible hidden grottos not usually entered by tourists. We left the main trail and climbed up for half an hour through heavy brush until we reached the grotto. We spent a lot of time going through the maize of ancient mud houses and examining the fragments of pottery which covered the ground. Then after resting for a while we decided to push on again towards the main trail which led down the cliff. My driver Kassim and his apprentice Karim stood on a lower ledge below the grotto and suggested that I jump down instead of walking down the long trail. I jumped the ten feet and thought nothing of it, never realizing that in doing so I had initiated a medical emergency. We finally got to the edge of the cliff, to that breathtaking view where all of a sudden you emerge from the shadows of a towering canyon where the sky rushes in on your senses and below the village of Irieli with its grass peaked houses and cylindrical granaries tumbles over the rocky crags and rises up the side of the far off cliff. Beyond the country races away from you, into the far off horizon, an undulating expanse of dunes and prairie covered with thorn trees and scrub. The excitement of the experience is intensified by the difficult descent, down vertical walls of stone boulders which are negotiated in some areas by sliding down patinated ladders. Echoes bounce off the walls of the cliffs and a cool breeze dances across your face and once down you sense a moment of triumph in having conquered a creation of nature.

The trail leads along the base of the cliff, past the whitened skulls of children sacrificed during the famine of 1917, under the overhanging grottos where the dead are still buried. It is an exhilerating experience to leave the twisting trail of the cliff and to enter into the calm atmosphere of village life. The trail passes the large shady palaver shelters of the Dogon, held up by exquisitely carved posts and skirts around colorfully decorated fetish houses and ancestor altars where millet and milk sacrifices are still made.

As we moved off the rocks and into the village I felt a mild pain in the left side of my abdomen. I fell slightly behind the others and while they examined the fetish houses and altars I sat down and rested thinking it a stomach cramp. Gradually, the pain intensified and although I didn't say anything to the others I fell out of the conversation. Helena Segy detected that something was wrong, but I told her it was nothing. But the pain grew steadily and persistently worse, a deep ache, radiating from the left flank down into the groin. By the time we left Irieli and entered the sandy plain I could scarcely walk. The clinical acumen of a clinician general disappears where his own illnesses are concerned and so I couldn't come to any definite conclusion as to what was wrong with me. I thought that perhaps it was a perforated intestine and visualized myself dying there on the cliff. Had it been on the right side I would have worried about an appendicitis. But at no time when I was below the cliff did I ever think of what it eventually turned out to be.

Like all humans, my primary concern was to get to a place where I could be helped. Sanga was ten miles and three hours away, two thousand feet up the cliff and across the plateau and beyond it Mopti was three hours away by road. At best it would take six hours for me to reach competent medical hands and with that thought before me I despaired and resolved that I would accept whatever happened.

The pain was the most excruciating I have ever experienced, but I kept telling the others it wasn't too bad and not to be worried. My pallid look and gestures told them the truth. What was to have been a leisurely ascent up the cliff now became a desperate effort to get to help. We started back up the cliff over a short cut I had learned many months before. It cut through the village of Pegue and then through a long cool tunnel. I remember now that as I crawled up through the village, bent in two, with Karim helping me, a woman came down the path screaming at us to stop. A sacrifice was being held over one of the ancestor shrines ahead so we had to back track and recross the village at another point. The sun had long since become an additional enemy and it beat down unmercilessly on us, rapidly exhausting everyone. Finally, we arrived at the tunnel where we rested. The rest wasn't palliative to my pain and I was unable to remain still. I lay writhing on the ground of the tunnel, holding my abdomen with my crossed arms. Ted and the Segys wanted to help, but they didn't know what to do and were I think more terrified than even I. Kassim told me later that he was sure I was going to die.

While writhing on the ground in the tunnel I made a very rash decision. I decided to go on ahead of the others with Kassim, greatly overestimating my knowledge of the trail. Before long Kassim and I were lost in a maize of tunnels and canyons. After wandering around for almost an hour during which I vomited five times we came to a large baobab tree. I sat down under it and although in terrible pain managed to see a man walking off into a grove of trees on the plain below. I told Kassim to descend the hardened volcanic slag onto the plain and to ask the man for help in taking us back to Sanga. When Kassim returned a short while later with the man he said, "This man doesn't speak either Bambara or French. He only speaks Dogon and that language you speak with the Americans at the embassy." It was incredible! The Dogon spoke English. He had traveled to Ghana many years before where he had learned English and knew enough to tell me that we were heading in the right direction to Sanga. As it turned out we were but a mile away. He said that there was a caravan of Tuaregs with camels a short way ahead and wanted to fetch a camel for me to ride on for the rest of the way. With the severity of my pain I would never have been able to remain on a camel and told him instead to give me a hand in moving along.

The McKinneys were in Sanga and put me on a comfortable bed in their rest house. It was while I was there that I urinated pure blood and at last realized that I was passing a kidney stone. Ignoring advice I insisted on returning immediately to Mopti where I thought I would be safer in the event any complications set in. The road trip back was agonizing and I spent most of it in the back of the truck writhing on the seat. The constant jolting of the truck precipitated repeated bouts of colic as the stone moved down the narrow ureter from the kidney to the bladder. When I finally got to Mopti I crawled up the stone staircase to the Szabo's home and virtually collapsed on their living room floor.

"You look like you're passing a kidney stone," exclaimed Rosey Szabo. I hadn't expected such words of medical wisdom from her but as I learned later she was not without experience in this sort of problem having passed several stones herself. She helped me to a bed in their back room while André went to the hospital to fetch one of the Russian surgeons. He confirmed the diagnosis and gave me an injection of morphine which finally ended the terrible pains which had begun twelve hours before. He was a kind man or so he seemed to me under the influence of a narcotic. He came from Samarkan and asked me many questions about medical practice in the United States. Before he left he reassured me and gave instructions to André for giving me additional injections during the night. It was a strange thing that many months later he himself developed a kidney stone and had to go down to Bamako for treatment. It is a common complication of living in a hot dry climate where water intake is often insufficient. Lastouillas had passed many kidney stones and I myself had treated many people in Bamako for the problem, although I never suspected it in myself when I was on the cliff.

I fell into the Szabo's home at an extremely difficult time. Joe Christiano, the deputy chief of mission of the embassy and his wife

Dorethea and their three children were stranded in Mopti with no place to stay. They had been scheduled to sail on the *General Soumare* downstream to Gao but when they arrived in Mopti they learned that the boat was going upriver instead. Finally, the boat's direction was changed again and it scheduled to go downstream, but with more passengers booked on it than could be accommodated. Then the sailing was delayed another day and so the Szabos had to accommodate nine guests in their two bedroom house plus themselves. Using cots and tents from my truck they put people up on the verandas and bedded themselves down in the living room.

By the next day word had reached Bramane up in Kona that I was very ill and he came down with surprising speed. He said that I looked bad and definitely needed an injection of Vitamin B 12. I thanked Bramane for his therapeutic advice but told him I had gotten enough injections for the day. In a hazy sort of way I remember him standing in my room as neat as a pin in his freshly pressed Chinese Mao suit and shiny black shoes. He was always impeccably dressed, spending a lot of time scurrying around getting his laundry done. Often I came on him in the remotest bush and found him dressed as if he had just stepped out of a show window. My illness thoroughly demoralized Bramane and in a way was the last straw for him. The day before he had received a telegram from Niafunke that Modibo was very ill with amebic dysentary and that there were no medicines in Niafunke to treat the disease. I told Bramane to have him evacuated on the single engined Air Mali bi-plane which went once a week to Niafunke. Modibo was finally evacuated out of Niafunke, twenty pounds lighter than when he went in there and spent a month in the Point G Hospital in Bamako.

I knew that after all the long months of harsh living it wouldn't take much of a set back to push Bramane to the limit of his emotional reserves. Alone, he couldn't have carried on at that point. And so if things were to succeed I had to remain on the scene, even if only as a stationary figure in Mopti, capable of descending into the arena as a last resort if things went wrong. The renal colic continued every day, especially if I moved around, a sure sign that the stone hadn't passed through the ureter yet. It was impossible for me to go to Lake Debo; I could never have withstood the trip. But Bramane went and carried on admirably, secure in the knowledge that back in Mopti there was someone who could in some magical way always overcome the teams' indifference and the intransigence of the nomad population. Bramane might have survived alone under the yoke and I wish now that I had forced him to do so for it would have given his character that aristocratic quality of confidence which he sorely lacked. He was in many ways a mighty and majestic creature who held his own opinions on most things and though he firmly believed in the necessity of what we were doing, he could never gather up the courage to declare to the vaccinators that he was a partisan to these ideas. Had he done so he would have isolated himself from his own people. So he felt more comfortable playing the role of the messenger and was never able to take on the mantle of leadership. In the final analysis, this worked out very well for Bramane because he could declare himself partisan to the vaccinators' complaints but at the same time set the example by obeying orders he said came from me. He moved among the people at Lake Debo with an air of mission and was successful as long as a higher authority was nearby, potentially able to inflict punishment if orders were not obeyed. Bramane's comfort and success at playing the role of the messenger hinged on my being around. He came into Mopti to report on progress and to get advice about changes in strategy. Then he crossed the river and went up to Lake Debo where my advice was presented as a new set of orders. Bramane embellished the scenario by reporting to the teams that I was moving around the lake. Those in the south thought I was in the north and those in the west thought I was in the east and everyone believed that at any moment I would descend to check on the quality of their work.

Within two weeks, the teams were right on the edge of the lake and began moving in a coordinated counter-clockwise fashion through the camps which ringed it. Mama Tangara went up to the eastern shore where there were heavy concentrations of Bozo fishermen and I dragged myself out of Mopti for a week and went to the southern shore of the lake where I met with the chiefs of the Dialloube and Sossobe clans. Within a few days, the bush telegraph brought the news of my presence on the southern shore of the lake to virtually all of the teams, something which delighted Bramane and he came back to Mopti to see if it were really true or an exaggeration of his own stories.

My health deteriorated after that and I developed an infection in the kidney where the stone had formed. With the Russian surgeon helping me I underwent antibiotic treatment, but without much success. A physician friend of mine came out to Mali to visit and when he saw me in Mopti he advised me to return to the States for treatment and removal of the stone. Dr. Milton Hadelsman and his wife Sophie had planned to visit Mali for almost a year and when I fell ill I didn't tell them, for fear that they would cancel their trip. Dr. Handelsman, a specialist in diabetes, conducted an interesting survey for the disease in Mali, in which I participated after my return to the country from the States. During the time he was in Mopti, I suffered the worst colic I had yet experienced and finally I agreed to leave. It was only with a lot of difficulty that I got back to Bamako. They propped me up on pillows in the back of the truck and Dr. Handelsman gave me large doses of morphine periodically as we drove for ten hours along the long road to Bamako.

When I next saw Dr. Handelsman it was from a patient's bed at the Long Island College Hospital in New York. There Dr. John Edson and Dr. John Ippolito had conducted a series of tests which showed that the stone was caught in that part of the ureter which leads into the urinary bladder. It took a month before the stone passed and from my hospital bed I read Bramane's letter describing the end of the campaign. Even from so far away I couldn't divorce myself from Mali. I had suffered too much there to put the country out of my life.

Chapter XIV
A Life at Home

When I returned to Bamako at the end of the rains it was with the medical advice to curtail my bush travel. For in the final analysis it was found that the severe jolting in the truck had caused a small hemorrhage in the kidney around which minerals had deposited, causing a stone. With only a half of Mali's population vaccinated, it would never have been possible for me to follow this advice to the letter, but as the new campaigns were being planned, I remained in Bamako for most of the time where I enjoyed a relatively quiet and interesting life.

Bramane's excellent work during the campaign in the inland delta merited a professional reward and we asked him what it was he wanted most. He told me that he wanted to go to the Centre Muraz in Upper Volta to take the year's course in infectious disease control. And so shortly after my return he left us. Jay Friedman also left Mali in order to work in Gabon and we all regretted his departure. His place was taken by Mark LaPointe who had several years of work experience in Guinea and Gabon. Some of the vaccinators resigned after being admitted to the national police force. In future years, almost half of our original vaccinators became policemen and often I drove around Bamako and was smartly saluted at almost every main intersection by uniformed ex-vaccinators.

During the months of recuperation, I enjoyed my home in Bamako and the life in and around it. It required three servants to run this home efficiently and for most of the time I was in Mali my household defied convention and remained remarkably stable. The staff consisted of Ahmadou, the boy-cook, Brahima, the gardener and Camera, the nightwatchman. Ahmadou always maintained that there were three imaginary elves known in Bambara as *wolklani* who lived on top of the suspended ceiling. There was also a pest control brigade consisting of a

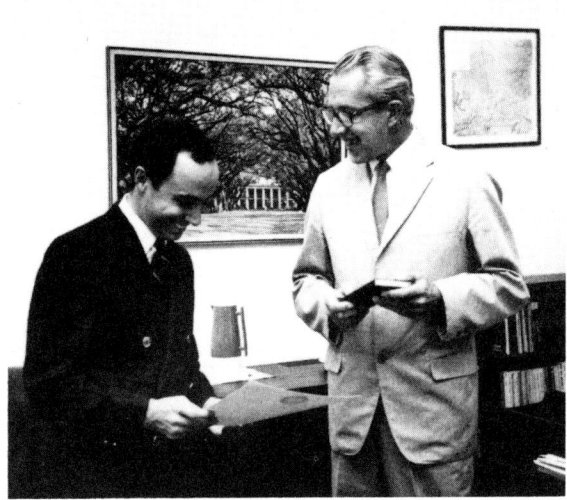

FIGURE 31. Ambassador G. Edward Clark *(right)* presenting the Meritorious Honor Award and Medal of the United States Agency for International Development to Dr. Imperato *(left)*.

pet rooster and his harem of African hens who kept the yard clean of insects. The battle against the insects never ended as long as I used insecticides and at night hundreds of millipedes would enter the house and crawl all over the floor and walls. Ahmadou suggested we put chickens in the yard and a week after they were there virtually all of the millipedes disappeared and never returned.

Meals were prepared by Ahmadou whose culinary expertise was a reflection of the lessons he received from his former employer, Mrs. Patty Baker, who was one of the best cooks in Bamako. He worked out of a small kitchen where he literally cooked himself over the stove in the blast furnace heat. But Ahmadou was a stoic and there was never a complaint. What his meals lacked in quality were made up for in quantity. If a soup were made one day then enough was boiled up to last for a week and if I complained about eating it for several days in a row then I was told that it would spoil and go to waste.

Whenever guests came to dinner Ahmadou was unassailable as a dignified butler buttoned up in my well worn white hospital uniforms. The red lettering bearing my name was never removed from the jackets.

"It shows I work for you," said Ahmadou with a burst of pride. When he appeared behind a tray of drinks wearing a broad white toothed smile, you almost expected a stethoscope to fall out of his pocket. Inconsistent with this intern look were the buttons from Woolworth's which Ahmadou enjoyed attaching to the lapels, Black Power, Don't Bug Me, Apollo 11 and Drive Carefully Doctor Barnard Is Waiting. Drinks were served with Ahmadou's size nine feet squeezed into my discarded eight and a half shoes, but by the time the desert came around the size nine feet were out of the shoes and stockings and comfortably wiggling in size nine and a half sandals.

Ahmadou looked fifteen years younger than his thirty six years, a well groomed person with a perpetual smile and tranquil expression. He was a meditative person, observant and sensitive and there was nothing which escaped his notice. Although I would have preferred that he prepare better meals and take better care of the house I am a realist and resigned early on to accept him as he was. Since the first day he smiled his way through the front gate, the others accepted his position as a combination major domo, translator and intermediary for the group. He functioned in those capacities for four years and there was never any great disharmony in the household. On the surface, he looks dignified and calm, a collection of reserve, but in reality he is full of fun and spirit and adds a stroke of liveliness wherever he is.

Ahmadou's goal in life was to be an important person, someone people will know and respect. In this there was no arrogant striving towards superiority nor even a tinge of vanity. It was humble desire to remold his world in Islamic greatness and perfection which in a sense was an obligation and a birth right since he came from a family of marabouts. He had a grand manner about him whenever he spoke about this and could philosophize his mission in life soundly and originally in the context of Islamic fatalism. He saw his ultimate role in the future as a man who prays in the purity of the mosque and whose thoughts are always about God. This made him aware of his apartness from others but there was never an intimation of condescension. His relation to the whole never suffered even though there was a conscious awareness of separateness. I think that this was because as a human being he was kind and considerate and thoroughly happy, devoid of vanity and pride.

Ahmadou's strivings in life were far too unlimited for him to remain a part of the quiet tranquility of his bush village of Boussin forever. At an early age, he went off to the town of Segou where he worked at being a driver's apprentice. Then he went to Bamako where he

A LIFE AT HOME 229

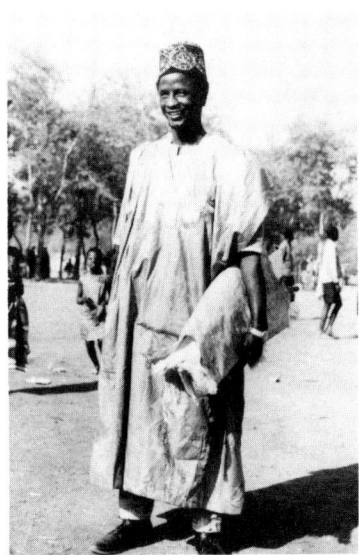

FIGURE 32. Ahmadou Sanogo dressed in his grand boubou and holding his sheep's skin prayer rug on the Moslem feast of Ramadan.

worked as a porter in the main market, carrying groceries for European women. Finally, he obtained a position as a servant in the Nigerian embassy and from there went to work for a French family who took him to Bordeaux with them for two years. Ahmadou was bright and willing to learn and under the tutoring of his various employers became a domestic servant of great skill and poise. When he returned to Bamako he went to work for Bob and Patty Baker and when they left Bamako, Ahmadou came to work for me.

His marriage to his wife was an arranged affair between parents and were if not for his deeply rooted trust in the traditions of his tribe and his faith in their value he probably would have refused. Amineta was a shy woman with a delicately shaped face and fine hands. Her complexion was light and her eyes full of modesty. Her form was slender and dignified and when she walked she had the air of someone deeply lost in thought. She was an intensely serious human being whose somberness was in clashing conflict with Ahmadou's gay and adventurous flair.

The pride of Ahmadou's life was his first born son Lassana. He had his mother's light complexion and his father's face and had he lived he would have been a handsome man. He was barely two years old when a measles epidemic came to Boussin. When Lassana died of measles Ahmadou's whole world came to an end. He wrapped his son's burning body in a white sheet and with his eyes blinded by tears carried him to the edge of the village and placed him in the small grave which the other men of the family had dug. His wife wailed and moaned and wept in the dark solitude of their mud house and the lament went on night and day for longer than anyone could remember.

In the years Ahmadou was with me, he often handled the boxes of measles vaccine which I kept in the freezer. He always gave them a hesitant and sensitive look and although I never asked him what he was thinking about, I suspected what it was. One day he brought in a bottle of the vaccine and put it down on the table in front of me. He looked at the bottle and gave a deep sigh. He looked up at me and said, "If my Lassana had gotten that he would never be dead." More than anything else in the world Ahmadou wanted another son. Since Lassana's death, Amineta had had a girl, Djeneba, but in Ahmadou's world little girls didn't count. The Bambara say that when a man who has sons dies then he is dead, but that when a man dies without sons then he is dead forever.

During the time Ahmadou worked for me, he suffered a terrible miscarriage of justice in my defense. One warm Saturday as he was preparing lunch a woman walked into the yard. From my bedroom where I was lying down I heard the footsteps on the gravel path and thought it to be a peddler. But then the footsteps came around the side of the house where no one had any business to be.

"Where are you going," asked Ahmadou in Bambara.

"Is the master home?" said the woman.

Ahmadou didn't answer her question. He posed another. "What do you want with him?"

Next I heard footsteps on the stoop and then the door opening. Ahmadou's feet raced across the veranda. There were shouts and scuffling and by the time I reached the veranda the woman was back on the gravel again. My initial reaction was, "Is she crazy?"

"No" Ahmadou said with surprising composure. "She's a prostitute out after white men."

The woman was poorly dressed and rather ugly, but full of a graceless vitality to execute her mischievous errand. With much shouting we chased her from the yard and watched her roam down the street and into the yards of several neighbors. An hour later she returned, having been turned out in every home and full of vengeance at having been thrown out started shouting that we had beaten her and caused her to abort her three month pregnancy in a ditch down the road. This fanciful lie was aimed at intimidating me to pay her off with money. An interested crowd gathered around her and for their benefit she embellished the story with all sorts of interesting details. The final version was that I had personally kicked her in the stomach.

I told Ahmadou to fetch a policeman never thinking that in doing so I was inviting trouble for both him and myself. The woman was taken off to the police station and locked up for disorderly conduct and we thought the matter closed. But later in the evening a policeman came to the house to say that Ahmadou was wanted for questioning at the police station. There he was arrested by order of the chief sergeant and charged with an act of violence. When Ahmadou didn't return to the house by midnight I went to the police station myself and learned of his arrest. The policemen who were convinced of his innocence did not lock him up as they had been instructed to do, but let him sit out in the yard with them. They told me that the sergeant had ordered his arrest in the afternoon but that they had delayed, hoping that he would forget the affair. But in the evening he returned and learning that Ahmadou was free had sent them to fetch him. The woman, they said, had been released by the sergeant. She was from the same tribal group as he and had rendered the sergeant some of her professional services.

This disgusting affair now took a turn for the worse. The following day the sergeant ordered Ahmadou locked up in a tiny cell with six other prisoners. Ahmadou later explained to me that the cell had only enough room for everyone to stand in. There was a tiny window in the door which let in a small stream of light and air. When I got to the police station with Djigui I found the sergeant there. He was a stupid brute, opinionated and proud and Djigui told me that there was no use in trying to reason with him. Djigui knew the man and said that he had been transferred from every post in which he had served because he was rash and cruel. But my inclination was to explain the affair as it had happened. It turned out to be a waste of time. He even threatened to arrest me, which was an arrogant bluff for it would have ended very badly for him if he had, and he knew it.

"The woman had a miscarriage," he said, "I saw the blood flowing down her leg." He then said he had sent her to the hospital for treatment. Though the policemen told me this was a lie I decided to check the hospital records just the same. I found that the woman had never been there. In fact not a single miscarriage case had entered the hospital the entire weekend. When I presented the sergeant with this information he became furious. He knew he was wrong and trapped because a foreigner had gotten involved in the case, something he hadn't foreseen. I wondered to myself how many innocent people had been arrested by this man and sentenced to prison terms because of his perjured testimony.

Because the following day was a holiday, I could not get to see the captain in charge of this police station. Quite by accident, I learned that his cousin was the chief sanitary engineer of the Ministry of Health who worked with us at the Service d'Hygiene in Bamako. I explained the story to him and he very kindly went off to see his cousin the captain who was out on his plantation near Bamako. When I met the captain at the police station the following morning he said, "There has been a terrible miscarriage of justice in this case. The one who is free should have been locked up and the person locked up should be free."

He summoned the chief sergeant before me and asked him to explain his conduct in the case. Under the cross examination, the sergeant's arrogance turned to wood. His defense was a series of monstrous lies in which he placed all of the blame on the policemen, saying that they had lied about facts of the case. It all ended with the sergeant being given an ultimatum to find the woman within a week. Ahmadou was released and the sergeant like a chamelion threw himself on his mercy and asked Ahmadou to help him find the woman. Eventually, Ahmadou found the woman in the market at Medina-Coura and brought her back to the police station where she was given a month of hard labor.

Behind Ahmadou came Brahima the gardener whom I first met in the front yard where he remained throughout the years. His vocabulary was limited to three expressions, ca va, oui patron and bon jour. He was definitely an outside man, an absolute disaster inside. Whenever he had to appear before me for an important request, he went to Ahmadou and memorized his lines behind the house. Ahmadou's French syntax was faithfully parroted, with a few forgotten words left out here and there. If Brahima were reproached for carelessness or for sitting for too many hours on the log in front of the house he got back into my good graces by presenting me with a gift. Occasionally, these ceremonies were graced by the presence of his wife who once handed me a dozen eggs and in the process dropped them on the living room rug. Although Brahima invested a fortune in water and tenacity into the garden, he was never able to get any flowers to grow because there were too many trees on the property. "Cut them down," I foolishly said, but he wisely retorted, "Aye, nkossobe, tle be diou kouyabi." And he was right because without the trees the house would have been an oven. The trees remained, giving their comfortable shade and flowers never bloomed. But in their place were a twisted jungle of leafy arrangements which Brahima watered all day long in the dry season. There was never an end to the sweeping up of the debris of leaves, pods and bark which fell from the trees in an unbelievable amount. The rest of the time Brahima spent washing my two ton Dodge crew cab truck and going on errands for Ahmadou who gave him a weekly dose of antimalaria medicine and saved his money for him in a big Mauritanian chest which stood in the living room.

Brahima was asked to come into the house and help out once and a while and where Ahmadou performed a job with grace and the exactness of a craftsman, Brahima was a chain reaction of turned over lamps, broken dishes, slammed doors and general disaster. I once asked Ahmadou if Brahima were dumb and he said, "Ah no, Brahima not dumb; he only very quiet," which wasn't an answer to my question.

Camera came with the house and was on the embassys' payroll. He had fought in the First World War in France at Verdun and on independence day wore his French army decorations on an old worn-out rain coat. He never won his war with somnolence in spite of many good resolutions. I discovered how soundly he slept one night when I was forced to break through two locks and a screen door since I had forgotten my keys. All of the dogs in the neighborhood reacted to the banging but Camera slept on. The only week Camera remained awake was the time the embassy was firing sleeping watchmen. I never thought he would survive the purge, but he did and afterwards Ahmadou confided to me, "Camera not so dumb. He bought little pills in the market which keep you awake and make you feel happy too."

All of the servants were Moslem but Camera belonged to a minority sect called the *Wahabia* who pray with their arms in a semi-folded position. Camera was liked and respected by the others as a person, but they disliked the way he prayed, saying that the Wahabia prayed for money which was a bad thing. Prayer time found Camera on a goat skin in front of the house, Brahima on a flattened out piece of cardboard in the garage and Ahmadou on the veranda or else on the living room rug. In later years, Ahmadou prayed on a sheep's skin he had taken from *Albert*. Albert was a sheep who had been presented to me at Walado, near Lake Debo, by the Peul Chiefs. Mark La Pointe and

I took him with us to Bamako where he lived in my backyard for several weeks. Later as he became accustomed to his new surroundings we let him roam out on the road. He got to recognize my truck and would come racing down the road after it whenever I returned to the house. Unfortunately, Albert made unbearable noises in the morning and created a terrible odor and after much soul searching I told Ahmadou he would have to go. Ahmadou and Brahima killed Albert in the back yard after the Moslem fashion which sanctified the deed and made it acceptable to us all.

The collection of discarded possessions was a highly competitive business in the house in which Ahmadou was the undisputed champion. His single room in the Bolibana quarter was a shrine of old objects. It was a small place, half of it taken up by a large table piled high with old medical magazines, newspapers and empty food cans. It was into this room that the broken phonograph player went, the faded curtains and the torn airline luggage. Ahmadou collected all of the drug company announcements which formed stacks on his table. "There must be a lot of paper in America," he once said as he carried in the sack of recently arrived mail. Whenever I asked Ahmadou why he kept all of this reading material he said it was for his friends to look at when they came to visit. Ahmadou couldn't read or write, but I did teach him some of the letters of the alphabet. Later he learned to read and write in Arabic which for him was more important since it is the language of Islam. He judged the quality of journals on the basis of the numbers of photographs they had and so medical journals were rated very poorly and *Paris Match* and *Life* highly.

The daily routine of the house included the visits of several mask dealers, known in Bamako as *commercants du bois,* wood dealers. The wood merchants were in the habit of coming to the house at meal time when they were sure I was home. I discovered early on that while I was getting some very fine old masks I was also eating cold meals. And so I struck on the idea of teaching the field to Ahmadou who after an apprenticeship of six months was able to judge authenticity and age in a mask. He then dealt with the traders, triaged the material in the yard and passed judgement on it. The fakes were sent away and only those objects he was certain of were taken across the threshold into the house. If an object interested me Ahmadou would bargain for it while serving a meal, walking to and from the kitchen into the dining room, carrying a tray of food while shouting prices to the trader out in the front. Ahmadou was able to obtain masks at prices lower than I could ever have hoped for. Over the years, I got to know all of the commercants du bois as did Ahmadou and often they would simply come by and talk with Ahmadou through the kitchen window. They admitted to him that there wasn't another European in Mali who knew the wood as well as I, an admission they would never have made to me.

The visits of my friends to the house were always very happy events and the servants knew it. Whenever I returned to Bamako from the bush it was always with a soul starving for news and intellectual stimulation. The visitors brought all of this with them and in return heard the tales of a wayfarer who had traveled through far away places and seen unusual things. To many, the house owed its charm to the African art collection which graced the walls and to its being the only stationary part of a great wanderer's life. In spite of its being un-lived in for long periods of time, it remained comfortable and unchanged. They had been in Bamako longing to get away into the bush, and I returned to my house longing for the comfort of clean sheets and a hard bed and the cool atmosphere of a high, well-ventilated parlor. While they dwelled upon their entrapment in Bamako, I sat by a campfire at night meditating on the joys of being back in Bamako. They often came even when I was away to see if all were well with the servants and Sonja Pate would send flowers and a baked cake over the mornings of my return from the bush.

Lew Pate was the director of the United States Information Service in Mali. He had spent many years in the jungles of Thailand, Laos and Viet Nam and was an avid collector of African art. Lew and Sonja loved southeast Asia and in later years they returned there. There was never an air of formality to our visits to one another's homes and we wandered in and out as steadfast as the orbit of a star. Our visits always troubled my Russian neighbor who was the Tass agent in Mali. He was convinced that both Lew and I worked for the CIA, a mistaken belief which prompted him to try and enter my house on several occasions under various pretexts. Ahmadou never allowed him in, I having told him that the man might plant a listening device in the house. Although the Russian lived only a few feet away we never spoke to one another. Once at a diplomatic reception he gathered up the courage to say to Lew, "Why are you always going to Dr. Imperato's house?"

"We have a common interest in African art," Lew replied without reflection and this only increased the Russian's suspicions all the more.

The Russian had a stamp of cleanliness on him which was surface deep, but beneath it was a deep rooted and well trained deviousness.

His conspiratorial mind was blind to the possibility that anyone might believe, think or act differently from himself. Once he invited Lew and Sonja to his home for lunch and tried to drench them with vodka and to provoke them into saying uncomplimentary things about Mali. But Lew and Sonja were temperate in drinking and discreet in their remarks, perceptive enough also to see the tape recorder playing behind a piece of furniture.

One day Lew came up with the idea of producing a film of the vaccination program using a Bambara minstrel as the chief character. A film had already been made two years before called, *Fighting Epidemic Disease in Mali* and it had been a success all over Africa. But Lew thought that a bard playing a *kora,* a twenty one string lute, and singing traditional songs could induce people to be vaccinated, especially in the Bambara country where we were then working. It sounded like an exciting idea and so I asked Badirou Sekou, the minstrel who gave me my kora lessons on Sunday mornings, to take the role. He was the leading minstrel in Mali and as far as he was concerned my house was a second home. Everything in it to which he took a fancy was his, but he was self-restrained in exercising his prerogative as a member of the bard caste where a foreigner was concerned. It is said that the bards have no shame for they will say anything and ask for anything. It is their accepted role in Bambara and Malinke society. But they are also the guardians of oral tradition and history, the makers of men's reputations and the intermediaries in disputes. It was outside of Badirou Sekou's usual role to teach a foreigner to play the kora but he came regularly on Sunday mornings whenever I was in Bamako and taught me to play several traditional songs.

In order to produce this film, Lew sent for Ed Hunter who came out from Washington, D.C., bringing George Bracher, a cameraman from Dakar, with him. Both of them had been to Mali two years before to produce the first film. Ed Hunter was an unusual man who was always deeply regretted by his friends whenever he departed and so much beloved and admired wherever he went. He would have cut the figure of a humanitarian in any age with his generosity, understanding and sympathy. The unique instinctive attachment which Ed Hunter felt towards other human beings had in the eyes of many brought him much grief in a world where concern was scorned as a fault and not praised as a virtue. But in Africa he was a noble pioneer, much admired by the Africans whose road had not parted from his, whose lives he always changed into a close comfortable corner of the world. He was an accomplished producer and director who executed his work with graceful calmness, free of that disturbing temperamentality factor so common to those of his profession. But he was a fine artist who in a calm and almost silent way captured the beauty and meaning of his subjects in the most telling way. I drove out with him to the north of Bamako in search of a site for the shooting of the film. It was a pleasant drive through the rain rejuvenated hills of the Beledougou during which we discussed the profound problems of life. Ed selected a beautiful setting for this film, the village of Sogoninikenye, which stood atop a majestic mountain overlooking a vally full of green pastures and smaller hills. He called the film *The Ballad of the Vaccinators* and it was full of gracefullness and serenity.

Meir and Marli Shamir were frequent visitors to my house. Meir was the Israeli Ambassador to Mali and his wife was an accomplished photographer intensely interested in Mali's culture. To me Meir Shamir was a kind of ideal, an adroit diplomat, a Renaissance man, responsive to all of the subtleties of art, music, history, and psychology and a man of great wisdom who could reason the predicaments and crises of the political world down to a logical conclusion. As the representative of Israel in Mali, he stood in a Moslem country where Arab presence and pressures were visible and strong. But Meir's soothing diplomacy and personal courage were an effective foil to the Arab ambassadors' frantic and nervous pressures on the Malians. He was a calm man who spoke with a measured baratone voice and engendered respect among those who heard his scholarly ideas. It was always a wonderful delight for me to discuss the happenings of the world with Meir for although he was naturally partisan to his own country he was virtually free of prejudices and would decipher out the motives and predict the future decisions of those who were making history on the world scene.

His wife Marli was a very close friend who worked with me on several of my ethnographic studies. The meaning of the country sank into one's soul on looking at her photographs for they conveyed the moods of the land and the people in an exquisitely beautiful way. She was a marvellous traveling companion who never complained of the dust and heat and the rough drives through the iron gray plains and valleys of northern Mali. She added those extra touches of refinement which my bush expeditions lacked and the staff always enjoyed her presence, behaving with the impeccable manners they knew a woman's presence demanded.

While I was working in the Dogon country, Marli came with me into the far off rocky mountains of Hombori where villages stand like rocky fortresses out in the wilderness. There is a strong atmosphere of fantasy about Hombori, for the place sits at the bottom of a great chain of giant ochre colored mesas, which stand scattered across a white sandy plain. They are overpowering monuments, three thousand feet tall. Few people visit them for it is so difficult to reach the place. I recall that it took us nine hours to cover the last ninety miles into Hombori, but once we were there it was a beautiful experience. The black vault of the nocturnal sky with its changing array of constellations swung back over our heads behind the towering cliffs as we sat out and ate one of Marli's delicious meals. Below us the moon flooded the white sands with an eerie light and the firewood burned like incense sending up smoke and sparks into the cool air. Marli caught the spirit of Hombori with her cameras as no one else I know.

Behind the domestic tranquility, and the three faces of my servants, stood an aggravating and nightmarish succession of boys and cooks

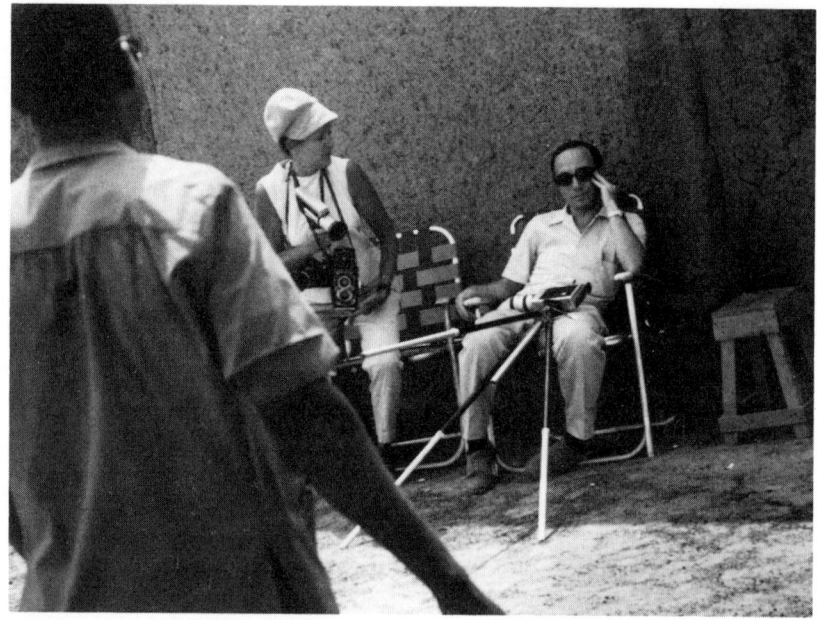

FIGURE 33. Marli Shamir *(left)* on one of her filming expeditions into the Malian bush urging a tired Dr. Imperato to help her start the next project. Djigui Diakite stands in the foreground. This was a surprise photograph taken by Modibo Keita during a trip into southern Mali.

and months of domestic turmoil. That trail of experience with Malian servants began with Dramaine who sold himself to me on the merit of his having worked for Americans. I think that in Dramaine's eyes all Americans weer credulous and kind even when being cheated. He was at my door asking for a job the morning after my arrival, fully aware I was an American. Dramaine pulled out a patinated bundle of reference letters whose quantity spoke for frequent displacement which should have aroused my suspicions. Not knowing any better, I saw nothing but excellence in the abstract qualities described, neat, cooperative, satsifactory and polite. Only later did I learn that the unwritten code in Bamako is that a fired servant is never given a damaging reference which will prevent him for getting another job.

Dramaine proved to be all the things the letters said he was, but it was what the letters didn't say which led to his departure. I was busy at the time getting the mass vaccination program started and was willing to let Dramaine run the house. Dramaine's four children were frequent visitors and grew healthy and plump on choice items from the storeroom, powdered milk, peach halves, diced pineapples, beef stew, sugar, rice, flour and cookies. They all disappeared at an amazing rate and I began wondering about the cause of this huge food consumption. Not all of the stolen items went into giving the Dramaine children pep and energy, but off to the market at Medina Coura where at five in the evening you can with luck retrieve stolen items. I might have overlooked the Dramaine children's eating my diced pineapples and peach halves, but selling the grocries on the black market was another matter.

It dawned on me also that I was paying five times as much for locally purchased items as everyone else in the Quartier Fleuve, except of course those who had Dramaines working for them. While the children came to eat in the unlocked storeroom, Dramaine padded the bills. Inevitably Dramaine was caught. One morning I woke at six instead of at seven and looked through the shutters just in time to see Dramaine making a pre-dawn foray into a freezer which served as a communal embassy depot in the courtyard. Three frozen Beltsville turkeys went into the box on the back of the bicycle and for this Dramaine earned another letter of recommendation.

The next boy came to me with an avalanche of praises from his former employers and taught me the lesson of taking someone else's judgement with caution. Camara was described as being scrupulously honest, faithful, polite, considerate and so devoted he would lay down his life on your behalf. He had worked for an American couple for a year and a half during which time he enjoyed both their confidence and their storeroom. Unlike Dramaine he didn't waste his time with the small time canned goods probably because he didn't have any children to feed. He concentrated on high priced easy to sell items like beer and whiskey. As I later discovered, he also went in for fancy clothing and divested me of the trousers of three of my best suits. My absence in the bush for long periods of time and the unlocked storeroom were just the right combination of circumstances to help Camara along. Whereas Dramaine's departure was calm and quiet, Camara's was a storm of shouts and threats in the presence of friends. Like so many of the vaccinators, he chose indignancy as his defense when accused. There was a firm denial and then a bluffer's threat to take me to court for defamation of character. He was the only servant for whom I refused to write a letter.

Guindo was efficient and honest, but fancied himself the best cook in Mali. When I suggested he spend some time in Mrs. Baker's kitchen, he refused saying she could learn from him. He was a Dogon and like so many of those people had a far away look about him and was given to long periods of brooding and outbursts of rage. In spite of the high opinion he had of himself, he did present some guests with an empty soup bowl when they asked for seconds and brought out an unopened can of peas after serving the meat. When I reprimanded him he pointed out that none of these mistakes were as bad as Camara serving peaches smothered with ice cubes instead of ice cream.

Guindo came into my employ in a storm of controversy since he had already agreed to work for a highly emotional woman. Because the idea of working for a woman didn't appeal to him he sought me out when he heard through the other boys that I was looking for someone. Guindo hadn't been in the house for more than an hour when the telephone rang and the excited voice on the other end screamed, "You stole my cook." There was no calming her and when I said I wouldn't buy back his uniforms since I had plenty of intern outfits on hand she hung up.

Guindo was sent over to her house to explain himself and to get released from her employ. There was a protest about her being mean, which she was, and a complaint about being too sick to go and to prove the latter Guindo fell to the floor and put on an hysterical seizure which would have bettered anything Sarah Bernhardt could have done. When he finally got to her door he stammered out, "I'm sick," and she being a mild hypochondriac by nature wouldn't let him in. Their conversation was carried on through a locked screen door and when her own boy shook Guindo's hand she ordered him to wash it off since as she put it, "He is full of microbes."

A lot of thinking went on in Guindo's head on the way back to the house and although he didn't know what microbes were he had at least figured out they were something bad and that his good name had been slandered. "I'm going to have her called before the Minister of Health. I'll sue her in court." It took several days to calm Guindo down, and in the end the matter was put to rest. Had I been left to myself I would have put up with Guindo's temperamental behavior and been philosophic about his self-esteem. But American women were oblivious to nothing and they insisted Guindo had to go. When defects of personality and character didn't move me they pointed out his physical shortcomings and produced a negative judgement from Mrs. Baker's culinary court. They said he had a face like an Easter Island Figure, and who could eat a meal at my house with an Eastern Island Figure serving.

The pressures for him to go mounted and I started looking for an excuse to fire him. It came the week he accidentally burned his finger on the stove in the kitchen. The injury was minor and I treated it myself. But Guindo insisted on going to the local dispensary. When he finally returned to the house five days later, he was completely healed. He said the infirmier had ordered him to rest and knowing Guindo as I did it was obvious that was the reason he went to the dispensary in the first place. When I took issue with him about his taking leave without my consent he stormed off to the dispensary and complained to the infirmier in question that I had said he had no authority to recommend sick leave. That wasn't of course what I had said and it put the infirmier up in arms against me. Guindo received a good letter of recommendation.

If ever I were tempted to complain about the servants who finally stayed with me I looked back to those early hectic months of domestic turmoil and realized how lucky I was. Brahima may have spent too many hours on the log out front; Ahmadou's pranks and Camera's sleeping got excessive at times and there may have been too much lively conversation and rippling laughter in the yard. But all of this was worth the devotion and honesty they brought along with them into the house.

Their families used to visit me in the quiet of a Sunday afternoon when little feet experienced for the first time the sensation of a carpeted floor and hesitant hands rubbed the soft cushions of the big sofa. When the children first came it was with that enormous power of imagination which only children can have. Whenever I spoke to them in Bambara they never answered, just stared at me with those infinitely patient faces and steady eyes. They were so quiet you could hear them breathe and detect the soft shuffle of their feet on the floor. They calmed their fears by keeping in physical touch with those they knew, with the shoulder of a sibling, with their mother's voluminous bou bou. I don't know what they thought of me when they first saw me but it must have been like meeting some friendly, kind and yet powerful being of whom they didn't know what to expect next. Packed inside of their minds were all of the good things their fathers had told them about me, but meeting the toubabou ke face to face for the first time created that dilemma which stems from the possession of foreknowledge and the lack of direct personal experience. When I finally got to know them, they would fill the house with ripples of laughter and brave to ask me questions and touch me.

The wives were as shy as the children, hiding their anxiety behind a screen of nervous giggles, turning their heads away with a gentle sweeping motion, their chins pivoted on their fisted hands. They ventured to cast a curious eye around the room but if they thought they were being watched their look darted to the floor. It took many months before the monosyllabic responses were transformed into a gentle flow of relaxed Bambara conversation. The atmosphere never became so animated nor so electrified that you craved a few seconds of silence, but gone was the uncomfortable subjective sense of making forced conversation.

I used to talk to Ahmadou about the time when I would no longer be in Mali and then suddenly he would become shrouded in an uncomfortable silence. But that silence didn't mean that he didn't have anything to say. Deep down all of them hoped and prayed that I would never leave, that somehow as some given moment a koranic miracle would take place and all the good genies from Kangaba to Gao in concert with God would arrange things so that their prayers would be answered. But they allowed for the possibility that the good genies would fail and faced that potential failure with that admirable sense of calm which Africans so often face profound changes in their lives. There was a dread fear of that final day when we would all go to the airport and only I wouldn't return. It would be an experience filled with a frightening finality as life's conclusive moments always are. Each of us would go down a different path in life and never meet again, but we would all take away with us the same warm memories which would in a unique way give us a common bond for the rest of our lives.

Chapter XV

The Song of the Minstrel

Our two years of hard work in the inland delta of the Niger virtually eradicated smallpox from Mali. It seemed incredible to many that such a momentous consequence should have come from only two years of work because health officials had been vaccinating people for years in the country and still the disease continued unchecked. We had immunized those people among whom the disease was entrenched and in doing so eliminated it. Even though we had no cases of the disease after vaccinating half of the country's population, we still had to vaccinate the remainder of the population. But by comparison to the inland delta these regions posed no great challenge to men who had come through the campaign in the inland delta.

It was just as well that the critical phase of the battle against smallpox was over for more serious upheavals and disease disasters now descended on the Malians. The diseases came with an almost ruthless brutality, totally unexpected and carried off thousands in their wake. All of the schemes for prevention and control which were eventually carried out did not lessen the hardship of those days. Yet the Moslem faith was strong and the Malians had a comforting sense of destiny. If they could, they would have bargained with fate, but they never became aroused when fate had its way. Behind it all they saw the workings of magic, seeking revenge, harvesting satisfaction through the infliction of death.

The political upheaval was also unexpected, but no violent alarm accompanied its happening. It ushered in days of joy and celebrations during which people sang and danced in the streets, more eager for the freedom it brought than for the blood of their former oppressors. It took place on a cool clear day in November as one of those dramatic events through which history accents its steady course. The president had gone to Mopti for the annual regional economic conference, taking with him a delegation of ministers and officials. While he maintained a veneer of popular participation in government through meetings and rallys, whatever democratic institutions Mali once had were by this time gone. He was a virtual autocrat, surrounded by pandering advisors and ministers who helped maintain his cult of personality. Had the coup d' etat removed the head of a democratic regime it would have been lacking in that dramatic quality which accompanied Modibo Keita's fall. As it was he was the government, the state, his will the supreme law,

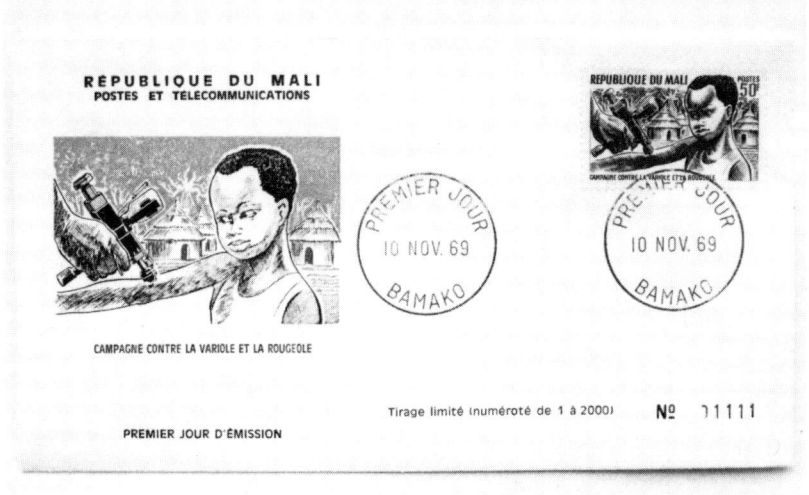

FIGURE 34. The first day cover of the fifty franc stamp issued by the Republic of Mali to commemorate the Smallpox Eradication-Measles Controls Program. The stamp was designed in France from a photograph taken by Dr. Imperato.

and when he toppled, all of the institutions he had created came crashing down with him. The Malian nation as it had existed from its birth was swept away and in its wake there came a frightening vacuum.

On the 17th of November, Modibo Keita boarded the *General Soumare* in Mopti. Most of the town was turned out to see him off, crowding the dock and streets which lay just below Henri Simone's semi-collapsed house. André and Resey Szabo watched the boat pull away from the shore and saw the president waving from the upper deck to a rather silent crowd. He was a very tall man, dressed in a brown Mao suit. He had handsome features and a pompous bearing and it was said that many trembled in his presence. I, myself, never met him; I only saw him from afar when he rode in his last May day parade in an open car down the Avenue de l'Independence. The people didn't applaud him, by then they could not bring themselves to do even that. But he looked straight ahead and waved as if a tumultuous crowd were greeting him.

It was dusk when the *General Soumare* glided up against the strong downstream flow of the Niger and headed for Segou. The president retired to one of the two deluxe cabins on the ship. They are comfortable cabins, with gray wall to wall carpeting, air conditioners, refrigerators and private baths. With him was his first wife, a proud and articulate woman who was very active in the political life of the country. She ruled over Mali next to the president with the majesty and confidence of a regal dowager queen. The rest of the boat was full of officials from Bamako and they sat out on the breezy open decks in clusters talking in hushed voices until the moon rose high over the river.

By sunrise, the boat reached the canal which bypasses the great dam and bridge at Markala and from there it steamed on into the broadened river in front of Segou. The officials of the political party in Segou had worked for days preparing a rousing welcome for the president, and as the boat edged its way into the dock, a great roar rose up and echoed out over the river. "Modibo, Modibo, Modibo," they shouted over and over again. Whereas Mopti had been silent, Segou roared with voices paid for by the political party. Soldiers from the Segou garrison were drawn up at attention on the dock and a line of obsequious officials, dressed in flowing finery of embroidered satin, lined the gangway as the president descended. It was unimaginable then to think that Modibo Keita would see the next sunrise from the inside of a prison cell.

As Modibo Keita was leaving Mopti, Mark LaPointe and I drove down to Bamako from San. We had spent a week in the hills along the Upper Volta frontier looking for signs of smallpox in company with Tom Leonard and Dr. David Vastine who worked out of Ouagadougou, the captial of Upper Volta, and Dr. Jean-Claude Latouche, the chief of the mobile medical service of this part of Upper Volta. On the 16th of November, we crossed over into Mali from Upper Volta on a remote mountain trail and fell on a group of villagers clearing a trail. "Modibo, Modibo, Modibo," they shouted in unison while clapping their hands as we passed. Even in so remote a place as this Modibo Keita was a god.

Mark and I had wanted to go up to Mopti on the 17th, but when we arrived at Tominian we learned that the road was blocked by the militia as a security precaution. So we had no choice but to go back down to Bamako. All the way to the capital the road was heavily guarded by militiamen who subjected us to an intensive search at every major town and village. It was the first time that we had ever been searched and we viewed it as a sign that things were going from bad to worse. We arrived in Bamako late in the evening and found that preparations were underway to welcome the president back on the 19th.

Up in Segou, a large political rally was held and the whole town was brought out in regimented groups to acclaim the "enlightened guide" as he then preferred to be called. They paraded him down the main street, beneath the cool shadows of the caicedrat trees where so long before I had watched the rain fall in a light drizzle on a quiet day. The town was hung with flags and banners splashed with slogans and photographs and filled with the roar of thirty thousand people. Sitting on the top of his pinnacle of power and glory did not so narcotize Modibo Keita that he was oblivious to the security of his regime. Up in Mopti, he had left Madeira Keita, his Minister of Justice and a doctrinaire Marxist along with a loyal regiment of troops and militia. Far to the northeast on the fringes of the Sahara in Kidal was Captain Diby Silas Diarra and a quarter of the Malian army. Diarra, a spit and polish soldier, was renowned for his cruel efficiency and thoroughness as an administrator and his harshness as a judge.

It was he who had finally crushed the Tuareg rebellion in 1963, with a ruthlessness which made even the hardest of Malians cringe. The Tuaregs have never been dainty opponents and their victories over the black soldiers were spelled out with mutilations and gore. Because the Tuareg consider themselves white, it was as much a race war as a political struggle. Then Modibo Keita put Diby Silas Diarra in charge and the trend of events changed. He repaid brutality with brutality, two eyes for one, napalm for guns and tanks for camels. Never did it slip into the world this micro-revolt in far away Mali, but to those who were there it was the country's parochial issue of the day. Once the revolt was crushed, Diarra launched his pacification program which included the organized and planned Bambarization of Kidal. He held power of life and death over everyone in Kidal and Modibo Keita sent his political prisoners up to him. The rigors of the sub-Saharan climate and forced labor provided ready explanations for the high mortality rate among the prisoners. The most famous of these prisoners, Fily Dabo Cissoko, was the leader of the short-lived opposition party. He was sent to Kidal and afterwards was conveniently moved out into the wilderness near Tin Essako close to the Algerian frontier. It was announced that he was accidentally killed during an ambush by Tuareg rebels, but it is now known that he was summarily shot on Modibo Keita's orders.

Down in Bamako, the city was guarded by regiments of militia equal to the army in strength. They were commanded by a strange and disturbed individual by the name of Diakité who was a Marxist and a man thoroughly loyal to the president. To prove this loyalty, Diakité had publicly shot one of his fingers off with his revolver in the Motel in Bamako. He was an unpleasant human being and once I had a bad run in with him in George's campement in Koutiala. He had come there to spend the night, his hand still bandaged from his loyalty demonstration. He was somber and sinister and drunk both with power and beer and spoke for most of the night in a mean and loud voice. I politely asked him if he could lower his voice since we were trying to sleep. He erupted with violence, exclaiming that this was "terre Malienne," and on it he could do as he pleased. The following morning he sat with a hangover in a large soft chair, dressed in a silken bathrobe and exhorted everyone to stand up as the commandant's flag was hoisted to the tune of taps across the road. I dared to tell him that he ought to practice what he preached, but he gave me no reply.

Seemingly, the president had nothing to fear. With the top officers of the army completely on his side, and his private militia at his back, it was unlikely that anyone would challenge his supremacy. But in spite of the recent coups in other African states, he did not measure correctly the true weight of the junior officers. On two previous occasions, they had planend to overthrow him, but nothing came of it. This time they would succeed.

Modibo Keita's revolutionary exhortations in Segou were greeted by choruses of rehearsed fidelity speeches from party officials, army officers, the militia and the children's organizations. Solidarity in speech characterized the day. From Bamako came the routine radio message from Ouloguem, the chief of security, "All is well."

All was not well, but neither Modibo Keita nor Ouloguem knew it at the time. Over in the army barracks in Kati the plan of operations for the coup d' etat were already finalized. Why had the junior officers decided to move? Certainly one could advance palpable arguments about the economic distress of the country and the deprivations of liberties, but none of this really touched the army officers who were well paid and sheltered in their comfortable camps from most of the regime's rigors which dominated life beyond the fence. But the growing menace of the militia alarmed them. It had become as large as the army and was being trained and equipped in such a way that eventually it would have been able to disarm the army, something which the soldiers now believed was part of Modibo Keita's plan for them. The militia had also become bold and reckless. Army officers were publicly searched and humiliated, a sharp blow to those who were sensitive about their dignity. But above all, they saw themselves threatened, as both individuals and as a group.

The notables escorted Modibo Keita to the boat and after all of the hand shakes had been given and all the farewells said, the boat sailed out onto the calm surface of the water, launched by the quiet waving of scores of hands. Because it had been a tiring day, the president retired to his room early.

As Modibo Keita slept on the *General Soumare,* fourteen lieutenants and captains gathered with five hundred men in Kati, twelve miles from Bamako. At midnight, they moved on Bamako in trucks, tanks and jeeps. Six cumbersome Russian tanks of World War II vintage rolled through the darkness along the almost deserted Lido road which enters the city from behind. Soldiers sped in trucks over the undulating paved road from Kati to Koulouba where they surrounded the camp of the elite presidential guard. After only a few moments of discussion, the officers of the guard joined the coup. A small contingent moved on the massive white presidential palace which fell without a shot being fired. Down below Koulouba at the back of Bamako, the garrisons of gendarmes and army troops in the sprawling camps joined the coup. Numbering close to a thousand men now, they rolled out into the town, seized the radio station, the airport and the railway yard. Then they marched on the militia camp. Although the militia outnumbered the attackers, they were no match for the army and after a brief skirmish surrendered to the soldiers. The noise of the skirmish at the militia camp was enough to alert Ouloguem who managed to send a frantic radio message to the *General Soumare*. "The army has launched a coup d'etat."

As this terrifying message fell into the ears of Modibo Keita's security aide, the army moved to arrest all of the government ministers in Bamako. Two of them managed to escape and sought refuge in the Russian embassy. Those arrested were taken to the headquarters of the Union Soudanaise, known then as the Permanance du Parti, which was but a few hundred yards from my house. Most people in Bamako slept through all of these events, but on the *General Soumare,* the president was awakened and given the news by a trembling aide. His reaction exteriorly was one of calm and he quietly told his aide to summon his advisors and other aides. By this time, Bamako was solidly in the hands of the revolting army officers. But Modibo Keita had no way of knowing this. His only source of information, Ouloguem, had himself been arrested. Although Bamako was now under the control of the junior officers, no one could tell whether the coup would succeed or not. Bamako was not Mali. Out in the rest of the country were large garrisons of troops and militia. If they remained loyal to the president, the coup would fail.

The *General Soumare's* lighted form glided through the darkness along the river, casting rippled reflections on the water. Some advised the president to turn around and return to Segou, others that they drop anchor in Nyamina which lay on the northern bank opposite them, but the president decided to sail for Koulikoro as planned. He reasoned that the militia would hold its own in Bamako and even if they didn't, the population of the city would rise up in arms in his support. It is truly amazing that Modibo Keita so misjudged the mood of his own people. Had he gone back to Segou there is a strong possibility that the coup would have either failed or else that some kind of compromise would have come out of the deadlock. For it to succeed, the army officers had to lay their hands on the president and now he decided to sail right into their laps.

At 4 A.M. the old Moslem men and women of Bamako went out to the mosques in the darkness to pray, carrying lighted kerosine lamps with them in their hands. They saw the troops and the tanks and reasoned that they were there for the welcoming celebrations for the president. Others, however, suspected that something was happening. News of this kind spreads very slowly at this hour of the morning and even after sunrise when people poured out into the streets, most did not suspect at first what was happening. The presence of soldiers around the town did not at first seem strange for they were always posted this way whenever the president returned to the capital. But the bridge over the Niger was blocked by tanks which altered many to the fact that a coup was in progress.

While I was still in bed that morning, I sensed a concentrated stillness outside the house. On a normal day I would have heard the roar of motor bikes racing down the street and the muffled chattering of children as they shuffled their way to school. But outside, everything was quiet, quieter than I had ever known Bamako to be. As was my habit, I unlatched my front door at 7 A.M. and shut off the globed light which stood atop the gate post. The street beyond the gate was deserted. I thought to myself that everyone had gone off to the Koulikoro to welcome the president back.

At 7:15 A.M., Ahmadou left his house in Bolibana and rode across town on his motor bike to my house. He passed groups of soldiers standing at the street corners and tanks and armored trucks surrounding the headquarters of the Union Soudanaise. Like many people, he thought that they were part of the welcoming ceremony for the president.

As Ahmadou served breakfast, I asked him why the street was so quiet and devoid of children.

"The president is coming back today," he said. "They have cancelled school so that they can line the road from Koulikoro." This was a plausible enough explanation, but by 8 A.M. Brahima had not come to work. He had never missed a day's work in all the years he was with me. He lived on the other side of the river and with that thought in mind I started thinking that perhaps something was happening. I asked Ahmadou if he had seen anything unusual on the streets.

"No," he said, "just some soldiers and tanks."

"You saw what?" I exclaimed. Ahmadou was thoroughly perplexed and looked at me with a blank stare. "A lot of soldiers and tanks," he answered in a calm voice. He didn't share my suspicions about a coup d'etat and went out into the yard to feed the chickens and to check on the hen who was sitting on six eggs.

"The chicks are hatching out," I heard him call out from the yard. I went out to have a look and then walked across the garden towards the gate and my truck. I had decided to have a look at things for myself. I had no sooner opened the gate than Mark LaPointe came racing up in his Volkswagon and before he had even stopped shouted, "There has been a coup."

Ahmadou looked dismayed and then he said, "Ils ont attrapé Modibo," — they have caught Modibo. It was in these terms that the majority of Malians would understand the events of that day. They knew nothing of the words coup d'etat. These were European words without meaning for them. But they knew that if a chief were caught then his power was gone, his talismans ineffective.

At 8 A.M, as Mark and I stood in the garden, the *General Soumare* steamed towards Koulikoro. Modibo Keita still had every intention of disembarking and going on to Bamako. His personal charisma had never failed in the past. Radio Mali, now in the hands of the young army officers, continued broadcasting after its usual shut down hour of 8A.M. No announcements were made, but the military conveyed the message of the overthrow in a direct manner which all Malians understood. They put Bassoumana Cissoko on the air, a blind minstrel who played a four-stringed lute. The two-fold significance of Bassoumana Cissoko's presence on the radio and the songs he chanted was not known to foreigners in Mali. He was by then a very old man, the dean of the Bambara minstrels who had refused to deform traditional songs in order to sing the praises of the president and convey political messages. Because of this, he had incurred the displeasure of the president and was rarely allowed to sing on the radio. That he should be singing on the radio after the usual broadcast hours was a message in itself. But the stronger message was in what he sang, songs prohibited by Modibo Keita, which told of the fall of chiefs, the rusting of iron, the decay of great trees, metaphores which reminded Modibo Keita of the finiteness of his power, which on this day announced to all that the president had fallen. As the minstrel of great events sang of the president's fall in indirect metaphores, the *General Soumare* dropped anchor in Koulikoro.

Since sunrise, the president and listened with fury to Bassoumana Cissoko's singing and determined that as soon as affairs were put right he would have the minstrel in prison. Before the boat landed, he summoned all the passengers and radiating great calm told them that a group of irresponsible army officers was attempting to take over the country. He reassured everyone that all would be well as soon as he got back to Bamako.

The officers had decided against arresting the president in Koulikoro. Popular reaction was unpredictable and the sight of the president being arrested might spark off an unwanted fracas requiring force to put down.

Instead they decided to arrest him on the lonely road leading out of the town. When the president descended the gangplank he was greeted by the officials of the town as if nothing had happened. Even a line of troops was drawn up as an honor guard. He and his advisors interpreted this as a sign that the rebellion had been unsuccessful. He delivered a speech and Madame Keita received a bouquet of flowers from a group of small children. Then he got into his Citroen sedan, and escorted by white-helmeted presidential guardsmen, started off for Bamako. A few minutes later the presidential convoy came to a road block out in the bush. An army lieutenant went up to the limousine and asked the president to get out. At first Modibo Keita refused, but finally he got out.

"Mr. President," said the lieutenant stiffly, "I request that you put yourself at the disposition of the army." Modibo Keita was under arrest.

The army took their prisoner to Bamako in a Russian armored truck which completely concealed him from everyone on the roadside. As the truck sped along the dirst road into the city, no one had any inkling who was inside. They passed under the tall caidedrat trees of Medina Coura and then went on towards the tree-shaded streets of the center of the city. At the party headquarters, the young captains and lieutenants waited for their prisoner to arrive. No single officer could have faced him alone and come off first in the encounter. They were nervous and tense, he calm and full of confidence. As he got out of the truck, one of them kicked him. It was meant to humiliate him, but he ignored the act and walked inside. They told him that he was no longer president and to this he replied that he would accept it if that was what the people wanted. "Go and consult the people," he told them.

They tried to force him to sign a resignation in order to add legality to their deed, but he refused. Then they threatened to parade him through the streets naked if he refused, but the threat had no effect. Finally, they took him away and said to him, "We will consult the people and you will hear what they have to say."

Modibo Keita was then searched, not for arms, but for talismans and charms, those objects which even the young army officers believed had supernatural powers to keep a man president of a country. He wore his share of these things as do most Malians, leather sacs filled with bits of herbs and bones and pieces of paper with passages from the koran written on them. Later, he was transported to an isolated portion of a military camp and locked up under heavy guard.

All of those who had been on the boat with him were taken into Bamako and held in the large hall of the political party headquarters, where they were kept for several days while the military interrogated them and decided on their fate. By noon, most of the ministers of the now defunct government were under arrest as were the members of the National Committee for the Defense of the Revolution and the superior officers of the army. Up in Mopti, Madeira Keita tried to rouse the town and launch a counter coup, but this attempt failed and later in the day he was put under arrest. Two ministers held out in the Russian embassy and the army surrounded the place, arresting them when the Russians, seeing how things were going, decided to get rid of them.

That the president and the top officials of his government were all under arrest was not known at the time to most of us. The radio kept playing the same music all morning and we sat wondering what indeed was happening. The diplomatic community buzzed with activity; ambassadors rushed about visiting other ambassadors, trying to gather whatever bits and fragments they could piece together. Rumors ran wild through the population. No one knew who was launching the coup d'etat, whether it would succeed and if it did succeed what would happen afterwards. All communication with the outside world was cut, telephone and telegraphic services suspended, the airport closed and the roads blocked. The lower portion of the town below the railway tracks was open and people circulated there if they wished, but north of the tracks where most of the key military installations lay, no one was allowed to circulate. At the Grand Hotel, four European ambassadors had been waiting for the past few days to present their letters of credence to President Keita. Now there was no president to present anything to and they were trapped in the town for many more days.

Bamako was quiet and peaceful, filled with an almost absolute silence and dramatic stillness. A great event made itself known not by any hammering noise and virile outpouring of audacious display but by silencing the movement and noise of city life. Never have I seen Bamako's streets so empty and quiet, its buildings standing like the mute hulls of a deserted town. Apprehension and fear muted the thoughts of most Malians. In one way or another, most of them had been politically active. What would happen to them now? Pragmatic hearts were not yet willing to commit themselves and so they remained silent.

At noon, the music stopped. There was an awkward pause followed up with a background noise of shuffling and shouting. Then a brusque voice said, "Venez, venez, parlez, parlez." We held our breaths. "They are going to make the president talk," we thought. But Modibo Keita's eloquent voice did not come on the air. Instead a shaky and stuttering staccato came over the air, announcing the fall of "the dictatorial regime of Modibo Keita and his lackeys." The Military Committee of National Liberation announced its name and function. It assumed all the powers of the state with Lieutenant Moussa Traore as its head. In a second of time, an unknown lieutenant had made world headlines. Who was this man and what did he stand for? No one really knew. Then the minstrel's music returned to the air, interrupted a half-hour later by announcements by one of Radio Mali's well known announcers, repeating the statement about the fall of Modibo Keita, the imposition of a curfew from 6 P.M. to 6 A.M. and the prohibition of public assembly. All of these announcements didn't rule out the possibility of a counter coup and some of Radio Mali's announcers aware of this possibility, refused to announce messages for the military. It was still to early to change colors.

The genuine possibility of the coup's failing posed a thorny problem for the newly-arrived American Ambassador, G. Edward Clark. If it did fail, then the Modibo Keita regime would almost certainly have made the United States the foreign scapegoat and severed diplomatic relations. We had to prepare for the worst possible repercussions such as the summary expulsion of Americans from the country and a physical assault on the embassy. And so, in the afternoon, we met at the embassy to discuss a plan of action for meeting all contingencies. But by sundown all was quiet, a subtle indication that the coup had succeeded. The following day confirmed this and the people of Bamako poured out into the streets shouting, "A bas Modibo, à bas le Milice, à bas Modibo, à bas le Milice." Mobs of men and women surged through the streets carrying thee ranches and hastily made banners, shouting the praises of their new heroes. Whatever anger there was, was vented against the militia more so than against the fallen president. The soldiers rounded up the militia, some of whom had fled and burned their uniforms. But they were caught and paraded through the streets barefoot and clad in their underclothes. The women and children paraded them through the city to the headquarters of the new military committee. There was no violence in this, only gross humiliation for the militiamen. Over the hills in Kati, the ex-president's jailers played the radio for his benefit. He heard the common people denounce him in the foulest terms in Bambara and the radio announcers who only a few days before sang his praises, refer to him as a despot and a tyrant.

Messages of support flowed in from the provinces, from the south and west and from the center of the country. But nothing came from

Kidal where Diby Silas Diarra announced his support for the fallen president. The military committee threatened to bomb him out if he didn't cooperate. His support was never genuine and nine months later he led an unsuccessful coup which resulted in his arrest and being sent to the salt mines at Taoudeni in the Sahara, condemned to life in prison at hard labor. For days and weeks following the coup d'etat, the country celebrated. In Bamako everyone held parades, the taximen, the horse cart drivers, the women and children, and from the bush whole villages came in with their masks and danced in front of the military's headquarters. But up in Mopti and Gao, the nomads thought that the country had dissolved and announced their independence, a notion which was rapidly corrected by the military. But throughout the land a uniform voice sang out with what pleased the hearts of the new military masters of Mali. It was a voice which had once sang out what Modibo Keita's heart had wanted to hear.

Chapter XVI
A Sorcerer's Revenge

In the weeks which followed the coup d'etat, the new regime proceeded to build up public and international credibility in its ability to run the country. At the same time, the military had to ease itself into the place of a highly charismatic national leader of international repute and this was no easy task. What did this group of young and inexperienced officers know about statecraft? Certainly very little at that time. The leader of the military junta, Lieutenant Moussa Traoré was a first among equals, chosen by the others to be the figurehead of committee rule. He was thoroughly unknown to the public and so the press notices took special care to emphasize his academic achievements and some obviously cursory training he had received in administration. But these scarcely qualified a man for being president of a country and could never have mustered national and international respect. Having power was one thing, but doing something effective with it was quite another. In order to run the country, the young officers formed a government composed of respected professional men and well known ex-ministers who had been sacked by Modibo Keita. In many ways, it was a strange alliance of forces, but for the immediate it served the purpose. It stirred just hearts to see public figures who had been disgraced by the former regime now elevated to their former rank. More importantly, they knew how to run the country and at the level of foreign affairs were skilled according to their fashion in dealing with other nations and international organizations. The ever rising popularity of Modibo Keita's former ministers and the military's gradual increase in ability and confidence led eventually to their dismissal.

The aftermath of the military coup was a euphoric rising of expectations for both a better future and the punishment of those who had made the past so miserable. It is always difficult to make adequate amends to those who have been unjustly imprisoned or to give retribution to the survivors of those who have been unjustly killed. Financially, the new government was in no position to do either, but most hoped it would at least bring the leaders of the old regime to trial and deal them a harsh sentence. Considered opinion, however, held that no such trials could ever take place because the new leaders of Mali were not untainted by the sin of close association with the old. The militia may have been monstrous, but it was the army which had trained them. Political prisoners had been jailed and executed, but it was the army which had been the jailer and executioner. The inference from these and dozens of other specifics was that public trials could never be held without the army coming out the looser in the affair. They, like all of the civil servants, had collaborated to a greater or lesser degree with the old regime.

No trials were ever held and public demands for them were calmed by explanations that inquiries were first being held. Within a year, Modibo Keita slipped quietly out of the news and out of people's thoughts and before long all demands for trials ceased. Although the military never published any reports about Modibo Keita, rumors ran rampant in Mali, dripping with the gore of human sacrifice and other deprivations at the palace. In the days following the coup, Bamako rang with tales of what had been found in the presidential palace by the military. Much of it echoed familiar passages from the *Sundiata Epic,* telling what Sundiata Keita, the Emperor of Mali, found in the palace of the sorcerer king of Sosso. People in Bamako said that a drum had been found in the palace covered with human skin and that next to it were two human arms which had been used as batons. The rumors also had it that the palace was full of jars of human fat, skeletal remains, the completely preserved bodies of young girls and albinos floating in vats of formalin. The rumors were not without their Arabian Nights refinements of magic carpets and looking-glasses. If there were any doubts about the validity of these stories, most of that doubt rested with the foreigners in Mali. As for the Malians, most of them believed these accounts.

But what is a serious historian to make of all these accounts aside from the fact that they ran rampant after the fall of Modibo Keita. Obviously, most of the stories are fanciful, but there is serious disquieting evidence that others may not be. There is too much evidence to dismiss them as mere rumor, and yet there is not enough hard data to conclude that they are absolutely true. When one cuts through the instinctive attachment to rumor which the Malians have, one sees that there are some convincing facts which lie beneath. The most famous of the stories involved the mysterious disappearance of an albino man who worked on the president's estate. Even if it were not for that fact that albinos are the sacrificial victims of choice in the Bambara animist religion, this story would be the most credible of the lot. The man in question had been out of work for many months. His closest friend was the night watchman at the market place in Bamako. One evening the manager of the president's estate came to the market place and seeing the albino talking with the watchman walked up to him and struck up a conversation. After ascertaining that the albino was out of work, the manager offered him a job on the estate. Naturally, the albino accepted and went off the next day to the president's estate. A few days later his friend the watchman went out to see him. Several weeks went by and finally the albino's wife decided to go out to the estate to see her husband since he had not come home in such a long time. When she saw the manager of the estate he foolishly told her that her husband had never worked there, that he knew nothing about him. Dumbfounded, the women went to the market place and poured this story out to the watchman. He then went off to the estate and confronted the manager, and was told that the albino had quit. Suspecting the worst, the watchman threatened to take the matter to the police. He never got to the police. That same night he was found dead in the market place.

The police was more indifferent to this murder than they should have been and this aroused the suspicions of the families and friends of the watchman and the albino. There was no question in their minds that the albino had been sacrificed and the watchman killed before he made any trouble about the matter. After the coup d'etat they demanded that an inquiry be made, but the matter was hushed up. For if the story were true, and most believe that it is, then its public disclosure would serve more to embarrass and disgrace Mali than to convict Modibo Keita of ritual murder.

Malians feared that the fallen president would somehow avenge himself on them and eventually they saw this vengeance in the devastating epidemic of meningitis which descended on Bamako in early 1969, a few months after his fall. It slipped quietly into the city, like a traditional magical curse, moving slowly in the beginning like the first gentle ripples on a soon to be turbulent sea, robed in the sinister clandestine clothing of a sorcerer's patient revenge.

In most instances, it is scientifically possible to trace the sources and the beginning of epidemics, chart their past course and predict their futures. But meningococcal meningitis, also called, cerebro-spinal meningitis, is a disease which defies such precise analysis. It occurs throughout the world as isolated cases and as epidemics. In Africa, cases of the disease occur periodically, but every several years large epidemics break out in that strip of hot dry land which lies just below the Sahara. This part of Africa is known to medical experts as the *meningitis belt* and it stretches from Senegal in the west all the way through Mali, the Niger Republic, Upper Volta and Chad until it reaches the Republic of the Sudan. On a map of Africa this belt is 4,200 kilometers long and roughly 600 kilometers wide and passes between the area which is bordered on the north by the desert and on the south by the forested country of the West African coast and central Africa. In this belt, meningococcal cerebrospinal meningitis is severe, especially in young children whose natural resistance and immunity levels are lower than those of adults. From the sight of these children, feverishly huddled in the dark hot corners of their huts, becoming quickly dehydrated and then comatose, shaken from time to time by convulsive attacks, striken down by the disease as by a thunderbolt, it is easy to understand why an aura of sorcery has surrounded meningitis in Mali for centuries.

Meningococcal meningitis is caused by a bacterium which enters the body through the respiratory passages and then passes through the blood stream to the covering of the brain and spinal cord, known as the meninges. Here it sets up an inflammation which produces high fever and pressure on the brain which eventually can lead to death. From 1950 to 1960, some 300,000 cases of this disease occurred in the *meningitis belt* and of these 50,000 were fatal. The clinical diagnosis is generally easy, the patients coming in with stiff necks, fever, varying degrees of mental confusion and headache. The spinal tap usually reveals milky pus in the spinal fluid from which the bacterium, *Neisseria meningitidis,* can be isolated in the laboratory with special techniques. The disease responds very well to treatment with a single injection of sulfa drugs, but in recent years certain strains of resistant organisms have developed which only respond to other antibiotics. If patients are not treated early on in the illness then a number of complications may develop such as hemhorrage into the vital adrenal glands, hemorrhage into the brain, or paralysis of certain vital nerves of the eyes and extremities.

Why is there a *meningitis belt* and why do these epidemics occur? It is known that this belt depends on rainfall, which exerts its influence either directly or indirectly by mechanisms which are as yet not fully understood. As a rule, the epidemics strike during the dry season when temperatures are exceedingly high and humidity low, when the harmattan blows hot air and dust off the Sahara. It is thought by many that when such climatic conditions prevail the organism is better able to infect nasal passages and then pass through the mucous membranes and invade the central nervous system. Generally, the bacterium causes only a slight infection of the nose and throat indistinguishable from the common cold or else it causes no illness at all. Thus many healthy individuals serve as carriers both during and between epidemics.

From the available data, we know that prior to 1950 waves of epidemics swept from one country to another in a fixed direction. In Mali such epidemics occurred in 1905, 1921, 1937 and 1944. From Mali, they spread eastward into the Niger Republic and then into Chad. Since 1950, however, there has been no real pattern of epidemics such as existed before, but instead a situation wherein meningitis is present at all times at a low level with periodic epidemics and outbreaks.

In the second week of January, 1969, five cases of meningitis were diagnosed at the dispensary in the eastern part of Bamako, in the old crowded quarter of Bozola. In keeping with regulations, the cases were taken to the Service d'Hygiene where the diagnosis was confirmed and then they were sent to the *lazaret,* an isolation facility on the edge of town. I saw these five cases as they were carried out of a truck and taken into the small examining room. Four of them were children and one an adult and in all of them the diagnosis was certain on the basis of clinical grounds only. Not much was thought of these cases in terms of an epidemic, but as an epidemiologist, I feared that they represented the beginnings of one. The following day, seven cases occurred and the day after, twenty-eight, all of them from the eastern part of the town where conditions of poverty, overcrowding and poor hygiene prevailed. The director of the Service d'Hygiene was an old man, unable to understand the epidemiolgic significance of a geometric progression of cases from one day to the next. But Dr. Paul Jean-Joseph, the director of the well-baby clinics in Bamako was as alarmed as I and together we went to see the Minister of Health, Dr. Benitieni Fofana and presented the situation to him. That day seventy cases occurred.

We all realized that we had the beginnings of an epidemic on our hands but no one could say how long it would last and how many victims it would claim. Worse still, it was a disease against which there existed little in the way of preventive measures and whose causitive agent was present in the nose and throats of healthy carriers. The very thought of organizing a fight against it was despairing because there was virtually nothing we could do to stop the disease. No official announcements were made about the epidemic for fear of causing public alarm, but over the next week the population of the city became aware that meningitis, or *kangwele* as it is called in Bambara, had hit Bamako. By the third week, the disease had broken out of the eastern quarters and spread across the city to the western quarters. An average of a hundred cases were occurring per day and fifteen deaths. For a small city like Bamako, this represented an incredibly high prevalence rate, equivalent to what four thousand cases and six hundred deaths per day would have been for the City of New York. If one thinks of that many cases and deaths per day in a city like New York, one can get an idea of the panic and terror which seized the population of Bamako. The disease struck mostly the young and the poor, but it did not spare the old and the rich. No one knew who would fall next. Out in the cemetery of Hamdallaye, there was a constant procession of funerals and the wailing of mourners filled almost every street in the city.

The lazaret lies out at the base of the Manding Hills. At that time, it consisted of three old cement buildings, capable of holding two hundred people. Within a week those facilities were exhausted and the ministry of health had constructed large straw mat shelters. They were airy and cool, but a great fire hazard. On the average, there were a thousand people housed in the shelters plus another thousand relatives and friends who were there to treat them and take care of their nursing needs. There was but one water faucet for all of these people, no electric lighting and six out houses. At night, the army of infirmiers worked by kerosine lamps and flashlight, performing spinal taps, giving injections of sulfa drugs and starting intravenous infusions. When I told Ambassador Clark about the conditions at the lazaret, he immediately authorized emergency funds for electrifying the place, for putting in new plumbing, to pay for the cost of the straw shelters and for the construction of a new cement block building. In addition, he had desperately needed medical supplies flown in from Europe and the States.

I knew that this epidemic would not end until it had run its course through the entire population. In such epidemics, the organism comes in contact with almost everyone. In most, it causes no illness or a mild upper respiratory infection which stimulates the development of protecting antibodies. In a smaller percentage, it causes meningitis. Thus as the organism infects people it also immunizes them and the epidemic finally ends when most of the population has been rendered immune. In former epidemics, the end had always occurred at the beginning of the rainy season in July and thus most Malians believed that wetting down the soil would help halt the disease. Certainly, the dust particles in the air helped spread the disease, but the relationship between the beginnings of the rains and the end of epidemics is considered by most experts to be coincidental. What happens is that the epidemics usually start at a period when temperatures are maximal and humidity minimal and take several months to work their way through the susceptible population. This end-period of mass immunity usually occurs slightly before the start of the rains. When I presented this view of things to the Malian health establishment they refused to believe it and launched a campaign for wetting down the streets of Bamako with water trucks. Every day the huge water trucks roared through the city, drenching the soil, but all this wetting down had no effect on the epidemic.

By mid February, the situation was desperate. Europeans and Malians sent their wives and children out of Bamako, to Dakar and Abidjan and to Paris and outsiders avoided coming into the city. The flights into Bamako were deserted, and the train from Dakar silent and empty. The schools were closed, the theatres shut down and all public assemblies banned. On the streets, people walked with cotton stuffed up their noses and koranic talismans around their necks to prevent getting the disease. We had by then adopted a policy of systematically giving sulfa drugs to all those people who had contact with a case of meningitis. But in many instances this failed to prevent the disease. This development plus the fact that many victims did not respond to treatment with sulfa drugs led me to suspect that some of the organisms were resistant. It was urgent that we confirm this suspicion so that the proper antibiotics could be given. The Laboratoire Biologie in Bamako did not have the necessary culture media for growing the meningococcus and testing its antibiotic sensitivity and so I sent an emergency telegram to the State Department requesting that these supplies be sent out. The Center for Disease Control had the materials in Bamako within forty-eight hours and I rushed them to the laboratory. At the same time, I sent a dozen specimens to the Center for Disease Control and within a week had a reply which indicated that half of the meningococci were resistant to sulfa drugs! They were, however, sensitive to two other antibiotics, penicillin and chloramphenicol. The bacteriologist at the laboratory in Bamako had not as yet come up with any results, and Ibrahima Diallo from the Service d'Hygiene went to see him. He learned that the bacteriologist, who had been trained in Czechoslovakia, had refused to work with "materials supplied by the imperialists." The culture media stood on the floor underneath a sink, unused. It didn't bother the bacteriologist when Diallo told him that his actions might have caused the death of hundreds of people had it not been for the work of the Center for Disease Control. Had we depended on him, we would never have learned that half of the people were infected with organisms which were resistant to the drug being used.

The people of Bamako grasped at every possible straw of hope during those terrible months. The marabouts did a thriving business in selling charms and talismans and were often responsible for patients being brought too late to a medical dispensary, because they advised people that their charms were sufficient for curing the disease. A new experimental vaccine was sent out from France which our vaccinators administered to thousands in the city with the jet guns. This vaccination program turned out to be a nightmare for Mark and I since contrary to the claims of the French pharmaceutical house which produced the vaccine, it was much too viscous for administration by jet injectors. The vaccine was as thick as curdled milk and clogged the chambers and gun heads each time only a few injections had been given. This required the guns being flushed out with distilled water after only a few injections had been given. The vaccine did not really have any effect on the course of the epidemic, but the highly publicized campaign organized for its administration had a tremendous psychological impact on Bamako's population.

By early April, the meningococcus had run through the entire population, creating a high level of herd immunity and gradually the number of new cases per day declined. The fact that the epidemic ended well before the beginning of the rains uprooted the long entrenched conviction that the rainy season caused epidemic meningococcal meningitis to disappear. In Bamako, a total of 6,712 cases and 759 deaths were recorded and in the entire country there were 11,626 cases and 1,221 deaths recorded. Because many cases were not reported nor brought to the attention of medical authorities, the true morbidity and mortality figures are probably much higher than the ones recorded. In Bamako, the cemetery at Hamdallaye was full of fresh mounds and as people passed them they murmured that the sorcerer had had his revenge.

Chapter XVII
The White Goddess

The meningitis epidemic greatly taxed the resources of the Malian Ministry of Health and required that we re-schedule our mobile health activities. We sent a large proportion of our personnel, supplies and equipment out to the lazaret during the epidemic to help in treating the sick and to assist in the administration of drugs to contacts of cases. Although the epidemic ended well before the onset of the rains, it wasn't possible for us to launch a new campaign in the few weeks which remained available for bush travel. And so it was not until the fall of 1969 that the vaccination teams moved into the mountainous western region of Mali which is known as Kayes. It was a pitiable part of Africa, sparsely inhabited by small villages afflicted with sleeping sickness and river blindness. There were no roads to speak of, only miles and miles of impassable rocky tracks winding their way between tiny hamlets in which a total of 700,000 people lived.

In those hamlets, people scratched out a living from the hard laterite soil by growing millet and peanuts, but every year witnessed a famine in the region because they couldn't grow enough to feed themselves. It was this part of Mali which the French first saw when they began their penetration of the West African savanna. This early French presence is marked by architectural remains in towns and villages and along the railway tracks which stretch east to the Niger. But the style and date of the buildings tell you that at some point in time the French realized that the land was barren and moved on towards the Niger. In many ways, it was a land which had been abandoned to nature and to time.

The Cercle of Kita is the portion of this region which is closest to Bamako and at the outset of the campaign I traveled out there to supervise the operations. I always measured the distance to Kita not in miles but in hours, for the track is extremely bad. Also, I always braced myself for hours of traveling in first gear and in four-wheel-drive with the truck moaning and groaning most of the way. The track cuts through a land of brutal desolation, of dry and ugly bush which is uninhabited because of simulium flies which transmit river blindness. There are no clear open spaces here, no patches of cool green, no heartening warmth of inhabited villages, nothing but woodland and tall grass. One passes the abandoned ruins of what once were villages and sees the millet and maize growing in wild clusters around the roofless shells of houses. Tall elephant grass flops and arches over the track and sends down showers of prickly seeds which add to the general discomfort.

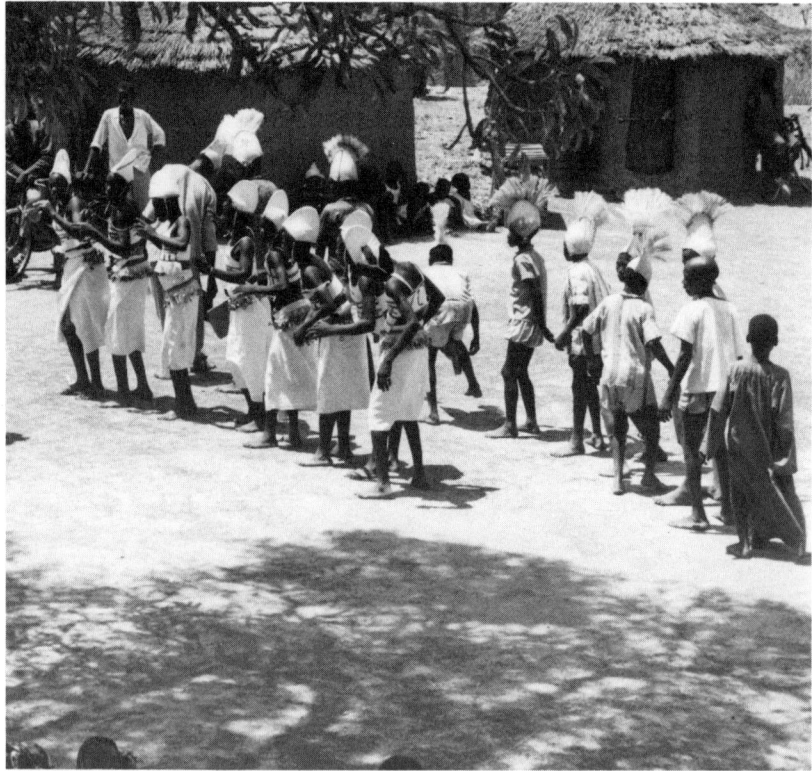

FIGURE 35. Young boys and girls of an age set association known as the *ton* dancing in a Bambara village to celebrate the arrival of a vaccination team.

There was a time, however, after the sun went down behind the thready remains of the Manding Hills, when the whole took on a more pleasing appearance. I always noticed the heavens more when I was in such places because there was little else around on the earth to distract me. The early hours of the night in the camp were filled with idle conversation and stories which had the added quality of being told in a wild setting in the bush. Whenever I traveled over the track to Kita, someone always brought up the strange story of the white goddess of Marena. I was among the few foreigners in Mali who knew the unusual story of this idol, for it was a well-kept secret known to only those people from the area and the men in Bamako who sell authentic art objects.

Djigui, who was from Kita, came from the village of Tiebassa which is not far from Marena, the village where the idol was kept, and was familiar with the details of the story. There is nothing very unusual about the village of Marena. When we went there to vaccinate the people it came on us out of the bush like any other village in this part of Mali, as a clearing filled with round mud houses and conical straw roofs. There are not many villages in this part of the country so when you come to Marena you have a sense of relief in discovering other human beings in the wilderness. The people assembled for vaccination beneath a silk cotton tree in the center of the village as orderly rows of boys and girls, men and women. They looked and behaved like people in any other village in western Mali, the children screamed and pulled away when their arms were seized by the vaccinators and some of them urinated out of fright. The women either laughed or moaned and at most the men only grimaced. From beneath the silk cotton tree I looked out towards the east and saw the jagged face of a mountain rising up some thirteen hundred feet. Its details were dim from the distance and its shape danced up and down in the haze and layers of heat waves. On the surface, it was just an ordinary bush village and a lonely mountain, but both of them held the memory of a tragedy which took the life of one man and committed three others to prison.

It all beagn when Lamine Kante and his son got off the train at Kassaro with the intention of going to Marena. Old Lamine was a well-seasoned hand at procuring art objects in the Malian bush and was teaching the business to his son. If one were intelligent and shrewd, it was a profitable business because there was little overhead and things which were purchased cheaply in the bush invariably brought a high price in Bamako. Lamine had never prospected for *wood,* as art objects were known in Mali, in this part of the country. His usual circuit included the cercles of Segou, Dioila, San, Bamako and Bougouni where the process of conversion to Islam left many statues and masks unused. In many villages, these objects had fallen into disuse and the younger men were quite willing to sell them to people like Lamine for a few hundred francs. Lamine, in turn, sold them to other Malians in Bamako who in turn took them to Abidjan or else up to Paris.

In order to compensate for the diminishing supply of authentic masks, Lamine and his colleagues hired village blacksmiths to reproduce old masks and to artificially age them. These were then taken to Bamako and sold to unknowing buyers. This was a thriving industry in Mali, particularly in the arrondissement of Sarro in the cercle of Macina where some blacksmiths work from books on African Art supplied by people like Lamine. Artificial aging was accomplished through a variety of techniques such as burying masks in termite hills where the action of the termites gave them the look of several decades. A final fake patina was achieved by using shea butter, palm oil, bee's wax and encrustations of ground millet mixed with sand, cement and sawdust.

The voluminous production of fakes in Mali led to the opening of a number of outlet shops in Bamako on the Avenue de la Nation which did a retail business for tourists and ex-patriates and a wholesale trade with shops in Dakar, Abidjan, New York and Paris. The owners of these shops used to descend on the Quartier Fleuve at noon and in the evening with their burlap sacs stuffed full of fakes which in Bambara are called *gnamagnama*. Occasionallly, these men came around with authentic objects, but this was rare since most of the authentic and old pieces were flown off to Paris where they were sold at astonishing prices. These *commercants du bois* never admitted that their wares were fakes, for they were convinced that foreigners wanted only old things. "C'est tres vieux, tres ancien," they always insisted, even though the mask may have been carved the week before. But they thrived on a clientele who were trusting and who could not imagine that business ethics were vastly different from those of an established shop in Paris or New York. Curiously, these merchants never sold the modern sculptures made from red kola nut wood or Yelimane ebony by the artisans in downtown Bamako. These carvings were exquisite and beautiful, but their creators were very proud of them and would never allow the merchants to sell them along with the tons of fakes which came in from the bush.

The business and social relationships among the commercants du bois were complex. They were formed into several cliques which were unstable in their composition because of constant squabbles and entanglements. Foul play in business, even among themselves, was the rule. When I first came to Bamako they sold me a full share of fakes but this buying pattern was abruptly changed when I met by chance a man who was one of the foremost mask dealers in Bamako. He was brought to my office by Boundiar because of an intractable amebic dysentary problem. At the time, Boundiar didn't tell me that he was a member of the elite group of dealers who sold authentic objects in Paris and New York. I treated the man and in two weeks he returned, completely recovered from his illness. When he visited my home for the first time and showed some interest in my then modest collection of fakes I asked him what he thought of them. "Burn them," he said.

I didn't burn them but over the next six months I served an apprenticeship under him and learned the intricacies of authentic and fake Bambara and Dogon sculpture. I was given practical examinations and taken to the center of town to the shops and asked to pick out the authentic objects from the piles of fakes. In time, I acquired all of my teacher's skills. It was the most unusual form of compensation I have ever received for a medical service, but I count it as one of the most important. Ahmadou Niono, who was my teacher, maintained that I was "plus fort que moi" in this field because I saw not only the authenticity in a mask but also its aesthetic qualities. Niono himself was unable to appreciate the aesthetic qualities of a mask to the same degree.

For all of the commercants du bois objects were either fake or authentic. If they were authentic, then they demanded an enormous price, even if the object were quite ugly by western standards. For most of them, the matter of beauty never entered into consideration where determination of price was concerned. They, themselves, often wondered what the white people did with all of these masks and thought it laughable that someone would want to hang them on their walls. Being Moslems, they were iconoclasts, who would never hang a mask in their own homes.

While Lamine had been doing a profitable business in selling fakes, he still went out and prospected for authentic masks. By that time, it had become a market of increased demand and diminishing supply and so people in Europe and America paid high prices for authentic objects. Lamine is no longer a wood merchant. Because of the tragedy which surrounded his attempts to procure the goddess at Marena, he went over to selling cloth in the grand marché. When he went to Kita in 1965, it was with the intention of finding an authentic statue of exceptional value. He knew that most of the people in the Fuladougou-Arbala area of Kita into which he was going were animists and their villages rich in masks and statues. But the risks involved in getting an ordinary mask out of a fetish village were inordinately high compared to what it could be sold for. To make it worthwhile, one had to go after a priceless item and from all of the accounts he had, the goddess at Marena was one. As he walked towards the village from Kassaro, he had visions of selling it in Paris for thousands of dollars.

On very sunny days the silk cotton tree in Marena throws a round pool of shadow across the ground where the old men sleep on goat skins or propped up against the butressed roots of the tree. N'Tyi was a respected elder of the village and often he idled away the hot hours of the day beneath the cool tree. He was sitting there the day Lamine and his son walked in off the hot dusty track.

"Ani oula," said Lamine, addressing the old men.

"M'ba ini oula. Ikakene," they murmured back.

"Toro te."

Lamine sat down with the old men and their lazy conservation drifted through a number of subjects and wore the afternoon on until dusk. He told them he was a cloth merchant on his way to Kita and was interested in spending a few days in Marena in order to make a few sales. There was no reason to doubt his word since he had a large bundle of cloth with him. They invited him to stay in Marena and gave him a house to stay in. Lamine's usual routine was to feel people out, to drop nuances and to tempt a few appetites with more money than the villagers thought existed. On this occasion, however, the information didn't come easily and he had to adopt a new strategy. He made up a story about his coming from a village in Dioila where there was a fertility statue called guandusu. He embellished the story with vivid descriptions of sacrifices he had made to the fetish, all of which greatly impressed the old men and loosened their tongues to talk about their own fetishes.

"Your guandusu is not like our koblenale," said one old man. "Our koblenale is standing and she is white and she lives on top of the mountain. She watches all of the people from up there, Marena, Bangassi and Galamadioi."

So it was that Lamine learned that the statue was worshipped by three villages and guarded by an old man chosen on an annual basis from one of the villages. This was contrary to what he had been told in Bamako, but that was of little importance because this particular year an elder from Marena was in charge of guarding the statue. N'Tyi became Lamine's key man because it was he who was in charge of watching over the idol, the man who had to climb the mountain once a week in order to make a chicken blood sacrifice on behalf of the three villages. Lamine talked at great length with N'Tyi about the guandusu fetish statue he claimed was in his own village, and the old man, feeling at ease with a fellow animist agreed to take Lamine up to the mountain.

They left three days later, over a narrow dusty foot path which led to the base of the mountain. The climb was hard, a trail of twisting stone, labyrinths and dead end passages. Anyone who didn't know where the goddess was kept could never possibly have found the location except by chance. When the yarrived at the cave where the statue was kept, Lamine saw that the entrance was covered by a sculptured door bolted with a lock. When the door was pushed open it fell back into the cave and hit against the stone wall, sending a loud booming noise down into the hollow chamber. The opening was small and they had to crawl on all fours in order to get inside. But once through they were in a large room some twenty feet deep and fifteen feet wide. Lamine now stood in that room, looking at the horizontal ray of light which slid in through the small doorway. He didn't see the statue at first because it was standing in the rear behind an abutment of rock. But when the old man pointed it out to him he lit a match and what he saw set his heart pacing out of control. He had never seen its like before in Mali.

N'Tyi bent down and cut the chicken's throat, but Lamine didn't take note of what he was doing. His eyes were fixed on the white idol. He knew he had to have it. It would make him a rich man for the rest of his life.

"Let us take her outside into the sunlight," said Lamine. "Then I will be able to see her better."

N'Tyi became angry. "No," he said. "She cannot leave the cave." Lamine pleaded with the old man, but he refused to take the statue out of the cave.

Lamine was in a frantic state of mind at this point. Here he had before him a sculpture which could easily bring a fortune in Paris and yet between him and that fortune stood a stupid old animist. For the first time in years, he lost his composure and was tempted to do something to the old man. His pleadings became almost childish. He promised to make N'Tyi the richest man in Kita. But N'Tyi wanted nothing to do with either taking the idol out of the cave or selling it. Lamine didn't want to leave the cave. It was like turning one's back on a once-in-a-lifetime fortune. But the old man crawled out, deaf to Lamine's ranting and entreaties. Lamine didn't observe silence for one moment on the climb down into the village and continued his appeal on into the night. But N'Tyi showed no signs of breaking.

The following day, a young man came to the village on his way to Bangassi from Negala and asked if he could spend the night. N'Tyi volunteered to give him a place to sleep for the night in an isolated hut on the edge of the village. Later on in the day, N'Tyi sought Lamine out and asked him how much he would pay for the idol. Lamine agreed to give two hundred dollars for the statue. This sudden change of mind in the old man didn't seem at all abnormal to Lamine. Old men were always changing their minds and in this instance N'Tyi had simply come to reason.

When Lamine, his son and N'Tyi took the goddess out of the cave and wrapped it up in burlap sacs only N'Tyi knew that this was the first time that the goddess had left the cave in over seventy years. Before the French had occupied the Fuladougou-Arbala, the goddess had often left the cave, every seven years, and had been taken down into the villages. But on these occasions, a human sacrifice had been performed. Lamine gave N'Tyi the money and started off on his way back to Bamako. Getting the large statue back to Bamako was no easy job. He couldn't travel by train or truck since the militia would have seen the statue and confiscated it. So he decided on a very bold plan of action. He walked back to Bamako, through a hundred miles of the Baoule wilderness.

N'Tyi had known that he had a duty before him if the statue left the cave. Thus, he waited until after midnight before going to the isolated hut where the young men was sleeping. The koblenale had left the cave and this sacrifice had to be done. Otherwise, he and his family would be under a curse for the rest of their lives.

Sudden death in the African bush, even among young healthy people is not considered out of the ordinary. But, what disturbed the chief of Marena and the remainder of the village, was why N'Tyi had buried the man himself in the middle of the night. If the man had died normally he should have called someone and then waited until morning before burying him. All of this and Lamine's sudden departure the day before aroused suspicions. The old men of Marena decided to go up to the cave.

When the discovery was made that the statue was missing, the village chief had N'Tyi locked up in a hut and then a delegation was sent off to the chief of the arrandissement at Sebekoro. News of this kind travels very quickly in the bush and by the afternoon of the same day the two other villages who worshiped the statue were aware of the theft. The reaction among them was explosive and they began preparing their gunpowder for an assault on Marena. The chief of the arrondisement had N'Tyi sent off under guard to the town of Kita where he was put into jail. Then he went to Marena with a contingent of militia which had been sent out from Kita to help him solve the problem of the stolen statue. Lamine, unaware of the chaotic situation he had left behind was by this time well out of touch in the Baoule forest. The militia managed to hold the revolt of the two other villages in check while the chief held meetings and tried to straighten out the affair. The villagers were not so much upset by the possible murder N'Tyi may have committed as by the loss of their idol.

The whole affair became complicated by the arrival of President Modibo Keita in Sebekoro. He planned to visit Bangassi after that but the whole population refused to come out to greet him unless their idol were returned. Furthermore, Bangassi and Galamadioi swore to attack Marena as soon as the president left. The chief decided to put the entire matter before the president as soon as he arrived. When Modibo Keita rode into the silent village of Bangassi he knew that something was wrong. Much to everyone's surprise, he proved to be very understanding and asked to meet with the elders of the three villages. He promised to find their idol if they would promise to put away their arms. He sent out an order to the police in Bamako to find the statue and in a matter of hours several detectives were on the train to Marena while others combed the alleys of Bamako. As the detectives rode on their way to Marena, Lamine struggled with his heavy load up the hills which mark the end of the Baoule forest. The following day he arrived in Kati and then from there walked to Bamako over the back road, arriving late at night. He put the statue under his bed and considered himself a lucky man.

Back in Marena, the police exhumed the body of the young man and took it to Bamako where a Russian pathologist examined it. It was found that the young man had been bludgeoned over the head with a blunt instrument and that his throat had been slit. Once this was brought to light, the detectives had N'Tyi brought to the main prison in Bamako where they got a confession out of him after confronting him with their findings. N'Tyi confessed to being wrong in selling the statue, but not in killing the young man. The statue had left the cave and he had done his duty and performed a human sacrifice. The police saw things differently as did the criminal court which sentenced the old man to life in prison at hard labor.

Lamine's mind was preoccupied with the details of shipping the statue to Paris when he was arrested. He found the story incredulous. How could N'Tyi have killed a man for a wooden statue? he kept asking himself. But Lamine was a Moslem and knew little of the mentality of the animist. In speaking with him now, one senses more indignation over his loss of treasure than moral shame for the killing he precipitated. He and his son were sentenced to a year in prison.

I am certain that one day the white goddess of Marena will leave the cave again, at a time when the people of the three villages no longer believe in her powers. She will be carried to Bamako and then perhaps to Paris where she will be sold to an African art dealer who in turn will sell her to a private collector or a museum. She will be placed in a glass case or on a pedestal in someone's salon. Those who look at her form will wonder where she came from. At most, the plaque will say, "Maternity fetish, Kita, Mali." But no one will suspect anything about N'Tyi and the young man who lost his life nor think about Lamine and they will not envision the mountain cave where the koblenale once stood.

Chapter XVIII
A Difficult Vaccination Campaign

There were no good roads to speak of in the Kayes region and the only paved stretches, amounting to less than ten miles, were in the regional capital, a town called Kayes. Much of the central and southern portions of the region are mountainous, the highest peaks being found in the southwestern area, in the cercle of Kenieba where the Tambaoura Escarpment thrusts its eroded mesas and jagged cliffs high above the rock strewed plains. There were tracks in this area, stretches of solid rock which took days to negotiate, wrecking havoc on the truck suspensions, tires and motors and on people's backs. Up in the north towards the cercles of Kayes, Nioro and Yelimane, the terrain was softer, with the white sand and thorn trees of the sahel dominating the landscape. But the tracks there were no improvement over those in the south because they had been built by the early French administrators over the rockiest areas possible so as to passable for their ox drawn metal wheeled carts during the rainy seasons. In areas where there were no rocks, the French road engineers had them brought in and laid out beneath the sandy road beds.

The Senegal River rises in the mountains of Kayes, principally from the Bafing and Bakoye which join at the small town of Bafoulabe and from the Faleme which flows into the Senegal at a point where Mali ends and the Republic of Senegal begins. The Senegal River is navigable below the town of Kayes, but above it, the presence of the Felou Rapids and the Gouina Waterfalls constitute a natural barrier to river traffic. By comparison with the middle Niger, the Senegal and its tributaries look deserted. Because of the presence of river blindness and sleeping sickness, there are few villages on the river banks. As a consequence, even canoes are rare and exceptional on most stretches, being used primarily for crossing the rivers and not for traveling up and down their lengths. Therefore, it was pointless to think of using the rivers for transporting personnel and equipment and so our only other choices were the tracks as bad as they were, foot paths and the railroad.

The Dakar-Niger railroad is a single track affair which runs for four hundred and twenty miles in Mali. All of this length of track, except for fifty five miles, lies in the Kayes region. It is often said by Malians that the reason why there are no roads in Kayes is because of the railroad. But the absence of roads has many more and complex reasons than this. The good intentions of road builders have been thwarted by the fact that the region is one of low productivity with a steadily decreasing population. The latter is due to the emigration of the Sarakole who have abandoned farming and herding for international trade and salaried jobs in the slums of French cities, especially Paris. We knew that the railroad would be of little use to us except for transporting the trucks and heavy equipment up and down the line on flat cars. And, even that was fraught with difficulties because of long and sudden delays in schedules.

In the summer of 1969, we received a shipment of eleven new Dodge W-100 single cabin pick-up trucks and three new Dodge W-200 crew cab trucks, all equipped with four wheel drive. They had come across the Atlantic from New York to Dakar on the *African Planet,* a ship belonging to the Farrell Lines. After sitting on the docks in Dakar for several weeks, they were carried up to Bamako by rail on flat cars and then carefully examined by our mechanics. As with so much of our equipment, these trucks stood for several weeks in the freight yards in Bamako while they were cleared through the formalities of the customs service. Because they were a gift of the Agency for International Development, they were admitted duty free, but before they could be released, a voluminous exchange of documents had to take place between the ministries of health, foreign affairs, the treasury and the customs service.

Our Malian staff referred to the small and large Dodge trucks as the *petits Dodges* and the *grands Dodges* respectively. It had always been our intention to use the new trucks in Kayes since the older vehicles would never have withstood the rigors of the roads. To save the new trucks from as much of a beating as possible, we shipped them up to the town of Kayes on flat cars, sending four apprentices along to guard them and the equipment stored inside. After many frustrations, the trucks left Bamako on October 29th, but didn't arrive in the town of Kayes until the 4th of November because the flat cars were parked on sidings along the way at frequent intrevals. By that time, the cereal shortage in Mali had become a chronic annual problem and to avoid famine, thousands of tons of red maize had to be imported from the United States. The freight trains carrying all of this grain up to Bamako from Dakar were understandably given the absolute right of way on the track. As a result, however, outgoing trains were held up on sidings and most other imports left on the docks in Dakar.

Since the rains ended earlier in the sahel than they did further south in the savanna, we decided to begin the vaccination campaign up north in the cercles of Nioro and Yelimane and from there to move southward into the cercles of Kayes and Kenieba and then eastward into Bafoulabe and Kita. But that year, the rains lasted longer than they normally did and by late September many of the tracks in Nioro were still covered with water. The delay in getting the trucks to the town of Kayes was in a sense fortuitous since the teams could not have driven them the remaining one hundred and fifty six miles to the town of Nioro because of the flooded tracks. Before the tracks were fully passable, Mark and I took our own truck up to Nioro overland, Modibo driving it through three hundred miles of some of the worst terrain imaginable. It took four days to get the truck through, but had we taken it up by rail to Kayes and then overland to Nioro, three weeks would have been required. With our truck in Nioro it was possible within a few weeks to move around the sahel and organize the immunization campaign.

We established eight teams, each headed by an infirmier from the Kayes region. Prior to beginning the campaign, we brought the eight infirmiers into Bamako for a month's training course and had them participate in the ten day vaccination campaign in Bamako in which 278,337 people were vaccinated against smallpox and 59,679 children against measles. This enabled us to give them supervised field experience in the use of the automatic jet injectors and in conducting a mass immunization program. At the suggestion of Dr. Ousmane Sow, the newly appointed Director of the Division of Socio-Preventive Medicine, we chose an infirmier from the cercle of Bafoulabe to be the field supervisor.

Teninko Togola was intelligent, honest and experienced, but his many years of service as the medecin chef of Bafoulabe had endowed him with an appreciable degree of pride and independence of action which made subordination somewhat beyond his grasp. He was always polite, but always in a cold and detached way which expressed better than any of his other actions the considerable discomfort he felt in dealing with us. While he wanted to be a good collaborator of ours, he nurtured unfounded fears of the future consequences of such a close association. Mali's Marxist past was still a vivid memory for people such as Togola and they wanted to have a good dossier in the event that past reappeared again in the future. In the eyes of those who thought this way, being associated with Americans was about the best way to tarnish one's dossier. Togola, therefore, gave more consideration to the future than to the brief immediate, a not unexpected choice in this matter. After the campaign in Kayes was completed, we sent him to the Center for Disease Control in Atlanta, Georgia for a course in epidemiology and infectious disease control. He learned a great deal during this course, but when he returned he fancied he carried the visible imprint of being a friend of the Americans and he did his utmost to undo this image. Many of his peers in the health services, who were jealous of his having been abroad, aggrevated his fears by bantering him with accusations of being a stooge of the Americans. Togola understandably did nothing to actively cultivate and sustain our friendship, but he worked well with us, giving visible testimony to everyone that the association was not one of his choosing, but one required of him by circumstance.

On November 1st, eight of our drivers went up to the town of Kayes by train while eighteen vaccinators and infirmiers left for Nioro by plane. Three days later, the remaining vaccinators and infirmiers left for Nioro by plane. The passenger train with the drivers arrived in Kayes before the trucks, but by the 5th of November, they were able to unload the Dodges from the flat cars and drive them over the hazardous road from Kayes to Nioro. We had set up gasoline depots in Nioro and Yelimane for the initial phases of the campaign and later on did the same thing in the other cercles in the region. Although all of the personnel and equipment, including vaccines, were in Nioro by November 6th, we were unable to start the campaign because Air Mali had left most of the vaccinators' personal baggage in Bamako. And when Mark and I flew to Nioro on November 8th, we sadly discovered that our baggage had also been left in Bamako. Like the vaccinators and infirmiers, we spent a week in Nioro with the same clothes on our backs and had to buy soap and towels in the market in order to keep clean. We had our clothing washed at night and because it is so dry in Nioro it always dried within an hour while we wrapped ourselves up in sheets.

This experience taught us that the only way to fly to Nioro was with our baggage in hand in the plane's cabin. We also discovered why our baggage was never put on the planes, even though the flights were usually only half filled. The planes used on this run were Russian Antinov-24's which are capable of carrying sixty passengers plus a considerable tonnage of baggage and fuel. Although the flights went north beyond Nioro to Nema and Aioun el Atrouss in Mauritania, the fact that they took on fuel in both Nioro and Aioun meant that the apparent overload was due to other causes. As we discovered, the cause was the Sarakole traders from Nioro who flew from Bamako with hundreds of pounds of merchandise packed up into metal valises known as *cantines*. Their generosity with the Bamako airport staff assured that these heavy metal trunks were put aboard. But this also meant that the modest quantity of baggage belonging to unsuspecting passengers such as ourselves was bumped off the flights.

The hot dry climate of Nioro and the absence of personal baggage only served to aggrevate the vaccinators' chronic complaining. On top of these complaints, they moaned that the Lomidine I had given them as a prophylactic against trypanosomiasis was making them ill, which it wasn't. The commandant of the cercle of Nioro was an army captain who, like so many of his fellow commandants, asked when the vaccinators would be leaving his cercle, even before they started working. He was in a very agitated state when I first met him in his office since a crew from the Nioro Service d'Hygiene had almost accidentally blown his house up by pumping in a highly inflammable insecticide gas while his kerosine refrigerator was still ignited. The commandant was an efficient administrator who did his best to insure the success of the campaign. His close associate, the mayor of Nioro, was a man by the name of Lieutenant Ly, who later became the mayor of Bamako. He, like the commandant, was conscientious and hard working, and gave Nioro an impressive new look. The public buildings and schools sparkled under fresh coats of paint, trees were planted, the sandy streets cleaned daily and new construction undertaken. Lieutenant Ly later changed the face of Bamako when he became mayor of the capital. Although the town of Nioro was small, with an average population of six thousand, it was a difficult place to administer because of the presence of two rival Moslem sects, the followers of El Hadj Omar and the Hammalists.

In terms of numbers, both sects were of equal strength and each had a separate mosque in which they prayed. A strong feeling of

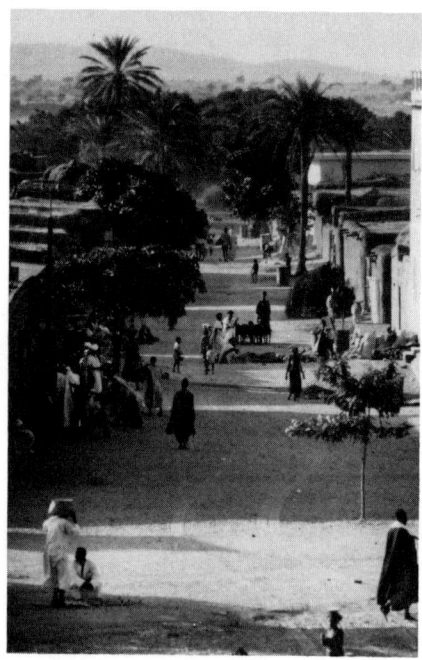

FIGURE 36. A view of the center of the town of Nioro.

antipathy reigned between them, expressed partially by a competitive fanaticism in religious practice and complete intolerance of one another's form of worship. In the early 1940's, this mutual intolerance led to a serious revolt on the part of the Hammalists in Nioro during which many people were killed. The leader of the Hammalists, known as the Sherif, was exiled to France where he later died. The Malian government has never given its assent to the numerous requests made by the Hammalists for bringing this Sherif's remains back to Nioro. The current Sherif lived in a large compound in the center of Nioro, a somnolent old man who sat out most of the hours of the day seated on soft pillows. He sat in the center of his compound in the shade of the tents which were pitched around him. He was suffering from hypertension when I saw him and his attendants proudly pointed out to me all of the medicines which his followers had sent from Europe, the U.S.A. and from other parts of Africa. As impressive as the mounds of medicines were in quantity, they weren't doing the sherif much good. His treatment plan was a rather unstructured affair, he swallowing a pill or two of a given color whenever it struck his fancy. I can't say that the Sherif radiated much dignity and this was a disappointment to me since I had imagined him to be otherwise. When Mark went to visit him one day, he had no sooner seated himself on a mat in front of the Sherif when a large rat raced across the courtyard and disappeared underneath the Sherif's voluminous robes.

The Sherif was a Maure and a descendant of the founder of the sect. Followers were required to provide the Sherif and his large extended family and entourage with all of their material needs in return for which they received a guarantee of paradise after death. Through this cornerstone practice of the sect, the Sherifs guaranteed paradise for their followers in the hereafter and paradise for themselves here on earth.

While we were in Nioro, a young graduate student in anthropology, Lucy Quimby, came out to Mali hoping to study the Hammalists in Nioro. I always doubted that the Malian government would give Lucy permission to go to Nioro to do this study since her mere presence there among the Hammalists would have upset the delicate religious balance in the place. As it was, the Hammalists quickly learned that Lucy was in Bamako and made capital of her intentions. They announced all over Nioro that there was a woman in Bamako who had been sent by President Nixon, the man who had placed men on the moon, to obtain for him some of the *sebe* (Koranic charms) made by the Sherif. In so doing, they scored a victory over the otherr Moslems and implied that the Sherif's power was so great that even one of the most powerful men in the world had need of his help. At first, the Malians said "no" to Lucy according to their usual fashion which is to give no reply at all.

The fact that they eventually did say 'no" indicated how strongly they felt about the matter. So Lucy went to the town of Bobo-Dioulasso in Upper Volta where she carried out an extensive study of Islam in the place.

The followers of El Hadj Omar were no less fanatical than the Hammalists. The iguana is a sacred animal among them, much as cows are considered sacred in India. Hundreds of these large lizards roamed the streets of the town. It is believed that they are all descendants of a sacred iguana which was brought back to Nioro by El Hadj Omar when he returned from his pilgrimage to Mecca. It is also believed that the iguanas verify the puirty of those who come to pray at the unimpressive mosque built by El Hadj Omar, hitting the impure with their tails. I never witnessed iguanas hitting people at prayer time, but I was present when one of our drivers accidentally hit an iguana with a truck in the principal market place. The popular reaction was unbelievably violent and the fact that we were returning from visiting the Sherif only made matters worse.

As difficult as the topography of the cercles of Nioro and Yelimane was, it was a pallid problem compared to the volatile atmosphere of religious rivalry which regined in the area. The hard core of fanatics of either group was relatively small. But they were surrounded by large numbers of people whose zeal for religiosity made them unreasonable in many matters, except business. The Sarakole, who comprise the bulk of the population of this area, viewed dishonest business practices as sound and could finger their prayer beads with total equanimity while trying to short measure someone out of a few centimeters of cloth. But the great wealth of these people did not come from chiseling on centimeters of cloth. It came from trading in kola nuts, diamonds and gold. Thousands of them had emigrated from the area to Sierra Leone and Zaire in search of diamonds and to Guinea in search of gold. In those places, they gained a reputation for being smugglers, which they are. They would periodically return to Nioro with their women and daughters covered with gold jewelry and parade their success and sing of their exploits before those who had remained behind. A man who had traveled widely was held in high esteem and a recitation of foreign places visited always drew the approbation of listeners. In 1971, the President of Zaire expelled several thousand Sarakole from his country on the grounds that their smuggling had metamorphosed over the years into a tentacle system of underworld activities. They were placed on planes and repatriated back to Mali, even though many of them had been born in Zaire. For a brief period of time, they constituted a social problem for the Malian government since many were without family ties in Mali and had no means of support. But the problem was short-lived because they eventually smuggled themselves back into Zaire.,

Over the years, thousands of Sarakole had migrated to the urban centers of France where they worked at menial jobs, lived in crowded slum conditions, but earned a wage considered enormous by Malian standards. Conditions of crowding, poor nutrition and poor environmental sanitation created the background for the present-day high incidence of tuberculosis among these immigrants. Many of them are smuggled illegally into France by well-organized groups of Africans and Europeans who extract a high price for getting them into the country.

The social and religious complexities of Nioro and Yelimane were the worrisome problems at the outset of the campaign. It was our good fortune that the medecin chef of Nioro was an exceptional man of great ability. Dr. Bakary Coulibaly was an accomplished surgeon who in addition to being a good administrator also understood the mentality of the local population. The hospital in Nioro which he directed was an impressive place with modern x-ray equipment, an up to date operating suite and administrative and housekeeping procedures which bettered those of the other hospitals in the country. Much of the physical plant and equipment had been provided by the European Development Fund. It was no easy task to operate a hospital of this kind which served an essentially tradition based population.

Dr. Coulibaly foresaw that we would run into difficulties at the outset because the Moslem month of fasting, Ramadan, was due to begin on the 11th of November. He feared the fanatical marabouts from both sects would proclaim to their followers that the injection of liquid vaccine beneath the skin would break their fast. And, if this were believed, then most of the adult population in both cercles would refuse immunization. As perhaps only he could have done, he called a meeting of the leading marabouts from both sects and after much diplomatic persuasion got them to commit themselves to the theological position that vaccination did not break the fast. It was a meeting which was full of discomfort with the opposite groups seated on large plastic covered chairs in two straight lines facing each other. But through it, Dr. Coulibaly was able to referee the ensuing debate which erupted between the two sides and in the end channel their opinions in our favor. This was no easy matter since these men held that even the swallowing of saliva broke the fast. When Ramadan began in Nioro everywhere one looked people were spitting. Even on the plane to Bamako, people spat throughout the flight into paper bags, generating a terrible stench in the cabin.

As soon as the teams began the program in Nioro, I left the town for Yelimane with Modibo and Dr. Mohamed Soumare, the regional director of health of Kayes. Dr. Soumare was a man in his late fifties and by Malian standards was considered old and wise. I never considered him as old, but wise he was, through years of experience. He was endowed with a refreshingly calm nature and was in spite of his deep involvement in the Marxist politics of the former regime devoid of any antipathy for Europeans. It was only eighty-four miles to Yelimane from Nioro, but because of the terrible state of the track it took us six hours to get there. The track ran through some very hilly country which was heavily wooded in many places and in some areas it completely disappeared. So often we drove up and down the hills and across the flat plains, making our own track as we went. A distinguishing characteristic of the Sarakole country is the paucity of villages, but what villages exist are very large with populations of a thousand and more. Interspersed between these large villages are the small hamlets of the Peul who comprise a small but important minority population in the area. Occasionally, one comes across a small band of Maure nomads who are disliked in this part of Mali because of their brigandage and raids on sedentary villages. The Maures primarily steal cereal and carry it back across the nearby frontier on the backs of donkeys. This stealing of cereal was so great that the Malian government maintained large garrisons of soldiers along the frontier in order to intercept the Maures. Fate dealt the Maures a hard blow in 1973 when hundreds of thousands of them were forced to flee southwards into Mali and Senegal because of the terrible drought. With most of their livestock dead from lack of water and food, they were forced to throw themselves on the mercy of the sedentary farmers whom they had pillaged for years. Not surprisingly, the Maures received little mercy from the farmers who themselves were in difficulty because of a poor crop. Severe starvation occurred among the Maures that year and were it not for all of the aid given by foreign countries and international organizations, many more would have died.

The Sarakole villages were surrounded by tall stands of an unusual form of millet which requires seven months to mature. Many of the fields had fences around them, an unusual feature in Mali where for the most part fields are left unfenced. We stopped at Kirane, the *chef lieu* of the first arrondissement of the cercle of Yelimane. It was a pleasant but isolated place located only a few miles from the Mauritanian frontier. The infirmier had no dispensary and treated people out of his small mud brick house. His name was Bekaye Samake and when I visited Kirane subsequently during the campaign, I witnessed how well he worked with the little he had. There were some very high mountains between Kirane and Yelimane and the region was full of dense populations of baboons and jackals.

The village of Yelimane is small compared to others in the cercle, but it was chosen by the French as their headquarters because of its strategic geographic location. The government buildings stand on a high and picturesque plateau which is at the end of a broad fertile valley. The mountains rise up to the east behind the government post, tall rounded peaks which are repetitive in both size and shape. During the rainy season, Yelimane is cut off from the outside world except for the flight which comes in once a week from Bamako via Kenieba and Kayes. At that time Air Mali used a Russian single engine bi-plane, an Antinov-2, which was some thirty years old. It carried a dozen passengers seated against the side walls of the non-pressurized cabin and heaps of baggage, including goats, sheep and chickens. I often used the Antinov-2 to fly to Kenieba and Kayes and to Niafunke and Timbuctoo. It always bounced up and down in the air pockets only a few hundred feet above the mountain peaks and it seemed miraculous to me that it never crashed except once. That time it went down in the Baoule wilderness where the uninjured passengers spent several days being bitten by tsetse flies while the pilot went off for help. There was a large hole in the side of the fuselage of the An-2 which was covered over by a piece of cardboard which invariably fell off when the winds outside were strong. The Malian pilots who flew the plane did so with the spirit of rodeo stunt men and got a hilarious charge out of every near miss with a mountain peak. The cockpit was always bubbling over with laughter and if you weren't a regular passenger on the flight you would have thought them all drunk. As fragile as this life line was for Yelimane, it was better than nothing and whenever the An-2 made one of its awkward and bouncy near crash landings on the strip, most of the village was on hand to meet it.

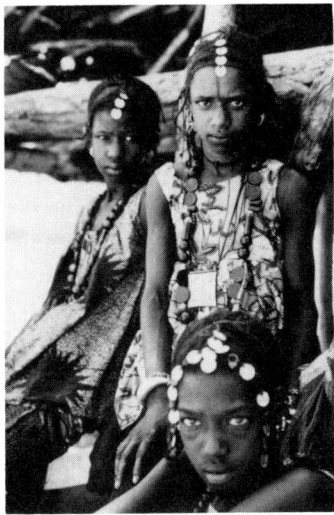

FIGURE 37. Peul girls at Youri in the cercle of Nioro.

There were approximately 65,000 people living in the cercle of Yelimane, distributed in four arrondissements, Central, Kirane, Marena and Tambacara. Dr. Soumare and I calculated that it wouldn't take the teams more than two weeks to vaccinate the whole cercle and so when we visited the arrondissements, we set the program up accordingly. As we knew then, the work in Yelimane was to be an easy two weeks in an otherwise six month period of arduous work. We met with all of the chefs of the arrondissements, the infirmiers in charge of the bush posts and the village chiefs, planned the day to day program and arranged for the logistical support of the teams. Once this was done, Dr. Soumare returned to the town of Kayes to plan the program in the cercle of Kayes and I returned to Nioro where a large number of problems had already developed with the teams.

The chief complaints in Nioro were flat tires and elephant grass seeds clogging the radiators of the trucks. These took precedence over the usual priority complaints of starvation, overwork and illness, and the fact that they did meant that they were real problems. The four ply tires on the small Dodges were too fragile for the terrain and not a day went by that the teams using them didn't get a flat. The drivers had their own repair kits and pumps, but the inner tubes gradually took on the appearance of quilts and got to the point where patches were placed on top of one another. Unfortunately, eight ply tires were not manufactured in a size which would fit the small Dodges and so our only resource was to provide large numbers of inner tubes. One of my most vivid memories of the Kayes campaign is of coming on teams in the bush and seeing the trucks up on jacks with the apprentices and drivers nearby, patching the inner tubes.

All over the region the narrow tracks were banked by tall elephant grass whose small seeds got into the radiator elements as the trucks rode by. The clogging reached the point where the engines overheated because no air got into the elements. The apprentices had to dismount the radiators and painstakingly remove each seed with their fingers, one by one. The delays caused by this problem were enormous until Modibo came up with the idea which solved the problem. We purchased fine wire screening in Nioro and placed it over the front of the trucks so that the seeds were deflected from the radiators.

I traveled into the southern part of the cercle of Nioro with Modibo and Togola in order to inspect the progress of the campaign in the arrondissements of Sandare and Lakamane. This region once formed part of the ancient Bambara kingdom of Kaarta. Although Lakamane was only fifty miles from Nioro it was one of the most isolated places I ever visited in Mali. It was in a sense a dead end, for beyond it lay a vast uninhabited region of wooded savanna known as the Sefeto, full of wildlife and tsetse flies. Vehicles rarely ever went to Lakamane and my truck was the first one to go over the track in over a year. The isolation of a place in Mali was measurable in my experience by the tenacity with which government officials there held onto a visitor. In Lakamane, the infirmier, the chef of the arrondissement and the two school teachers held on to us for dear life. There were no more than five hundred souls in Lakamane and the village itself was nothing more than a small clearing in an otherwise dense expanse of virgin woodland. Much to delight of the officials in Lakamane, the vaccination team which covered the arrondissement was forced to spend five days in the village, not by intent but because all of their tires went flat and the inner tubes were irreparable. They were finally rescued when someone from the village came to Nioro on horseback with the news of their problem.

The people in Lakamane were both Bambara and Kassonke, the latter being an ethnic group which numbers 75,000 and which is of Peul origins. The Kassonke are reputed for their singing ability and for their orchestras of large drums and according to many Malians for being extremely lazy. There was nothing lazy about the reception which the Kassonke gave us in Lakamane. The village chief and elders came in to see me at the head of a delegation carrying more food than an army could consume. After them, the teachers and the chef of the arrondissement came with their wives, also carrying food. All of them had one wish and that was that I stay as long as possible. I would have stayed longer than I did had it not been for the incredible rat problem in the village which made sleeping at night an impossibility. Lakamane's rat problem wasn't brought to my attention until I was getting into my cot which was set up in the infirmier's house. He lived in a large unfinished cement block building which had been meant to be a storage warehouse for kapoc until it was discovered that there wasn't all that much kapoc in Lakamane to be stored. The infirmier had made the abandoned government folly as livable as he could. He was very solicitous about my comfort and with much self-consciousness told me that there were a lot of mice in the village at night. "They make a lot of noise," he added after mustering his courage. The name for both rat and mouse is the same in Bambara and so few Malians distinguished between the two when speaking in French. They usually refer to both rats and mice as mice. For me, the difference was important because whereas African mice are rather innocuous, rats are not, especially when they're hungry.

"Don't worry," I assured him. "I'm accustomed to mice." These words comforted him and he went off to the far end of the warehouse to sleep. Once I extinguished the pressure lamp the room filled up with rats. I saw them crawling up the walls, scampering across the rafters and climbing up the legs of the cots. With my flashlight I made the species identification and the simultaneous decision that I would sleep in the cabin of the truck. Modibo and Togola were already asleep, but they didn't sleep well for long and spent a very bad night because of the racket made by the rats. The infirmier and the village chief were embarrassed when they learned that I had slept on the front seat of my truck even though I assured them that I was in the habit of sleeping there. The village chief apologized for the rat problem and asked that I get the Nioro Service d'Hygiene to come to Lakamane and poison the animals. I told the chief that the Nioro Service d'Hygiene had almost blown the commandant's house up during a disinsectization operation and that I wouldn't want to predict what might happen if they got involved with rat poison. There must have been a paucity of food in the surrounding bush for all of these rats to have descended on Lakamane at night, but the chief maintained that it was because of the large marsh which lay on one side of the village. According to the chief's modified theory of spontaneous generation, the rats formed from the mud at the bottom of the marsh under the influence of a sorcerer. I was never able to solve Lakamane's rat problem and when we left there it was with a feeling of relief and desire for a good night's sleep in Sandare. After spending several days in Sandare we drove up to Gogui, an arrondissement which lies to the north of Nioro at the tip of an excresence in the otherwise linear frontier between Mali and Mauritania.

When the teams finished vaccinating the cercle of Nioro they moved on to Yelimane and then down to the cercle of Kayes where Dr. Soumare had already planned the program for the cercle's eight arrondissements. Once the campaign was underway there, Mark and I traveled back and forth between Bamako and the town of Kayes on the Dakar-Bamako express which was usually delayed for anywhere from a few hours to a day. On the average, it took ten hours of traveling to cover the 318 miles between Kayes and Bamako, but overall it took almost twice as long because of delays. The Senegalese trains were more comfortable than the Malian ones and the service better, but both were the same when it came to delays. I felt that both of them lacked that margin of safety which you sense rather than see as a passenger. They took the curves at a faster speed than one thought wise and I once remember how our compartment filled up with smoke and flames as the train plunged through a roaring bush fire. Trains were often derailed and it wasn't uncommon that freight trains spilled most of their contents all over the bush during such derailments. Miraculously, the trains were always put back on the tracks, the freight re-loaded and the trip begun once again. A serious accident involving a passenger train occurred once in 1970, between Toukoto and Kita, when over a hundred persons were killed.

Once the teams began working in the cercle of Kayes, my participation in the campaign there gradually diminished. An outbreak of yellow fever occurred near Faladie, some sixty miles from Bamako and later cases appeared in Kati, a large town only twenty miles from the capital. Two missionary sisters at a mission near Diamou in the cercle of Kayes also died at the same time from what appeared to be yellow fever. The appearance of yellow fever in humans in Mali after an absence of three decades generated great concern, for people still remembered the frightening epidemics of previous decades when thousands died. By this time, we had vaccinated most of the adult population in Mali against the disease as part of our mobile health activities. But, children below ten years of age were not vaccinated because we used the Dakar neurotropic strain of vaccine which causes a severe meningoencephalitis in roughly 0.5 percent of children vaccinated. The pediatric populations of both Bamako and the affected areas were susceptible for the most part. This coupled with the fact that the vectors of urban yellow fever were present in Bamako and Kati, gave us real cause for concern about a possible epidemic. Ambassador Clark had 100,000 doses of the 17 D chick embryo vaccine flown out from the U.S.A. for use in a special vaccination campaign. Although this vaccine causes virtually no adverse reactions, it is extremely fragile, especially in the hot ambient temperatures of Africa and must be stored at freezing temperatures and used within an hour of being mixed with the diluent. The use of so fragile a vaccine in the rough hot African bush required special care in refrigeration and handling.

While Mark directed the campaign in the cercles of Kayes, Kenieba and Bafoulabe, I assisted Dr. Ousmane Sow in organizing a yellow fever immunization campaign in Bamako and in the arrondissements of Negala,

Kati and Sebekoro. We deployed six vaccination teams for the operation and within two months vaccinated the threatened population. Simultaneously, mosquito control measures were implemented in Bamako and Kati and in the villages in the affected areas. As a result of these efforts, the epidemic was quickly brought under control. We placed Boundiar in charge of the vaccination teams since he was an old hand at dealing with yellow fever outbreaks. In doing so, we pulled him out of his semi-retirement, but were careful to put him back into it when he began showing signs of causing trouble. There was much disagreement at the time about the value of disinsecting the trains coming into Bamako from Kayes. Those in favor of it argued that potential mosquito vectors would be destroyed in such an operation, but others, including myself, argued that the mosquito vectors were easily capable of flying on their own from Kati to Bamako. Hence, the spraying of trains wasn't really going to add very much to the control effort. It was decided to spray the trains and unfortunately most of the spraying took place at night when supervision was lacking. When Mark and I returned from Kayes to Bamako one night, the train was stopped at midnight at Kati and suddenly laborers from the Service d'Hygiene descended with motorized insecticide pumps. Without warning they blasted the train full of a dense fog of insecticide, both inside and out, sending everyone running for cover from the choking fumes. Walking down the aisles of the cars, they knocked on the compartment doors and when the passengers opened, they shouted "Disinsectization!" and then blasted the compartment and any passengers who happened to be in it with a suffocating cloud of noxious fumes. Many passengers fled the train in panic, but because the station at Kati is in a narrow canyon, there was no place for them to flee to. So dense was the cloud of insecticide that neither Mark nor I could see the lights of the train from twenty feet away. With everyone either coughing, vomiting or screaming, the engineer blew the whistle, meaning that he was going to start moving. Although no one could see the train, we all headed in the general direction and climbed aboard. Those who got to the steps first pulled the others aboard. Mark and I managed to pull several old people on board who were so blinded by the smoke that they couldn't find the steps. It was almost impossible to breathe on the train and everyone hung halfway out the windows, gasping at every patch of fresh air which flew by next to the moving train. Mark climbed onto the roof of the car by way of a ladder and I rode on the steps. When the train disembarked its passengers at the Bamako station the terminal took on the appearance of a disaster area. Everyone was suffering from insecticide intoxication and some so seriously that they had to be taken to the Gabriel Toure Hospital which was scarcely equipped to handle the problem. My clothing was so saturated with insecticide that it killed every insect in the house overnight. The disinsectization program for trains was discontinued the following day after I spoke with Dr. Sow and the Minister of Health.

Once the yellow fever epidemic was brought under control, we took four of the six vaccination teams which had been formed and put them into the cercles of Segou and Niono, the two remaining areas of Mali which up to that time had still not yet been vaccinated against measles and smallpox. The combined population of this area was 300,000, but compared to the Kayes region it was an easier place to work in because the terrain was flat and the tracks good. Even up in the

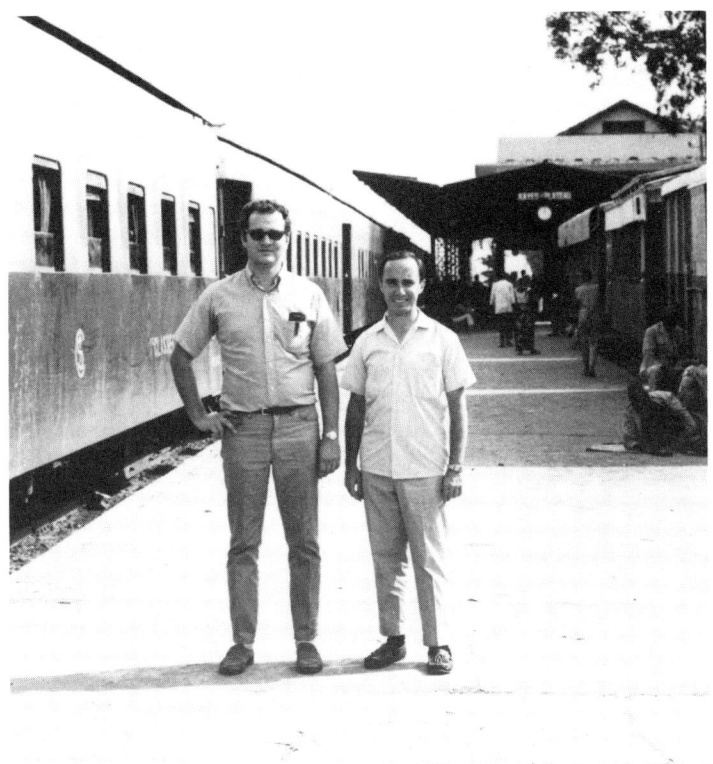

FIGURE 38. Mark LaPointe *(left)* and Dr. Imperato *(right)* standing on the platform in the town of Kayes. The train was delayed six hours that day.

Office du Niger in Niono where canals and irrigation ditches crisscrossed the land, the teams were able to move with amazing rapidity. Djigui and Kassim worked with me in Segou and Niono while Togola and Modibo remained in Kayes with Mark. I set up my heaquarters in the cercle of Segou, in Ahmadou's village, Boussin. To make it comfortable I brought out some furniture from Bamako, a chest of drawers, chairs, a table, a water filter and a complete set of cooking utensils. All of these things were carefully put into a house in Ahmadou's family compound and my tent pitched in a corner of the yard. Although the house was comfortable, I found it better to sleep in the tent and so I rarely used the house for that purpose. The house would heat up during the day and wouldn't cool off until the early hours of the morning, making it unbearable when it came to sleeping. But it was a better place to sleep in when it rained since the tent leaked like a sieve. As good as this bush camp was, we never solved the problems of the bathroom. Ahmadou's family did all they could to remedy the situation, but in the end I simply grew accustomed to what was already there. The bathroom was a prototype of its kind, an area about ten feet long and six feet wide, closed off by mud walls five feet high. The toilet consisted of a round hole in the ground above a deep cesspool and a smaller hole in front which served as a urinal. If nothing else, this toilet demonstrated ingenuity in design, but in order to use it one had to be ever conscious of physical positioning and take careful aim when using the urinal part of it. This was no easy matter since the earthen floor was slanted to permit the runoff of bath water to flow out through a small hole at the base of one wall. To defecate, one had to squat over the hole while taking aim at the urinal hole at the same time. There was nothing to grab on to but I learned through experience that it was best to bring along a heavy stick in order to obtain the necessary leverage. The walls were sufficiently high enough so that one was not visible, as long as they stayed in the squatting position. But squatting for a long time used to impede the circulation in my legs and cause enough discomfort that I needed to stand up for a short while in order to continue the operation. My standing up caused no end of problems since I would become visible from certain parts of the village. This bothered Ahmadou and his family more than it did me personally. Even when squatting one could be visible if anyone in the immediate area went on top of their roof, which they often did to get any number of things which were stored there.

This same bathroom was used for bathing and the women of

Ahmadou's family always placed straw mats on the earthen floor which made it reasonably comfortable. Because these mats were sturdy I could walk on them and squat on them while taking a shower from the large tub of water which was placed in the center. Showering, or tub bathing as it is more correctly called, was no easy matter either because the water attracted large numbers of bees. Because Boussin is situated in an area which lacks permanent surface water, bees congregate around the wells and wherever they are able to find water. Whenever I awoke in the mornings and took my morning shower from the large tub in the bathroom, I always found the place full of bees. African bees are extremely aggressive and it doesn't take much to provoke them. While bathing in Ahmadou's bathroom, I was always completely exposed and so I learned early on to give the bees a wide berth. But even when the water was removed and one crouched over the hole in the ground, the bees buzzed around and not finding any water would come down on any exposed part of the anatomy. After several months of this futile struggle I finally found that the only solution was to bathe at night after sundown.

The teams working in the Kayes region gradually moved eastwards towards the cercle of Kita where they arrived in the month of March, 1970. When Modibo arrived in his home town, his family decided that it would be a good time for him to get married to his fiancee, Astan Cisse. It was a gala affair, made all the more colorful by the presence of the vaccination teams. The wedding had been planned for some time in June, but Modibo's family changed their minds once he arrived in Kita. As it turned out, I was away in Segou when Modibo and Mark tried to reach me about the change in date. When I finally did arrive in Kita, the festivities had quieted down and life was going on as usual in the Keita family compound. All of the teams were looking forward to returning to Bamako because the campaign of the previous months had been extremely tiring and it showed on them physically for the first time. The cercles of Kenieba and Bafoulabe had proven especially hard because many of the villages were located on the tops of mountains accessible only on foot. The teams had also been greatly bothered by tsetse flies in the arrondissements of Faraba, Oulia and Koundian and I was happy that I had given them pentamidine before they left Bamako. The cercle of Kita was also full of tsetse flies, especially those areas close to the Baoule River and its tributaries. The vaccinators and drivers always became passive and quiet under prolonged severe hardship and their passivity in Kita spelled out what it was that they had just been through.

We had them rest in the town of Kita for several days before sending them out into the bush again for the final phase of the Kayes campaign.

Before going out, some of them accompanied me on a climb to the top of *Kita Kourou,* the large mountain which rises up some 1,800 feet behind the town. It took us several hours to reach the top after climbing through canyons and hidden ravines and up sharp inclines. The mountain is full of grottos, many of which contain prehistoric designs on their walls and its slopes support a varied flora, different from that found on the plains below. We came upon luxuriant growths of *kinkeleba (Tecla sudanica),* a plant long used by the Malinke and Bambara as a diuretic and anti-pyretic. The kinkeleba of Kita Kourou is renowned for its efficacy and is sought by people from as far away as Gao and Mopti.

From the top of the mountain, we had a spectacular view of the countryside. Off to the west in the Gangaran, long thin gray columns of smoke rose slowly up into the sky from sites miles apart and bent with the prevailing winds over the yellow and green plains. In anticipation of the soon to arrive rains, farmers were setting fire to the brush, clearing the land for cultivation. The wind blew gently on top of the mountain and echoed its passage through the ravines below. Down below us was a deep green valley, enclosed in the horse shoe shaped center of the mountain. Through the center of this valley a stream flowed, banked by bull rushes and tall acacia trees. The valley had once been the site of the original village of Kita, called Kita Badinka. We descended the mountainside into the valley, along broad slippery paths of flattened elephant grass made by troops of baboons. On the nearby slopes, the baboons watched us in silence and with passive inquisitiveness. There was only one family living in Kita Badinka, in three small houses which stood in the center of what had once been a large settlement. We spent a short time there and then began the ascent up to the top of the mountain again. The climb up the inner face of the mountain is exceedingly difficult and in a way we were lucky that we came on a group of smugglers who showed us an easy way up. They had walked from the Gambia through Kenieba and Bafoulabe and used the mountain as a cache for their contraband. When we got to the top again, it was very late in the afternoon and one could feel the evening air beginning to drift through the trees. Off on the eastern horizon, clouds formed and dissolved and let fall streaks of black rain against the pale blue sky. A season had ended and another had begun.

Chapter XIX
Cholera

By the end of 1970 we had vaccinated the whole country and in the next year planned to establish the maintenance activities whereby newborn children would be vaccinated by local dispensaries. Close to four and a half million people had received smallpox vaccinations and a million children measles inoculations. Our task now was to insure that the young newborns were vaccinated, for if they weren't, then both diseases could establish themselves again within a few years. Compared to the rush and bustle of the mass vaccination campaigns, the work was now steady and quiet, a restful calm after a great storm. We had no way of knowing at the time that it was in reality a calm before a new and terrible storm.

In the summer of 1970, travelers coming into Mali from neighboring Guinea told of the appearance in the country of a new form of dysentery which killed most people in a matter of hours. Because of the rapidity of the disease, the Africans had given it the name *Apollo,* after the space flights to the moon. The appelation seemed to me out of place, but to the Africans, Apollo symbolized speed more than anything else. It was impossible to substantiate these reports because few people traveled either into or out of Guinea, a country which was run by a radical Marxist government. Very little news ever came out of the country through the tight wall of censorship and so we presumed the disease Apollo to be typhoid fever. But throughout the summer the few travelers who did manage to get out of the country reported that the disease was epidemic and to their knowledge not typhoid fever.

By August, the disease reached the capital of Guinea, Conakry, and at this time the Guineans requested the help of the World Health Organization.

A special team of experts was sent out from Geneva, among which were two world authorities on cholera. They spent ten days in the capital and on the evening of August 26th left Conakry for Paris via Bamako. During the ten days they had been in Conakry, the Guineans held them incommunicado with the outside world and thus we had no way of knowing what they had found in the country. The chief of this team was a personal friend of the Malian Minister of Health, Dr. Benitieni Fofana, and on the evening of the 26th Dr. Fofana went out to the airport in order to meet with him and ascertain what was taking place in Guinea. Dr. Fofana was told that the disease in Guinea was cholera, a highly contagious and highly fatal form of dysentery endemic to Asia but unknown until that time in Guinea. This news was terrifying because cholera is a disease which thrives in the unhygienic conditions which exist all over West Africa. The World Health Organization experts had isolated the bacterium which causes the illness, the *cholera vibrio*, all over Conakry, even in the sea water along the beaches where concentrations of one thousand organisms per milliliter of water were found. They weren't able to trace the source of the epidemic because the Guineans wouldn't let them out of the city and greatly hindered their epidemiologic investigations in Conakry. But the suspicion was strong that either the Russians or a Guinean had brought the disease in from the Soviet Union where a major epidemic occurred a short while before.

Although the disease was confirmed as being cholera and thousands of cases were in the hospitals in Conakry, the Guinean government refused to officially recognize the existence of the disease. Likewise, they refused to officially notify the World Health Organization in accordance with international sanitary regulations and prohibited the use of the word cholera in the country. Anyone heard using the word was subject to imprisonment. Then they organized massive parades in the city in which the popular militia carried banners which read, *Cholera is an imperialist disease*. The chief of the World Health Organization team told the Guineans that if they didn't officially recognize the existence of the disease in their country then the organization would. The Guineans said that if this were done they would resign from the World Health Organization. They had already resigned from a number of international bodies, except the United Nations, and it seemed immaterial to many if they added the World Health Organization to their list. The dilemma posed by the existence of a lethal contagious disease in a bordering state which denied its existence and refused to give any information about its progress and distribution in the country was enormous. Cholera existed nowhere else in Africa at that time and now it lay on the other side of an artificial political frontier, miles from Mali's doorstep. At any moment, it could have spilled over the frontier into Mali.

On the morning of August 27th, Dr. Fofana called me on the phone and asked that I come up to the Ministry of Health at 10 A.M. for an emergency meeting about the cholera epidemic in Guinea. Then he told me about his airport meeting of the previous evening and that the Apollo of the travelers was not typhoid fever, but cholera.

The meeting was held in the minister's office and was attended by representatives from the Ministries of the Interior and Foreign Affairs. Dr. Fofana summarized his meeting of the previous evening and then went on to say that the purpose of our meeting was to come up with a comprehensive plan of action for the prevention and control of the disease and for treating cases if they occurred. Then he called on me to talk to the majority of non-medical personnel present at the meeting about cholera and what it might do in a country like Mali.

Cholera is an acute contagious disease characterized by profuse vomiting and diarrhea due to the presence in the intestinal tract of the cholera vibrio and the toxins it produces. The word cholera comes from the Greek word for *a flow of bile*. In untreated cases, the mortality rate is from fifty to seventy percent and death occurs from dehydration in a matter of hours after the illness begins. Cholera has probably been present in an endemic form in central China and in the Lower Bengal area of India since antiquity and has from time-to-time spread in epidemic form across India to Europe and the Western Hemisphere. In the nineteenth century, five pandemics (world epidemics) occurred, four of which reached the North American continent. We have no way of knowing whether any of these pandemics reached West Africa, but it is possible that they did. Historically, the disease has spread along the routes of trade and travel, being carried by infected individuals. The devastating nature of outbreaks is well known to the medical world. In 1947, for example, cholera was introduced into the lower Nile Valley from where it had been absent for forty-five years. In one year, twenty thousand people died of the disease.

The epidemiologic characteristics of cholera were first studied by an Englishman, John Snow, who conducted a painstaking personal investigation of two outbreaks in 1854 in London. The most dramatic of these outbreaks was the one associated with the Broad Street pump.

Snow demonstrated how the disease was caused by contaminated water supplies delivered to the pump. Snow's book, *The Mode of Communication of Cholera,* is a classic of medical detective work, demonstrating a superb degree of data collection and the use of inductive reasoning to develop, test and confirm a theory. Twenty nine years later, in 1883, the German bacteriologist, Koch, identified the causative agent of the disease, the *cholera vibrio,* in the excreta of patients in Egypt. Since that time, we have learned that under favorable conditions the organism can survive in water and on the surfaces of foods for extremely long periods of time. The bacterium does not occur naturally in any animal species except man and is found in large numbers in the vomitus and feces of victims. Under the "sanitary" conditions which prevail in Africa, transmission is virtually assured. All authorities agree that the prevention of outbreaks can only be accomplished by improving living conditions in regard to water supply, fecal disposal and personal hygiene. In times of epidemics, spread can be markedly curtailed by scrupulous cleanliness on the part of those who have contact with cholera victims and their dejecta and infected articles. The boiling of water and all foods and good environmental hygiene are the cornerstones of prevention and control. We knew that such measures could never be implemented in Mali and had to prepare for the consequences.

The available cholera vaccines are known to protect only sixty percent of those who receive them and this protection is only good for six months. So, vaccination is not an effective tool in long-term prevention and control. However, it can be used for the temporary protection of population groups under threat of immediate infection. To explain such subtle refinements to a panicked and uninformed African public accustomed to vaccines which give unequivocal protection for years proved to be an impossible task in the future. The treatment of cholera cases is relatively simple, consisting of the replacement of salts and fluids by intravenous infusions. Individual cases require from five to twenty liters of fluids and salts and once these are given they recover. The prompt administration of such large volumes of fluids in a well equipped medical center is an easy task. But to treat patients scattered across the rugged wilds of the African bush is another matter.

The World Health Organization team had told Dr. Fofana that the type of cholera present in Guinea was a variant known as *El Tor.* This variant had first been isolated in 1905 at the El Tor, Egypt, quarantine station from Mecca pilgrims. From that time until 1937, the El Tor vibrio was found widely scattered in both the Middle East and India among well persons and in rivers and wells where clinical cholera was absent. The presence of this organism in the absence of human cholera led people to believe that it was not disease producing. Then, in 1937, a serious epidemic of cholera broke out in the Celebes and was found to be due to the El Tor vibrio. Since that time, the disease has smoldered in the Celebes. But in May of 1961 it spread for some unknown reason to central Java. In July it was in Sarawak, in August in Macao and in September in Hong Kong and the Philippines. By the end of 1961, El Tor cholera had swept through the Philippine archipelago causing 7,000 cases and a thousand deaths. It was now clear to everyone that El Tor was not an innocuous organism, but one with epidemic potentials to spread over wide geographic areas and the ability to cause serious disease.

By 1965, El Tor had spread westward to Pakistan and Iraq. Then in 1967 it moved across the Persian Gulf into Iran and the Arabian peninsula. In 1970, it crossed over into the southern portion of the Soviet Union. And then it hit the West Coast of Africa in the Republic of Guinea. How did the disease get to Guinea? Because no one was allowed to conduct a proper epidemiologic investigation, we can only piece the story together with scraps of indirect evidence. One could argue that the sea water near Conakry became contaminated with the organism from a ship carrying cholera victims. The bacterium thrives in salt water and can survive in it for months. However, if this were the case then the first cases among Guineans would have occurred along the shoreline, in people having contact with the ocean. This, however, was not the case. We had learned from travelers that many months before the disease appeared in Conakry it was already wrecking havoc up north in the bush. This means then that the disease began inland. If this be so then it is only logical to ask how did it get there and where did it come from. We know that it would have had to be brought in by a traveler coming from an infected area of the world. The likelihood is very strong that the disease was brought in from the Soviet Union. Being a socialist state, Guinea maintains very close ties with the Communist bloc. Most Guineans who travel to Europe go to eastern Europe and the Soviet Union. Also the maporrity of Europeans coming into Guinea are from that part of Europe. Cholera was present in epidemic form in the Soviet Union at the time that the first reports of Apollo drifted into Mali. Thus it is probable that either a Guinean or a Russian came to Guinea while in the five-day incubation period, went to their bush post where they came down with the clinical illness and thus started the epidemic.

With the presence of cholera in Guinea confirmed, we set about drawing up a plan of action to meet the crisis when it occurred. We were all unanimous in the opinion that sooner or later cholera would appear in Mali; it was simply a question of time. The measures we decided to implement were seen not so much as a solid defense against the disease but as a strategy which would delay the appearance of the disease and give us time in which to prepare. All airplane flights between Bamako and Conakry were terminated. River travel on the Niger between Bamako and the Guinean port town of Kouroussa was stopped as was the importation of all food products from Guinea. All travelers entering Mali overland from Guinea were put under surveillance at the frontier in quarantine stations for a period of five days. This measure was of questionable efficacy since people could traverse the frontier at will between the widely scatterd control points which were on the main roads. Travelers entering Bamako by air who had been in Guinea during the five days period prior to their arrival in Mali were placed under daily surveillance for a week.

Many of the older Malian physicians argued for the establishment of a *cordon sanitaire,* a sanitary ribbon along the frontier. What this amounted to was the vaccination of all villages a mile deep along the frontier. Personally, I thought it a useless measure since such a medical Maginot Line would never prevent the introduction of cholera into Mali. However, the Minister concurred with this proposal, more as a concessionary gesture than because he believed in its efficacy. Because world supplies of vaccine were limited we decided to limit vaccination to those areas in imminent danger of being hit by the disease. The Malian government made official appeals to the World Health Organization and to individual nations for donations of vaccine and received sufficient quantities to carry them through the early part of any crisis. More importantly, we obtained thousands of liters of intravenous solutions from France which were distributed throughout the country to cholera treatment centers which we hastily set up. The lazaret in Bamako and those in other major towns were readied. Special cholera cots were constructed in large numbers, consisting of impermeable rubber covers with large holes in the center through which feces passed via a sealed tube to a bucket of disinfectant below. Once all of the preparations were made, we watched and waited.

By September cholera had moved down the coast into Sierra Leone and from there it crossed over into Liberia with itinerant seagoing fishermen. By early October it was in Monrovia, the capital of Liberia and I flew down there to appraise the situation. At the time of my visit, the disease was restricted to an area of the city occupied by fishermen, but later on it broke out of this limited zone and spread throughout the city. I telegraphed my findings to Bamako and received a reply that there was still no cholera in Mali. A month later cholera cases occurred in Abidjan, the capital of the Ivory Coast, primarily among Dyula merchants who had come from Liberia. One of these merchants died in Abidjan and his relatives transported his body a hundred miles north for burial in his home village. Along the way they stopped with the body at various villages where ceremonies were held for the dead man. In all of these villages, cholera broke out five days after the body had passed. The disease was now moving north towards Mali.

The optimists argued that cholera would spare the dry savanna and remain down in the humid coastal rain forest. Others said it would come to Bamako first. But I thought that when it did come to Mali, it would appear in Mopti, because that town lies at the northern end of the great trade route between the inland delta of the Niger and the coast. This supposition was not accepted by most. They watched for cholera in Bamako.

On the morning of the 20th of November, the radio telephone at the Ministry of Defense was cluttered with messages coming in from the various cercles concerning routine administrative problems. By early afternoon the messages stopped and the operator took things a bit easier. At 4:35 P.M., the signal rang, meaning that a field post was trying to reach him. When he threw the switch he heard a voice through the static saying, "Hello, Bamako, Bamako, Bamako. Ici Mopti, ici Mopti."

The operator in Bamako shouted into his speaker, "Hello, Mopti, Mopti, Mopti, je vous ecoute."

From the governor's office in Mopti, the radio operator shouted, "There is cholera in Mopti!"

With those words the great suspense was shattered. The telephone operator at the Ministry of Defense conveyed the message to his superiors who in turn telephoned the Minister of Health. In spite of our preparedness, we were in a way benumbed and paralyzed by the terror of this news. Now that cholera was in Mali, right in the heart of the country, on the Niger River, we became phenomena of fear. It was a role not of our own choosing, but one inflicted on us by an ignorance of not knowing what to do next and by the knowledge that whatever we did would little affect the determined course of events.

The 19th of November was a Thursday, the day of the weekly fair in Mopti. It had started out as a normal market day, the dikes and stalls gradually filling up with people until by noon the river front in the center of the town teemed with thousands of merchants and buyers. They had come in on foot, on donkeys and horses, in scores of trucks and canoes, from villages in the flood plains and towns along the main paved road south to Bamako. Sanitary conditions were at their worst in Mopti on market day. Thousands of people urinated and defecated in the river and at the same time drank its waters. The cholera vibrio was now in these waters but no one could see it.

Late in the afternoon, a Dyula merchant was carried into the Mopti hospital in a severe state of dehydration and collapse. The medecin chef, Dr. Seydou Diallo, took one look at him and realized that the man had cholera. He rushed to the governor's office and sent a radiotelephone message off to Bamako. An hour later, seven more people were carried in and they too were suffering from cholera. Their illness had begun earlier in the afternoon just before they had gone to the river's bank where they defecated. A few hundred yards downstream from them several women and children were drinking water from the river.

The cholera vibrio had been seeded into the waters around Mopti on a day of the week which was most ideal for its dissemination throughout the country. Before any quarantine measures could be implemented, the thousands of buyers and sellers were on their way home and with them went the bacterium.

Fatumata Diallo was a fair-skinned woman about forty years old who was married to the police chief of the gendarmerie at Diafarabe. She rarely went to Mopti, but on Tuesday, the 17th of November, she decided to go to the market in order to buy some wool for weaving a blanket. She took the youngest of her three children with her, a boy of ten years named Seydou. Early that morning their canoe glided out of Diafarabe and two days later it arrived in Mopti, pulling ashore near the bustling fish market. Fatumata and Seydou walked around the market looking for the women from the village of Fatoma who sold the finest quality wool in the inland delta. Shortly before noon, they finally found them down near the river's edge. Once Fatumata had purchased her wool, she bought some millet cakes for Seydou and herself and went down to the river bank, to the cool shade of the fig trees to wait out the long hours until the canoe left for Diafarabe. As she sat there, she chatted with a group of women from Sarafere, a large village a hundred miles downstream from Mopti. They too were waiting for a boat to take them back home. As the afternoon grew on, they waded into the river and took a drink. Upstream from them a group of Dyula merchants from the Ivory Coast waded into the river.

An apprehensive lull filled the four days which followed the appearance of the first cases in Mopti. Although no new cases appeared during this time, we knew that many people were incubating the disease. On Saturday, the 21st of November, we sent three vaccination teams up to Mopti in order to vaccinate the town. On the previous day the town had been put under strict quarantine, no one being allowed either in or out. This measure was hardly effective since hundreds of people moved out of the city under the cover of darkness in canoes. That Saturday afternoon, Fatumata Diallo and her son Seydou arrived home in Diafarabe. As their canoe approached the broad sandy shore, her husband and her two other children came running down to the water's edge. Fatumata and Seydou were exhausted from their journey, for traveling in such small canoes is a very tiring enterprise. On Monday morning Fatumata suddenly vomited for no apparent reason. Then the diarrhea began, continuous streams of it, flowing out until she dropped from exhaustion on a straw mat in the courtyard. Her husband ran to get the local medical assistant who suspected cholera as soon as he looked at Fatumata. There were no intravenous fluids in Diafarabe and so he tried to give her fluids by mouth. But her vomiting was continuous and she couldn't hold anything down. No one in Diafarabe had ever seen this illness before. Fatumata, who had been fully well a few hours before, now lay on a mat motionless, her eyes sunken deep in their orbits, her skin dry and shriveled. Towards noon she stopped breathing and her husband and children stood by motionless as if they had lost the faculty of speech.

Down the river in Mopti, the lull was ended by a massive epidemic. By late afternoon, thirty three cholera victims had been carried into the lazaret. Here everyone was prepared and only five died. Down in Sarafere, the women who had gone into the river with Fatumata were dying of cholera. We had feared that the disease would spread with rapidity, but never did we imagine that it would move up and down the Niger as quickly as it did. By the 26th of November, the disease was a hundred miles further upstream from Diafarabe in Macina and by the 4th of December two hundred miles on up the river from there in Koulikoro which was but thirty five miles from Bamako. Downstream, the disease spread with frightening speed through the swamps and lakes of the delta and hit all of the villages along the way. By the 27th of November, it was in the town of Goundam where it claimed five hundred lives in a week's time. We sent vaccination teams all over in an effort to stop the outbreak, but as we all knew in advance, vaccination did not have much of an effect. One of my drivers, Zamble Kone, whom I myself vaccinated, contracted cholera and almost died in the cercle of Bankass. Fortunately, by that time, intravenous fluids were present in most of the bush posts and so he was treated by the local medical assistant. But then he went to Mopti to recuperate and there he contracted typhoid fever. He was finally evacuated to Bamako where we hospitalized him at the Gabriel Toure Hospital. He then suffered a perforation of the small intestine, one of the serious complications of typhoid fever and had to be operated on. In spite of all this Zamble recovered. When I saw him after the surgeons had closed the intestinal perforation, I never thought he would survive.

As soon as cholera came to Koulikoro, panic swept through Bamako. Again, many fled the city, as they had done during the meningitis epidemic and Dyula and Lebanese merchants sold cholera vaccine on the black market to terrified citizens. I had advised the Minister of Health to vaccinate Bamako at the last possible moment so as to profit from the maximal effect of the vaccine on the population when the epidemic struck. Had we vaccinated before that time then many would have lost some of the immunity given by the vaccine and would have been susceptible by the time the epidemic arrived. On the 6th of December, we deployed ten vaccination teams throughout the city and during the next few days delivered 234,610 vaccinations.

With such a good percentage of the population of the city vaccinated, it was unlikely that the disease coming up the river would cause a serious outbreak in Bamako. The road and the railway to Koulikoro were blocked for two weeks, reducing the possibility of the disease getting into the city. To our surprise, the disease only caused 158 cases in Bamako. It was as if a solid wall of defensive immunity had been built up. The disease spread to the north of Koulikoro, traveled around the back of Bamako and then came back to the river again. At this point, it didn't continue on up the river because there are few villages upstream from Bamako on account of the tsetse fly. Rather, it began traveling along the railway, westwards to Kayes. At Bafoulabe, it hit the Senegal River and traveled down it towards the Senegal frontier.

Downstream from Mopti, the disease caused the worst health disaster anyone could remember. It spread through the isolated villages of the inland delta, carrying off half the population. Sarafere's population of 828 was reduced to 436. This terrible mortality rate was not reduced until we sent mobile treatment teams through the area. Throughout the inland delta, those who buried the cholera victims contracted the disease and died themselves five days later. In Mopti, all of the mentally disturbed people who roamed the streets in rags were carried off by cholera. By January, not a single crazy person was left in the town.

Throughout Mali, people were exhorted on the radio and by health education teams to boil their drinking water and to practice some rudimentary sanitary procedures. For those who did, the reward was to escape the disease. Of the five thousand Europeans in the country, only three contracted cholera and they were individuals who lived in the bush ignoring rudimentary health precautions. In spite of all our measures, the disease marched on down the river towards Timbuctoo. Beyond Timbuctoo lay the great Niger Bend and a dense population of a million Songhoi people living along the banks of the river. In an attempt to soften the blow of the disease in this area and to protect as many lives as possible, I left Bamako on the 15th of December with eight vaccination teams and headed for Timbuctoo and the Niger Bend.

Chapter XX
Timbuctoo

Our race down the river with cholera was one in which the betting odds were against us. For the disease had already swept its way through the swampy world of the inland delta and ahead lay nothing but a clear stretch of river and a million people. It took us three days to reach Timbuctto from Mopti, driving through the land of the great lakes from N'Gouma to the shores of Lake Niangay and Lake Do, on to Bambara-Maounde and then to Rharous. Once there, we crossed the river on barges and drove back towards Timbuctoo. That trip along the shores of the lakes suddenly brought us into the presence of a disaster whose magnitude we could never have imagined. All around the lakes thousands of people had died of cholera. "How many have died here?" I would ask in the villages, but most often the reply was a mute expression of despair. Despair seems to be the only refuge in the wake of such a tragedy. Yet, I knew that we couldn't despair and my mind was overtaken by a terrifying fear, a fear of our being too late, a fear of our whole effort being ineffective. The distances across the flat flood plains seemed infinitely long even though I had gone over these tracks many times before. My impatience with our progress had no rational basis, only an emotional compulsion that we arrive at our destination in time to prevent the same disaster we were now witnessing.

The great disasters of Africa always come as a sudden surprise to the Africans even when they have been announced in advance. For the Africans will not believe that it is so until they see it themselves. And so, in Timbuctoo, life was going on as usual even though a few miles up the river thousands were dying from a disease which would soon be in the city itself.

The sun rose early the morning after our arrival, turning the gray mud buildings into a fluorescent scene of shimmering yellow. The thorn trees were full of the spirited songs of yellow and red weaver birds and a brisk cold wind whipped gusts of sand around the corners with a howl. We began vaccinating the city immediately, in the quarter of Dyingerey Ber. The women and children came out of the buildings and down the narrow streets by the hundreds and after them came the men. They clustered themselves in front of the vaccinators and refused to form lines, for they were here not only to be vaccinated, but also to see everyone else shot with the jet gun. The Songhoi women had decorative coiffures studded with silver coins and amber beads and braids which came down underneath their chins where they were attached with a metal band. Most of the children had their heads shaved in a pattern which reflected their ethnic group and social background. Towards the end of the session, the Maure noblewomen came out of their houses with their black slaves. They were enormously fat women covered with yards of rich blue silk cloth. They were not veiled, but whenever they met a stranger, they covered their faces by pulling the edges of their robes together. Their jet black hair, studded with amber stones, gold coins and three dimensional triangles of silver stood out in sharp contrast to their light brown skin. Their palms and feet were dyed an orange black color with henna and also their knuckles and they decorated their faces with local mascara called *kohl wa*. In the two succeeding days, we vaccinated the remainder of the city and in the end reached 12,346 people which was as accurate a census of the town as had ever been taken. We remained in Timbuctoo for a week, helping the medecin chef set up treatment facilities in the event cholera came to the town. During this time we sent some of the teams out into the rural areas surrounding the town in order to vaccinate the nomad camps and sedentary farmers along the river banks.

While I was in Timbuctoo, I visited Frank and Eleanor Marshall, American missionaries who have a station in the town. The Marshall's house was a modest one story cement block building surrounded by a small vegetable garden and several delicate acacia trees. It was a warm home where one felt welcomed and at ease as soon as they stepped inside the front gate. The Marshalls had been in Mali since 1953 and in Timbuctoo since 1959. Frank and his brother Dave were well known in Mali for the excellent work they had done with the Niger River fishermen in the inland delta. They had trained large numbers of fishermen in modern techniques and in the maintenance of outboard engines. Along with other missionaries in this part of Africa, they

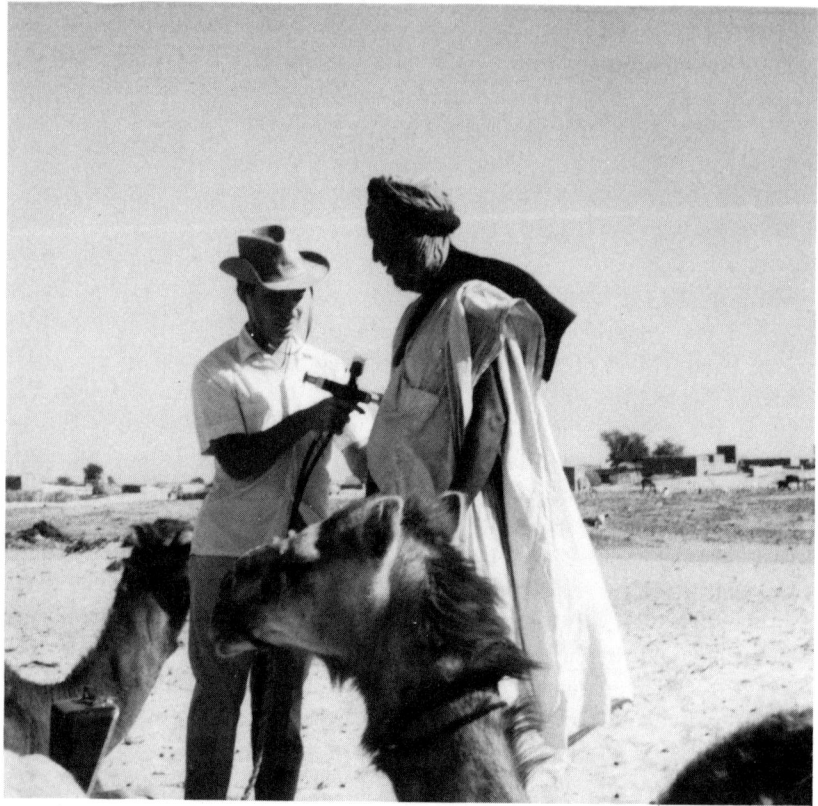

FIGURE 39. Dr. Imperato vaccinating a Maure nomad on the edge of the city of Timbuctoo.

operated a houseboat called the *Niger River Gospel Boat* and with it were able to reach many remote villages where they rendered sorely needed medical care. Although the Marshalls could write a fascinating account of their life in Timbuctoo, I think myself that the more interesting account would be about the numerous visitors who have come to the city since they have been there.

I had visited Timbuctoo many times before and on each of these visits it seemed to me that the renown of the place was not in what was physically there nor in what had been there, but rather in what had taken place there. It was sad, I thought, that so many of the foreigners who came from afar found the town a disappointment. All of the centuries of history and civilization were preserved there in a

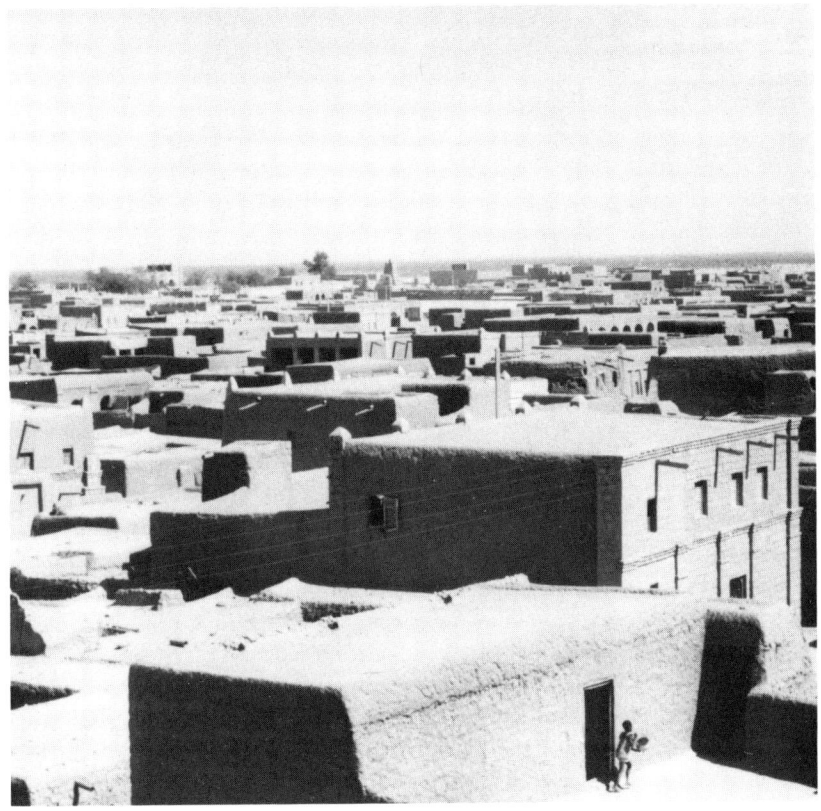

FIGURE 40. The city of Timbuctoo as seen from the minaret of the mosque of Dyingerey Ber. Most of the buildings in the city are built of mud brick.

language different from stone monuments, royal tombs, castles and palaces and great museums. But most of them did not understand that language. They saw before them a mass of dingy mud buildings lying on the edge of the Sahara where the Niger laps at the silky white desert sands. But they did not see the story of the place preserved in its present day ethnic diversity, in oral traditions and ancient arabic manuscripts, and went away thinking the town greatly overrated. I found it futile to explain all this to them for they wanted to be shown what they expected to find and would settle for no other alternative.

The first recorded history of this part of the world exists in Arab chronicles written about the year 1000 A.D. At that time, the Ghana Empire was the center of political dominance in the Western Sudan.

Ghana was strongly influenced by the Arabs who had invaded North Africa in the eighth century and then crossed the Sahara into the savanna country of West Africa. In 1076, the captial of Ghana, also known as Ghana, adopted Islam as its official religion. This city was then the center of the caravan traffic between West Africa and North Africa. At this time Timbuctoo was only a seasonal camp of the nomadic Tuareg who left their desert oases in January and descended towards the river where there was sufficient water and grass for their flocks. During these early decades, the Tuareg frequenting this site left some of their utensils and grain there as they do today in their dry season river camps. All of this property was entrusted to a woman by the name of Buctoo. The name, Timbuctoo comes from the two Tuareg words, Tin, meaning "that belonging to," and Buctoo.

As time went on, some people established permanent residence at the site, traders came from the west out of the Ghana Empire and Songhoi people came from the east out of Gao. Eventually, a village formed and then a town, peopled by a mixture of races from all over this area of West Africa. In 1336, the emperor of the Mali Empire, Mansa Moussa stopped at Timbuctoo on his way back from Mecca and had the great mosque known as Dyingerey Ber built by his Andaulsian architect, Ibrahim es Saheli. It is thought by most scholars that es Saheli introduced baked brick into the western sudan. The mosque he built in Timbuctoo still stands today, although it has been much renovated over the centuries. Until the time of Mansa Moussa's visit to Timbuctoo, the city did not have much of an intellectual elite. By order of the emperor, the local scholars were sent to study at Fez in Morocco where they acquired a learned character and brought themselves into contact with the main stream of Arab scholarship. Although the city was Moslem and possessed an elite group of scholars and Koranic theologians, the surrounding rural population was animist and not at all under the control of the city.

By the middle of the fifteenth century, the power of the Mali Empire had wanned and in 1468, Sonni Ali Ber, the emperor of the Songhoi Empire of Gao marched westward out of Gao and captured Timbuctoo. From there, he marched on Djenne and then defeated the Mossi in the south and in doing so brought all of the country in the Niger Bend under his control. Sonni Ali Ber died in 1492 and was succeded by one of his generals who usurped the throne. This general, Askia the Great, expanded the conquests of his predecessor and organized the empire in a way which gave it administrative cohesion. Timbuctoo became a center of trade and learning, both of which prospered under the military and political protection of the Songhoi emperor. The judge of Timbuctoo, known as the *cadi,* became the supreme judge for the entire empire and holy men and students of the Koran came from all over the Moslem communities in the western sudan to study at Timbuctoo. The city reached its zenith in this period of great peace.

Much of the commerce of Timbuctoo depended on the extraction of rock salt from the mines hundreds of miles to the north in the Sahara. Although the mines were under the control of the Songhoi, they were geographically closer to Morocco than to the sudan. During the early part of the sixteenth century, the sultans of Morocco tried to foment trouble with the Songhoi over the mines. At this time, they had been driven out of Europe and now looked south across the Sahara as an area of expansion. The dispute over the mines provided them with an excuse for invading the Songhoi Empire. The Moroccans sent four military expeditions across the Sahara between 1543 and 1591, only the last of which succeeded in reaching the southern limits of the desert. This expedition which was headed by an Andalusian eunuch by the name of Djouder was composed of about nine hundred men, most of them Europeans who had been captured by the Moroccans in various wars. They were equipped with firearms and easily defeated the Songhoi army at Tondibi on the Niger near the present day town of Gao. The Songhoi were so desperate against this superiorly armed force that they tried to trample them with herds of cattle during the battle, but with no success. The Moroccans brought the order and prosperity of the sudan to a sudden end. All of the vassal people revolted and anarchy reigned. Djouder entered Timbuctoo, confiscated the wealth of the city and distributed it to his soldiers. He then arrested the most influential learned men, massacred some and sent the remainder off to Morocco. Many of them did not survive the desert crossing. Having thus disposed of the custodians of Timbuctoo's intellectual life and culture, the Moroccan invaders settled down to ruling the sudan. They made Timbuctoo their administrative and military center and had as their head a pasha who resided in the city. During the first two decades, the pashas of the city were named by the Sultan of Morocco, but later on as ties with Morocco weakened, subsequent pashas were elected by the Moroccan troops stationed in Timbuctoo and by their descendants, the Arma.

The invaders intermarried with the local population and their descendants became the distinguished ruling class of the city. Eventually, internecine struggles occurred among the Moroccan descendants and led to a state of absolute anarchy. In time, the Arma came to rule the city on the sufferance of the Tuareg nomads who had hovered on the outskirts of the place as all these historical events were taking place. They themselves did not like living in the city; they only wanted to loot it from time to time and were careful not to go to extremes and destroy the commercial life of the city in the process. Within the city, the Arma exploited the rest of the population. In the late nineteenth century the Bambara king of Segou conquered Timbuctoo, but his hold did not last for very long. Within a few years, the Tuareg wrested it back from him. Then the Peul emperor Cheikou Ahmadou marched out of his new captial at Hamdallaye and captured the city and when his empire fell to the Toucouleurs the city came under the rule of the new conquerors.

That Timbuctoo existed was well known to Europe by the nineteenth century. But what Europe didn't know was what sort of city it was and the mere thought that it existed on the other side of the Sahara in an Africa otherwise devoid of cities sent imaginations to work. Because no Europeans had ever seen Timbuctoo notions about the city were based on the descriptions of Arab chroniclers and travelers who had either been there or else had spoken to other Arabs who had been there. The lack of direct European observation of the city and its location across a hostile Moslem world and miles of desert generated an aura of mystery about it and the notion that it was the end of the world. This latter idea had been carried through in popular language usage, especially in the United States, where the word Timbuctoo is often used in the sense of a far away place at the end of the world or else as a nowhere. That the use of the city's name in this way had its roots in the western world's concept of the city some one hundred and fifty years ago is unknown to most. There was, of course, nothing mysterious about Timbuctoo, except to those who hadn't been there and they wove descriptions of the city which made it out to be an African El Dorado. Between 1588 and 1853, a total of forty-three Europeans attempted to reach Timbuctoo, twenty-five Englishmen, fourteen Frenchmen, two Americans and two Germans. Of these five reached the city. The first of these was a Frenchman, Francis Paul Imbert who accompanied his master, a Portugese renegade, who was sent to Timbuctoo by the governor of a province of Morocco in 1670. Very little is known of this journey except that they did arrive in Timbuctoo and later returned to Morocco. In 1805 the celebrated English explorer, Mungo Park, began his second journey into the interior of West Africa, traveling down the Niger from Sansanding. In 1806 he approached Kabara, the port village of Timbuctoo which lies on the river some twelve miles from the city. There he met with hostile bands of Tuareg nomads and consequently was never able to enter the city. He continued on down the river into what is now Nigeria where his raft either capsized or else was attacked at Busa. Park's journals, however, were recovered and in them he gives a description of Timbuctoo which is unfortunately quite inaccurate, based on his own ideas of what the city was probably like.

In 1810, an American sailor, Robert Adams, was wrecked on the coast of Cape Blanco which is to the northwest of Timbuctoo. There he was captured by Arab nomads and enslaved, a not unusual happening at that time and, according to his account which was published in 1816, taken to Timbuctoo. The validity of Adams' claim was much debated at the time and has been ever since, but today most scholars in the field accept the fact that he did visit Timbuctoo. His descriptions of the city and the surrounding countryside are too accurate to have been obtained second hand. Certainly, his descriptions of the city contain gross exaggerations in terms of size and wealth, but Adams was an uneducated man who was probably intimidated into catering to popular notion in order to make his story believed.

In 1827, Major Gordon Laing, an English explorer set out for Timbuctoo from Tripoli and succeeded in reaching the city. On his way back to North Africa, however, he was ambushed and killed by Arabs and his journals lost. In 1824, a Frenchman, Rene Caillie, set out to reach Timbuctoo from the West Coast of Africa. He was at the time only twenty-four years old. Caillie had gone to the French colony of St. Louis in what is now Senegal in 1816 where he had worked at a variety of petty jobs. His greatest ambition in life was to visit Timbuctoo and this ambition was in a sense an abnormal obsession which drove him relentlessly on towards the achievement of this goal. During his early years in Senegal, he had the opportunity of traveling into the interior of the Senegal River basin which enabled him to learn of the problems posed to Europeans in this part of the world. He rapidly realized that his only hope of getting through to Timbuctoo was in his disguising himself as a Moor. This was not to be a simple costume disguise, but one of life style and so for over a year he learned Arabic, studied Islam and the way of life of the Moors to the point where he easily passed for one. Then he set out for Timbuctoo, relating to everyone that he was returning to Cairo from where he had been kidnapped by the Christians. In 1828, Caillie reached Timbuctoo and remained in the city for two weeks. He was disappointed by what he found, a small mud city of some twelve thousand inhabitants who were poorly fed and dressed. He returned to France to claim the ten thousand franc prize which had been offered by the Geographic Society of Paris to the first man to describe Timbuctoo. There were some who doubted his story, especially since the Timbuctoo he described was not the Timbuctoo of legend and fancy. But there is no doubt that he visited the city and from him we have the first detailed description of not only Timbuctoo, but also of that portion of the interior of West Africa.

In 1853, Heinrich Barth, a noted German explorer traveled from North Africa down into northern Nigeria and from there across what is now the Niger Republic to the Niger River. He then went north to the west of Hombori through the dry country of the Gourma and reached Timbuctoo. Barth was a scholarly man and a superb observer and in his three volume account of this journey entitled, *Travels and Discoveries in North and Central Africa,* is found the earliest and best descriptions of that part of Africa. In 1880, another German explorer, Oscar Lenz, visited the city for sixteen days and with him the period of peaceful exploration came to an end.

Although the first French gunboat reached Kabara in 1887, it was not until 1893 that the town was taken from the Tuareg by the French military under Boiteaux. The Tuaregs, however, managed to re-take the city and annihilated a brigade commanded by the famous French soldier-explorer, Bonnier. It was finally Joffre, who later became a Marshall of France, who took the town in 1894. After this the apparatus of colonial administration was brought into the town, missionaries came, scientists and ordinary travelers. The great sleep of centuries had been ended.

In spite of the arrival of the western world in Timbuctoo, there was much about the place which remained unchanged. The salt caravans still come down from Taoudeni in the Sahara, each camel carrying a large tombstone size bar of salt on either side of its hump. These bars of salt sell for about three American dollars in Timbuctoo, for six in Mopti and for ten in Bamako. There used to be two large salt caravans per year, called the *azalais,* containing up to ten thousand camels. But in recent years, truck convoys have replaced many of the camels and salt caravans rarely number more than two hundred camels.

In recent years, a modern airport has been built and in 1966 an electric power plant was installed. Bright fluorescent street lamps now throw patches of white light onto streets which passed centuries in darkness. There are over forty electric water pumps in the town and a new black tarmac road which stretches like a ribbon over the white sands to the river port of Kabara. There is a movie theatre and a gasoline station and three flights a week to and from Bamako.

There was in Timbuctoo at the time a remarkable man whose name was Eliot Elisofon. He was producing a film for the Westinghouse Corporation which was later called, *The Bend of the Niger*. Eliot first came into my life because he was sick and when I told him the diagnosis his reply was, "Wow!" an exclamation which I later learned he used for reacting to extraordinary phenomena of all kinds. For others, he himself was an unusual phenomenon, a complex man with many talents who could not be neatly summed up and classified but only described in great detail. But such descriptions rarely told the full story because he was a category without precedent, a man who could have walked against the landscape of any era and found renown just the same. Among other things, he was a well known *Life* photographer, painter, African art historian, writer and explorer. He had been to the top of the Mountains of the Moon in Central Africa, to New Guinea with the late Michael Rockefeller and into almost every jungle in Asia and South America. By the time I had gotten to know him, he had already lived three lives in one and was starting on a fourth. The kinetic drive and ambition charged up inside of him were enormous and in the quiet somnolence of Africa he was like high voltage electricity rushing down the fragile wires of a pocket transistor radio. He burned everything up in his path. But, he was essentially a creator of beauty, who on film and canvas and in his writings brought the aesthetic wonders of Africa as he saw them to millions of people.

Eliot did not enter people's lives slowly, but came in as a crashing tornado, carrying everyone off on his course and towards his goals. It was this turbulent exterior which terrified my African staff and the announcement of Eliot's impending visits always put a look of terror onto their faces. The turbulence created by Eliot's presence cast a shadow over his associations with the many people who never got to know him well. But over the years, Eliot visited Mali on three occasions and was a guest in my home and during those visits I got to know him well. Our common interest in African art and ethnography were the common grounds on which our friendship grew. I found that beneath the frenzied exterior was a warm and generous person who over the years became a loyal friend.

The artist in Eliot drove him to create and so he always tried to create on film Africa as he wished to see it and in so doing often missed documenting the Africa that was there. He and I were always in hot dispute over this matter and it brought him into continual conflict with the Africans. The way he wanted masked dances performed for his cameras was the way he would have painted them on his own canvas. But it was usually at variance with how they were actually performed. Eliot wanted the dancers out in the sun and against an acceptable background. But they were accustomed to dancing in the shade next to a dense background of onlookers wearing T-shirts, sun glasses and wrist watches and leaning on bicycles. Eliot wanted nothing of T-shirts, sunglasses and wrist watches in his creations and so off they came and out went the bicycles. The polite tolerance of Africa permitted this once in a village, but not a second time.

The Malians pronounced his name as "Monsieur Elisophone," and he took great delight in hearing this. Whenever he came in from the airport it was usually in a convoy of taxis loaded down with camera equipment and with a film crew in tow. He would plunge through my front gate and crunch his way across the gravel walk to the veranda. He was always in an open neck shirt and khaki trousers with a red or white handkerchief dangling from his belt. There was a delicate bounce to his walk, an unexpected trait in so large a man. Ahmadou was the first object of his domestic onslaught for Eliot would go into the kitchen, examine the meal, pronounce it unsatisfactory and then proceed to cook himself. He was an excellent cook and on this point he was never modest. I never heard him say to Ahmadou, "I'm a better cook than you," but he did say, "I know of only a few people who can cook better than I." Eliot often insisted that we eat out at the *L'Aquarium* where Monsieur Gatineau, the proprietor, always gave him a visa to the kitchen. There Eliot modified our order as he saw fit and gave advice to the chef who took it in good humor. Back in New York, Eliot took quite naturally to bringing complete meals into hospitals, whose menus he considered totally inadequate and unworthy of human consumption. When our mutual friend, Lester Wunderman, an expert on the Dogon and an Africanist, was ill with malaria at New York University Hospital, Eliot made a daily pilgrimage from his home on East 27th Street to the hospital his arms loaded with soup and main course dishes.

It was in the *L'Aquarium* in Bamako that Eliot acquired one of his best pieces of African sculpture, a Senufo maternity figure. It stood in one of the front windows of the restaurant, an object which Monsieur

Gatineau had placed there to fill a large open space. Eliot was an experienced connoisseur who recognized an authentic masterpiece the moment he saw it. And the Senufo maternity figure was such a masterpiece. But for Eliot to make Monsieur Gatineau's space filler his prized possession required great operative tact, because Monsieur Gatineau also knew that Eliot was an authority on African art. When Eliot told Monsieur Gatineau that the statue brought back cherished memories of his mother, Monsieur Gatineau's heart melted and when he finally sold it to Eliot it was after they had spent an hour speaking about their own mothers and about motherhood in general. But after a few weeks, Monsieur Gatineau had reason to regret the sale he had made in a

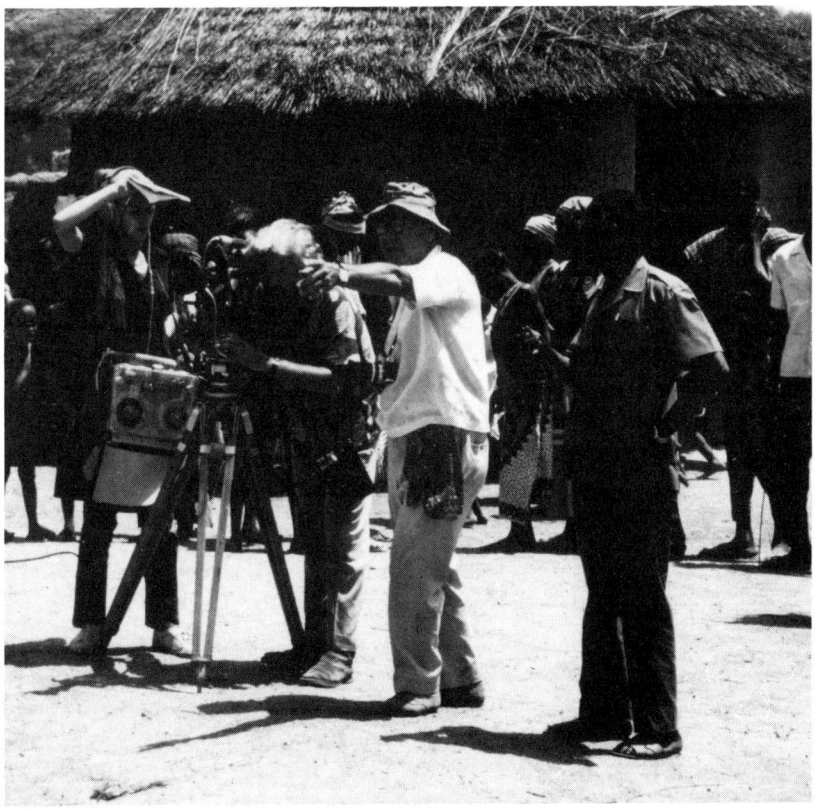

FIGURE 41. The late Eliot Elisofon *(in center with hat on) directing* cameraman George Bracher. To Eliot Elisofon's left stands Djigui Diakite, our chief vaccinator.

moment of deep emotion and whenever Eliot returned he always chided him about having pulled a fast one on him.

Eliot Elisofon died suddenly in New York in 1973, leaving his fine collection of African art and his photographic collection to the Museum of African Art in Washington, D.C. The last time I saw him was at my home in New York on a cold December night before he was leaving for India and I for Africa. To those who knew him he will always be remembered as a genuine and loyal friend.

When I last saw Eliot in Timbuctoo, he was in the middle of a herd of camels and a group of Tuareg nomads. He pointed out with pride the famous life preserver kit he always carried and said, "I'm prepared for cholera too." When he said that he wasn't thinking of himself, but of everyone around him for he had enough tetracycline in that kit to treat a ward of cholera patients. The nomads and camels were all comfortably lying down in the shade of several thorn trees. But Eliot was standing out in the sun, making what seemed to me like a futile effort to get them all to join him. Djigui shook his head. "He will never get them to move," he said. But as the film later showed, Eliot's efforts as usual ended in success.

Once we had completed our vaccination of Timbuctoo and the area surrounding it, I was anxious to move the teams out along the banks of the Niger, up towards Dire and Goundam and down towards Gourma-Rharous, Bourem and the Niger Bend. But we were delayed for a few days, waiting for the flight from Bamako to bring vaccine supplies. Dr. Lamine Keita, the medecin chef of Timbuctoo, had housed our thirty-two vaccinators and eight drivers in a rest house built next to a waterhole, beneath a thick cover of dolm palms and thorn trees. Those who couldn't sleep inside, slept in large tents we erected or else outside. Keeping so many idle men out of mischief in so small a place as Timbuctoo wasn't easy. So I put them to work cleaning and repairing the jet injectors and had the drivers fix up their trucks.

There is not much in Timbuctoo to hold one's attention for long, unless he is interested in those things which are not seen on the surface. The market place is small and inactive compared to those in the savanna and the products sold in the greatest quantity, salt, cereals, spices, dates and milk, very much reflect the fragile subsistence level at which these people exist. There was a profusion of watermelons in the market because they grow well in the sandy soil around the town. It was a remarkable sight to see a score of canoes filled with mountains of watermelons sailing up the Niger towards Mopti where most are sold.

What attracts the eye most in Timbuctoo is the ethnic diversity of the town's inhabitants, a diversity which is seen not only in physique but also in mode of dress. To the trained eye a person's cultural identity is immediately known and his social status as well. The three principal culture groups in the town are the Arabs, called the Maures by the Malians, the Songhoi and the Tuareg. The Tuareg are composed of three classes, the Imochar (nobles), the Imrad (serfs), also known as the Daga and the Iraouellen (salves), commonly called the Bella. The Tuareg nobles wear veils and cover their heads completely with their turbans of indigo cloth. The Daga men wear plain black cotton cloth, a long piece of which they wind about their heads in a partial turban, leaving the top uncovered. The same piece of cloth is wrapped over the mouth, forming a veil. By comparison with the light-skinned nobles and serfs, the black-skinned Bella are poorly dressed. On the whole, they are short and mesomorphic in build with broad faces. It is said by Malians that the Bella are a treacherous people, given easily to murder and theft. Although this is less true of the Bella today than it once was, other groups still feel uncomfortable with them around. Such antisocial acts were not peculiar to the Bella alone, and in reality they simply carried out the orders of the nobles who left the dirty work

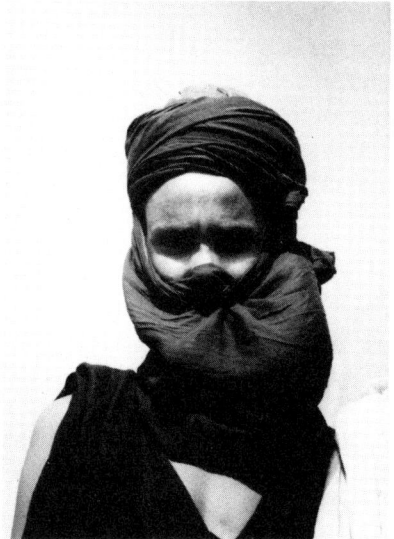

FIGURE 42. A young Tuareg nomad in the inland delta of the Niger near Timbuctoo.

to them. This is not to say that the nobles would not stoop to steal and murder if it took their fancy. They were fully capable of it because pillaging was a necessary way of life in their harsh desert world where getting the best of a victim was the key to survival. But if at all possible, they left it to the Bella.

The Songhoi of Timbuctoo are composed of the Arma who are nobles and their serfs, the Gabibi. The Arma are a black people with fine facial features and are descendants of the sixteenth century Moroccan invaders who married Sudanese wives. Their serfs are often indistinguishable from them in physique, but are less finely dressed. The Arabs are socially stratified into nobles and slaves, the latter being black Africans descended from enslaved Sudanese negroes. The Berabich are Arab nomads who are socially equal to the Arab nobles, although their material possessions are considerably fewer.

The social classes which exist in Timbuctoo lack a present day legal basis, but the weight of centuries of tradition is behind them. Their breakdown has been gradual, hastened by the education of the younger generations and by extended contacts with the outside world. But for many families, the traditional relationships are still respected to a certain degree. It is doubtful, however, that even so strong a force as tradition can keep alive for another generation, even as a vestige, this ancient social system.

The tourists who came to Timbuctoo at that time were housed in a four-room campement built up on an elevation near the Bandyinde quarter. There was a lovely seasonal pond behind it, located down in a depression, and beyond it a large white sand dune topped by spreading acacias formed the horizon against an almost cloudless sky. When the Niger rises, water flows up through a canal which connects to the pond, a ribbon of blue water, meandering across white sand and shaded by graceful acacia trees. It is thought that this canal was built by Askia the Great in the latter part of the fifteenth century.

The campement was being enlarged at the time we were in Timbuctoo, a new two story building being built out of gray stone behind the original structure. The building got off to a bad start because one of the main walls collapsed before it was completed. But eventually a spacious building rose with moorish arches, doorways and terraces and a large courtyard in the center. In spite of the greater comfort provided by the new building, tourists still complained. They complained about the heat which no one could alter and the lack of water, unaware that it had been drawn up out of wells, transported and then put up into tanks on top of the roof. There was sand in the bread and this often surprised them even though they were in the midst of a sea of sand. Sand was also in the bread at Nioro and Nara and in Rharous and Ansongo, but not ever visiting these places, they thought it peculiar to Timbuctoo which it wasn't.

The mud brick mosques and the homes of Laing, Caillie and Barth did not draw many compliments. And, occasionally, when a tour guide slipped under the hammering interrogation of an experienced tourist and let it be known that the plaques identifying the three explorers' homes were on recently built houses in areas representing an educated guess, a groan of disappointment rose from the crowd. When the plane carried tourists on to Gao or back to Bamako, they were hot, dehydrated and tired, somewhat disappointed in what they had seen, but pleased to be in possession of the ability to say, "I've been to Timbuctoo."

Two days before I left Timbuctoo, Dr. Malhamane Diarra, the regional director of health of Gao came overland around the Niger Bend from Gao to meet me so that we might travel together to Gourma-Rharous and to Bourem to supervisce the vaccination and health education campaign. Dr. Diarra was an elderly man who had been working in the Gao region since Mali became independent and he knew all of the river people and desert nomads well. It was our plan to drive along the left bank of the Niger and to then cross the twelve mile wide river in order to reach Rharous. It took us a day to get all of the teams ready for the departure. We sent two teams up towards Dire and the area around Lake Faguibine. One of the teams was to start their program in the arrondissement of Ras el Ma which lies at the tip of the lake. This arrondissement's name in Tamashek, the language of the Tuareg, means, "the tip of the spear," because Lake Faguibine is shaped like a spear head and Ras el Ma lies at its tip. The six remaining teams were to leave with Dr. Diarra and myself for the campaign in the Niger Bend.

As the evening of the last day drew near, Djigui came in to tell us that word had arrived that cholera was already in one of the Bella nomad camps on the outskirts of the town. I mounted a camel with Djigui and an infirmier and rode out over the undulating thorn bush covered sands. As we rode along, the air became uncomfortably cold as the sun fell behind the round dunes on the far horizon. Low stratiform clouds laced the sky, turning all shades of pink and orange and from the town behind us the drums rolled up and down with the wind and floated across the dunes. The glowing warmth of the late afternoon had turned into cold darkness by the time we reached the camp. The camp was composed of several small oval huts built of bent sticks and woven straw mats and the wind whistled its way through and around them. The chief of the camp came out to greet us when he heard the soft approach of the camels. He took us to one of the huts where a small boy lay on a patinated leather cushion. I had only to look at him once to know that he had cholera.

Chapter XXI
Into the Niger Bend

There are two tracks which lead eastward out of Timbuctoo, one being next to the river and the other running parallel to it but over the higher ground of the dunes a few miles to the north. We took the higher road since the lower one was still flooded in many areas. It is pleasant country to drive through, extremely hilly, the dunes being covered with an unexpected growth of tufted grass, dolm palms and thorn trees. The track is marked every few miles by small concrete blocks because otherwise there wouldn't be any way to distinguish it from the rest of the sandy landscape. The air was crisp and clear, the sky cloudless and high above us eagles drifted up and down in the wind currents in a lazy sort of way. The number and variety of birds present wasn't unexpected, but it was a real delight to see them on such a beautiful morning. Small groups of camels browsed among the tall acacias and large herds of goats and sheep walked slowly through the thorn trees towards the river. We came across a band of Tuaregs mounted on horses. They were dressed in flowing robes which caught the wind and blew up into large dimensions. Aside from them, we didn't see any people until we arrived in a small camp called, Ber. The seven trucks in our convoy followed one another at a considerable distance to avoid the dust clouds which were constantly forming.

Ber had only recently been established as an arrondissement, but the camp itself consisted of only several Tuareg tents and a rectangular mud brick building which served as an office and home for the chief of the arrondissement. He was a Tuareg and arrived on his white camel a few minutes after we pulled the trucks into the shade of the thorn trees. The Tuaregs do not like to live in houses and I wondered if the chief actually lived in the building. As it turned out, he did and he didn't, because he also had his family tent erected out behind it. His wife served us tea on the soft sandy floor of the house as we discussed the cholera prevention program. It was a bad time of year to vaccinate the nomads because they were widely dispersed away from the river, water and grass being abundant even high up in the sahel. Because of the rapidity with which cholera was moving down the river, we decided that we could only vaccinate the riverine population and could not spare the time to go up north after small scattered bands of Tuaregs. From the epidemiologic point of view, the nomads were fairly safe for the moment since the disease was confined to the river. We left a team behind in Ber to vaccinate the arrondissement and instructed them to meet us in Bamba in a week's time. Before leaving, we set up a cholera treatment facility with a stock of intravenous fluids and antibiotics and carefully instructed the medical assistant in the treatment of cases.

Beyond Ber the track passed through some very sandy areas where four wheel drive had to be used. We continued on over the dunes and in most places made our own track as we went. Finally, we got to a place where the track broke off to the right and ran over a man made dike towards the river. The dike passed over riverside flood plains and was in a very bad state of repair, being completely washed away in places. It ran for over two miles towards the river. The village of Gourma-Rharous lay on the other side of the twelve mile wide river. The commandant there had been informed by radio telephone the day before of our arrival and so Dr. Diarra expected to find the cercle's launch on the banks waiting for us. There was no launch either on the river bank or anywhere in sight on the river itself and the Sorko fishermen who were repairing their nets in the shade of straw huts told us that they hadn't seen or heard the launch all that day.

Our plan was to leave two teams on the left bank of the river for the night along with our own truck and to cross the river in the launch. The following morning we hoped to have the two teams and their trucks ferried over to Gourma-Rharous on a barge. We sent the three remaining teams on to Bourem, with instructions that one remain in Bamba to work there during the week we would be in Gourma-Rharous. Dr. Diarra had already passed through Bourem and Bamba on his way to Timbuctoo, met with the local administrative and health authorities and set up the itineraries for the teams. The infirmiers at the head of the teams were all thoroughly familiar with the clinical management of cholera by this time and were instructed to train the local medical assistants in treating cases. The health education goals, perhaps the most important of our mission, were more difficult to achieve, but the infirmiers made considerable progress in virtually every village visited. People boiled their water, washed their hands and were careful about handling cholera patients once the disease appeared.

We waited along the river bank for a long time, but saw no sign of the launch. Finally, towards sunset, Dr. Diarra decided that we should attempt to cross in a canoe, an unwise decision when I think of it now since it was sundown and the river twelve miles wide. But Dr. Diarra was not the kind of man one could argue with. So off into the Niger we went, in a small twenty-foot-long canoe, loaded with baggage and paddled by two young boys. It seemed to me that the river would never end once we left the shore, and after an hour of paddling we didn't even reach the main stream, still being in the center of what was a sort of inlet. We passed a large island where wild horses roamed, their domesticated ancestors having been trapped there during the high water mark. There were also crocodiles on the banks of the island and Dr. Diarra, who never once lost his presence of mind, suggested I photograph them. Photography was the furthest thing from my mind since every movement in the canoe tilted the sides sufficiently so that it took on water. Just as the sun was setting over the center of the river, we heard the launch coming towards us and after much shouting and hand waving, managed to catch the attention of the crew. It was with a feeling of being rescued that I jumped onto the launch and when I later saw the expanse of the river and the swiftness of the current I realized that had we made it across in the canoe, we would have come ashore miles below Gourma-Rharous. Canoes of the kind we were in often capsize, even when being manned by experienced oarsmen. In 1972, two Europeans from Mopti went up to Diafarabe with an experienced oarsman with whom they had traveled the Niger many times before. So confident were they in his ability, that they unrolled their sleeping bags on the bottom of the canoe, zippered themselves inside and fell asleep. The canoe moved along the quiet river. Suddenly, they came to a curve in the river and there ahead of them loomed the *General Soumare*. While the oarsman was able to avoid being hit by the steamer, the canoe was caught in the waves made as the boat passed and capsized. The two men, tightly zippered up in their sleeping bags went down to the bottom of the river and through some miracle, woke up, got out of the bags and surfaced. There they found the oarsman holding onto the capsized canoe for dear life, shouting that he couldn't swim. They rescued him and then swam

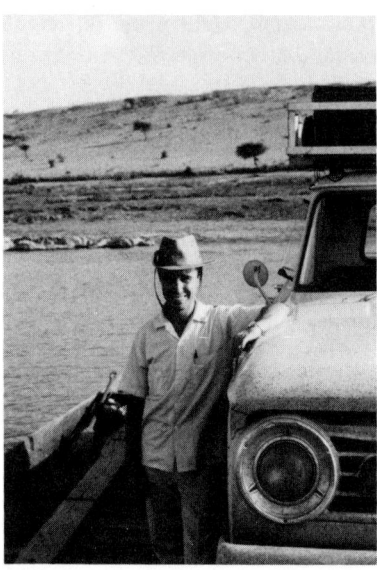

FIGURE 43. Dr. Imperato with his Dodge truck on a barge crossing the Niger River near Rharous. In the background are the sand dunes of the Gourma.

ashore. Although it was night, there was enough light generated by the passing steamer that its crew should have seen the canoe capsize. But the steamer sailed on down the river. Once ashore, the men had to undress and dry off their clothing and wait out the cold night until the following morning. Just before noon, some Bozo fishermen came by and picked them up. The two men involved in this near tragic accident, Monsieur Carola and Monsieur Hermant, vowed that they would never set foot in a canoe again, and they never did.

Gourma-Rharous, which is also called simply Rharous, is a large village which is longer than it is wide, stretching along the top of the high sandy river bank. Behind it to the south is a large sand dune which constantly encroaches on the village. The sand drifts with the prevailing winds and in the period of one month accumulates to a depth of two feet in places. Behind this dune are fifteen others, running parallel to one another for a distance of over a hundred miles to Gossi, a waterhole which is the center of the gourma. Dr. Diarra never stopped talking about the sixteen dunes of Rharous, especially to Mark LaPointe who had been to Gourma-Rharous in 1968 with Dr. Ousmane Sow and myself.

The night of our arrival, we sat out under the stars, holding a meeting with all of the officials of the cercle of Gourma-Rharous, the traditional Songhoi and Tuareg leaders and the Moslem clerics. We explained to them as we had everywhere else, that the prevention of cholera lay in the practicing of good personal hygiene and that vaccination was at best a secondary and less efficient means of prevention. Although cholera had wrecked havoc in the region of the lakes, it had not yet arrived in Gourma-Rharous because this area was separated from it by an unpopulated expanse of sahel and desert.

At dawn the following morning, we sent the barge across the river to ferry the trucks and equipment over. It wasn't an easy undertaking because there was a strong breeze on the river whipping up the already strong current. Cheick Tawaty, one of our drivers who never impressed me as being a sage at anything, drove his truck off the barge before the barge had docked and promptly went right into the river. Dr. Diarra who was at the river bank when this happened came to give me the news at the dispensary where I was with the infirmier setting up the cholera treatment facility.

"Your driver, Cheick Tawaty, is in the river," he said, "and his truck is in there with him."

We had had trucks fall into the river before and always managed to fish them out, but because Cheick Tawaty was involved, I became apprehensive. I need not have because the truck was in only five feet of water and upright with Cheick Tawaty snugly roosting high up on the roof rack. There was a standard foremat to Dr. Diarra's tongue lashings and Cheick Tawaty having heard it so often knew what he was in for when Dr. Diarra got back to the river bank. "Espèce d'imbécile!" the old man shouted across the water. "Tu es un filou. C'est anarchie totale et intégrale," he added for good measure. Having called Cheick Tawaty an idiot and a cheat, Dr. Diarra ended by pronouncing his well known summary view of the vaccinators and drivers, "It's total and integrated anarchy." Anarchists they were and certainly at times their anarchy seemed almost total, but that it was well coordinated I doubted. They didn't have the organizational ability for that.

Although solidly stuck in the mud, with several camels pulling, the truck came up out of the river in short order. In the meantime, the barge went over to the left bank to fetch the other truck. The village was vaccinated that morning and later in the afternoon, we sent the two teams off with *gourmiers* (desert guards and guides) to vaccinate the villages and camps along the river. Cheick Tawaty and his team were sent down towards Lake Do and Lake Garou, against his rather violent protest. He didn't want to go into the area because when we were working there two years before, several of the teams were charged by elephants. We gave Cheick Tawaty a choice between Lake Garou and the elephants and Ansongo and its equally aggressive hippopotami. Figuring that his chances were better on land than on water, he opted for Lake Garou.

The program in the cercle of Gourma-Rharous was planned so that the riverine areas were vaccinated first, followed by the areas in the gourma, that waste-land of semi-desert which lies inside of the Niger Bend. The word gourma in the language of the Tuareg means, "the place where the well is," but is used by most people to mean the land on the right side of the Niger in the area where the river bends. It was this area just at the bend and below which concerned us the most because here the river breaks up into many channels and flows through a confusing tangle of marshes dotted with island villages. These villages are difficult to reach, even by canoe. Although we had outboard motorboats at our disposal which could have speeded up our progress through this area, they couldn't be used because the borgus grass and bull rushes got caught up in the propellers and broke them. So the villages had to be painstakingly reached by canoe.

The two teams in Gourma-Rharous were to move southward into the gourma towards Gossi and from there they were to visit all of the waterholes to the east, arriving on the Niger across from the town of Gao. They would then pass into all of the villages which lie on the 125 mile stretch between Gao and the Mali-Niger frontier.

A week after our arrival in Gourma-Rharous, we left, departing one morning in the launch just as the sun was coming up over the top of the borgus grass which edges the vast sweep of this part of the Niger. It was cold on the river and a strong wind whipped up white caps out in the middle of the stream. Our truck had been ferried over the day before and was waiting for us when we arrived on the opposite bank. Also waiting for us, unexpectedly, was a vaccinator from the team which had gone up towards Dire. He had been taken to Timbuctoo by the police from Dire because he had become psychotic. Had Dr. Keita been in Timbuctoo, he would have sent him on by plane to Bamako, but he was out on the river, treating cholera cases and setting up depots for intravenous fluids. So the policemen from Dire, on hearing that we were due on the left bank from Gourma-Rharous, decided to bring the vaccinator to us. With near complete

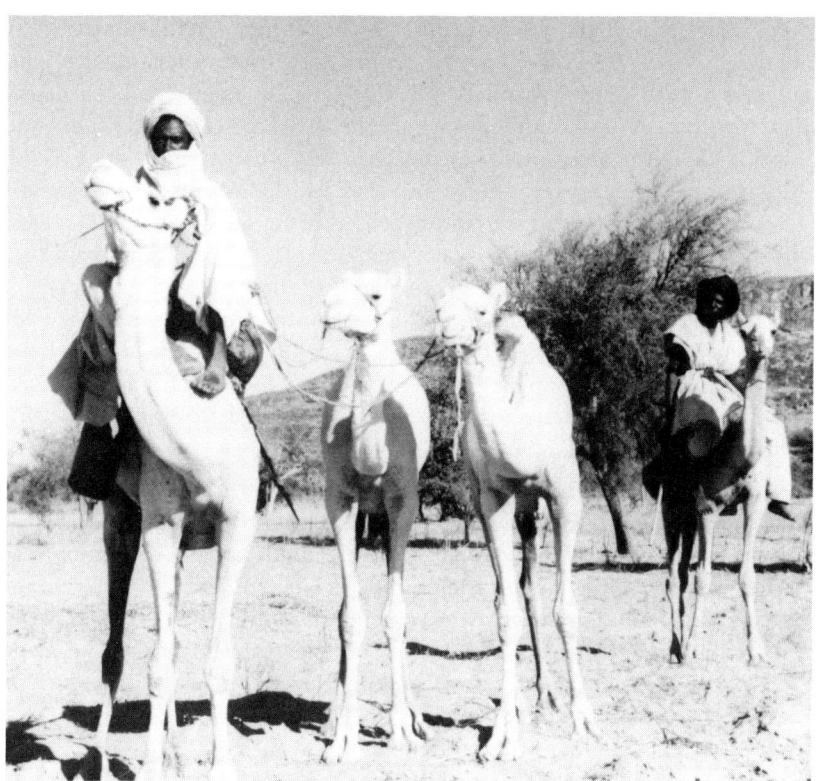

FIGURE 44. Bela nomads on their camels near Hombori.

conviction, the policemen said that the vaccinator had been cursed by a water genie who lived at the bottom of a whirlpool in the Niger near Dire. According to them, the vaccination team crossed the Niger in a canoe in an area I know to be dangerous because of cross currents and whirlpool formations. When they reached the middle of the stream, the oarsman warned them not to touch the water. "There is an evil genie who lives here," he said. "If you touch the water, his curse will fall on you and you will become crazy." The vaccinator ignored the warning, scoffed at it and to prove his disbelief, took a wad of cotton, dipped it into the water and washed off the case of his jet injector. The oarsman fell silent at this as did everyone else in the canoe. The vaccinator then washed his hands and face with water.

Once on the other side, the team vaccinated the village and the vaccinator seemed normal to his teammates and everyone else. However, during the night, he woke his teammates up, ranting that he was hearing voices and seeing monsters. At first they tried to reason with him, but to no avail. He demanded that the oarsman take him back across the river, but the man refused, saying that the same curse fell on anyone crossing the river at night. If anyone had any doubts about the validity of this curse, they were already dispelled by the vaccinator's behavior. The vaccinator talked incessantly, not making any sense and ranted all night long. In the morning, they took him to a Bozo marabout who was reputed to be skilled in removing the curse of the water genie. He pronounced incantations over the vaccinator, rubbed his head with water containing ink washed off a board containing passages from the Koran, and gave him amulets to wears. None of these tried and tested remedies had any effect, so the team leader decided to have the vaccinator taken back to Timbuctoo.

There is a strong belief in genies along this stretch of the Niger and they are believed to either reside in a number of fixed locales or else to move from place to place. In the main square of Timbuctoo, there is a gigantic statue sculptured in bronze, which depicts the famous genie on horseback who is believed to ride the road between Timbuctoo and Kabara. The fact that belief in this particular genie should be materialized in bronze and in such large proportions attests to the strength of the belief in Timbuctoo.

It was obvious to both Dr. Diarra and I that the vaccinator was psychotic. Why? We couldn't say. But we couldn't exclude the possibility that he had been given a hallucinogenic product by the villagers or the oarsman. Such a possibility would have been more likely had all this happened in Sikasso, a region of Mali where poisonings of all kinds are extremely common. The policemen said that poisonings were uncommon in Dire, but Dr. Diarra contradicted this on the basis of his first hand knowledge.

I gave the vaccinator an injection of a tranquilizing agent and within a few minutes he quieted down. We put him in our truck and took him with us to Bamba, the policemen leaving us at the fork in the track and returning to Dire. It took us a few hours to reach Bamba, the track passing through some broad sand traps and over some large dunes. We were fortunate that we were driving up the western sides of the dunes since they faced the prevailing winds and were hard compared to the eastern sides which were soft with shifting sand. Bamba is a picturesque little settlement composed of rectangular mud brick houses, Tuareg tents made of cowhide and Bella huts made of plaited straw mats. Informed of our impending arrival from Gourma-Rharous, the chief of the arrondissement came out to meet us elegantly dressed in his finest embroided boubou and black tassled fez.

We found our two teams in Bamba. During the previous week, they had completed the vaccination of Ber and the one which had gone on to Bamba had already vaccinated half of the arrondissement. We spent most of the day in Bamba, helping the infirmier set up a cholera treatment facility. And then towards late evening we started for Bourem where we planned to remain for several days. We left one team in Bamba to complete its program in the riverine villages and nomad camps and had the team from Ber accompany us to Bourem. There are large sand dunes to the east of Bamba and the track passes through the flat areas between them. The trucks sank up to their axles in the soft sand, despite our driving in four wheel drive. We were finally able to get them out by using the sand tracks, six foot strips of perforated steel which were once used in the Sahara as part of runways during World War II. Forty miles from Bamba the Niger narrows to a width of only three hundred feet in a rocky pass known as the Tossaye Pass. For several miles, the banks of the river lose their sandy character and become unusually rocky with layers of black marble.

Bourem stands high up on the sand dunes, overlooking the Niger Bend and the vast expanse of country around it. The massive fort built by the French of deep maroon colored mud brick dominates the village and from its top one can see the Niger coming out of the far horizon and making its great sweeping bend. The river is very wide at Bourem and breaks up into many channels which flow between islands of borgus grass. Its banks too, are edged with borgus grass and bull rushes, spread out in wide marshes of deep green. To the northeast of the fort is the Tilemsi Valley which stretches up towards Kidal and the mountains known as the Adrar des Iforas. The Tilemsi Valley once contained the eastern portion of the Niger which drained the mountains to the north. But today, it is dry, dotted with a few waterholes which are a life line for the Tuareg and Maure nomads moving between Kidal and the river. But centuries ago, early man flourished here in the Tilemsi, he leaving a legacy of rock paintings and drawings which gaze out today on the barren dry landscape where once water flowed.

The sands of Bourem vary in color from yellow to deep red and each year after the rainy season, the women repaint their houses both inside and out with solutions made from these sands. These brightly colored sands are also in great demand up the river in far away Segou. Each year barges are loaded with sand in Bourem and dragged up the river to Segou where the sand is sold and used for painting the exteriors of the town's mud brick houses. There is a surprising cover of thorn trees in Bourem and overall the village has a very pleasant appearance, especially at sundown when the sun sets over the river and imparts a pleasing glow to the fort and mud houses.

In some ways, Bourem reminded me of Nioro because it is a cercle from which over fifty thousand people have emigrated in the past decade. There are only forty-two thousand people now living in the cercle, less than half of what was once there. Most have migrated down the river to the cercle of Ansongo and into the Niger Republic, because of chronic crop failures. The local people say that the flood waters pass Bourem more quickly than they once did, leaving them with inadequate quantities for irrigating their riverside plots. This is true because of the erosion of the Tossaye Sill, a natural dam of bedrock which controls the flow of the Niger above Bourem. With the erosion of this sill, the flood waters are no longer held back, but flow on towards the bend with great speed and then downstream into the Niger Republic and Nigeria. For the past decade, the populations along the middle Niger have not been able to produce enough cereal to feed themselves and each year when I was in Mali, U.S.A.I.D. brought in thousands of tons of American maize which prevented famine in this region. In 1972, the rains failed in the sahel, causing the terrible drought of 1973 in which approximately forty percent of Mali's livestock perished. The severity of the famine in the Gao region was greatly lessened by an airlift of grain to Mopti, Timbuctoo and Gao, by the U.S. Air Force.

Most of the cercle of Bourem's population of sedentary Songhoi farmers lives on islands in the Niger, accessible only by canoe. Campaigns in this cercle were always slow and tedious because so much time had to be spent traveling on the river from one island to another. We arranged this campaign in such a fashion that the two teams which arrived in Bourem before us began on the river. The team from Ber then vaccinated the arrondissement of Almoustarat where most of the Tuareg nomads are to be found. The commandant of Bourem was himself a Tuareg and he knew every inch of the country well. The morning after our arrival he went out with the team to Almoustarat to begin the program among the nomads.

With the program operating smoothly all along three hundred miles of the river from Goundam to Bourem, Dr. Diarra and I moved on to

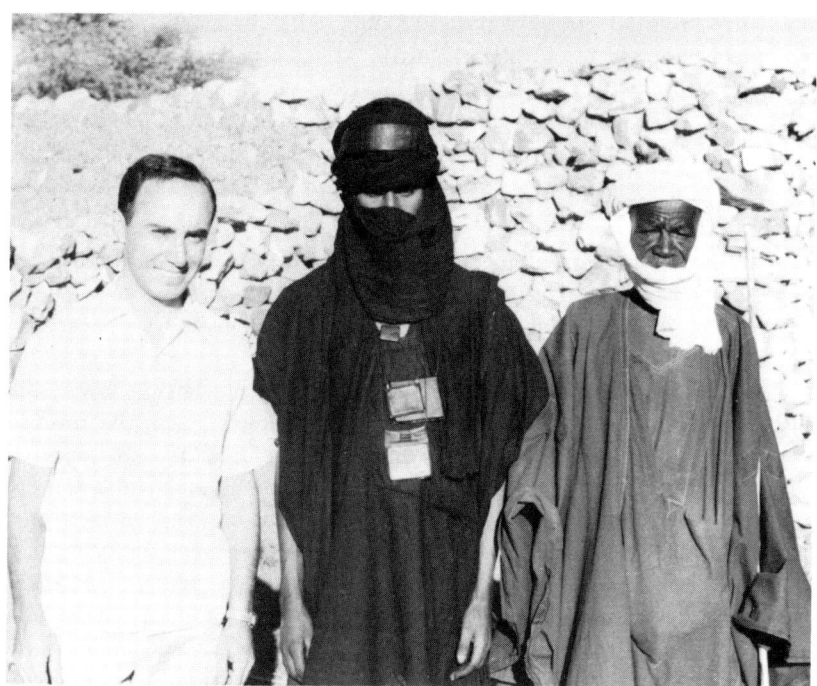

FIGURE 45. Dr. Imperato *(left)* with a Tuareg nomad *(center)* and a Songhoi chief *(right)* at Hombori. The Tuareg wear indigo colored cloth which gives their skin a blue hue and for this reason they have often been referred to as the blue men of the Sahara. The Tuareg also wear many Koranic charms.

Gao which lies sixty miles to the south of Bourem. Although the vaccinator from Dire was manageable because of tranquilization, we were anxious to evacuate him to Bamako. The day after our arrival in Gao, he was taken to Bamako on the scheduled weekly flight and hospitalized on the psychiatric ward at Point G Hospital where under the care of Dr. Faran Samake, Mali's only psychiatrist, he went into remission in several weeks and was discharged.

The track from Bourem to Gao was fairly good, passing through picturesque plains dotted with acacia trees. The banks of the Niger were edged with a deep green marsh of borgus grass which was in sharp contrast to the yellow colored sand dunes which rose up high on the horizon to the west. We came across a large caravan of sixty-four camels walking single file over the top of a large sand dune. On either side of their single humps were tombstone shaped bars of salt, strapped on with cord and strips of leather. The salt was from the mines at Taoudeni and was being taken south to Menaka and Anderamboukane. Anderamboukane lies close to the Mali-Niger frontier, several hundred miles to the southeast of the town of Gao. The Tuareg there raised armed resistance to the French during the early part of this century, an event which is now immortalized by the minstrels of Anderamboukane.

On the way down to Gao, there were many Bella camps of a dozen or more straw mat huts along the left bank of the Niger. And their large herds of goats and camels grazed by the thousands off the tops of the thorn trees on either side of the track. In recent years, the constantly increasing goat populations of this part of Africa have inflicted irreparable harm to the ecology of the sahel. For their owners have allowed the herds to overgraze the land and have cut down the trees in the process. Sand dunes have emerged where once there were grass and tree covered hills and close to the banks of the Niger, the dunes have begun to drift into the river bed. Modern veterinary practices have been delivered to these herds since independence by a well budgeted veterinary service. This has led to a decreased animal mortality rate and an increased number of births which together have caused an incredible goat population explosion. Like sheep and cattle, goats are rarely sold and are for the most part outside of the modern economic life of the country. Their main purpose is still prestige, they being a possession which is paraded before the establishment for the ego satisfaction of their owners. One can convincingly argue that the benefits of modern veterinary science should not have been delivered without the simultaneous development of a modern livestock industry. The delivery of the one and the failure to develop the other resulted in ruination of the ecology.

Some weak attempts were made to develop a modern livestock industry in Gao but to date they have been unsuccessful. The Yugoslavians built a modern abbatoir in the town of Gao, but it has never been used. And so the herds increased in size year by year and the pride of their owners swelled. In this region, the bellies of small children also swelled from protein malnutrition, for surrounded as they were by livestock, they were rarely fed any meat. Then in 1972, the rains failed in the sahel and in 1973 the worst drought since 1917 set in. The scarce reserves of the ecology had long ago been depleted by the dense livestock population. The grass and trees which once covered the dunes had been destroyed and in their place there was now only hot sand. The inevitable happened. Millions of animals died. A great cry went up from many Africans that they had lost a precious economic resource. But those familiar with the scene took issue with their claim because the bulk of the livestock while a potential resource was not an actual one. It was estimated that forty percent of Mali's livestock perished in this drought. Yet this did not mean that there was forty perecnt less milk to drink and forty percent less meat to eat. The remaining animals were more than sufficient to provide for the needs of Mali's human population and that of those countries to which Mali exports its animals and their products.

We entered the town of Gao from the north where the truncated pyramidal form of the tomb of the Askias rises high above the low mud brick houses. The tomb is about a hundred feet high and was built about 1525 for the burial of the first king of the Askia dynasty of the Songhoi Empire of Gao. The base of the structure is a square, each side of which measures about thirty feet and protruding from the surfaces of the structure are numerous twisted poles used as scaffolding by the masons who re-surface it after the rains. A stairway leads up to the top of the tomb on the outside and passes through a narrow tunnel before emerging onto a small balcony from where one can see the entire town and the surrounding countryside. I always wondered what was inside of this huge edifice. Some say that it is hollow and others that it is solid, but most believe that there is a golden canoe inside plus a vast treasure belonging to the kings of Gao. A truncated pyramid of mud brick stands on the banks of the Niger below the Sahara, a burial place for kings and their earthly wealth and this always stirs up in my mind speculation about the idea for it all having originated with Moslem pilgrims passing through Cairo on their way to Mecca.

The rest of present day Gao is fairly recent in construction, with wide sandy streets and rectangular blocks of courtyards and mud brick houses. Unlike Timbuctoo, the skyline is fairly low because two story buildings are rare and in place of Timbuctoo's gray color, there is a light brown hue to everything. One does not sense a preservation of the history of the past in Gao as in Timbuctoo for the old city was abandoned and destroyed long ago and what one sees today was largely built after the arrival of the French in 1898. The center of the town is called Gao-Dioula and it contains all of the administrative buildings built in a neo-maghrebian style by the French. Dr. Diarra lived in the

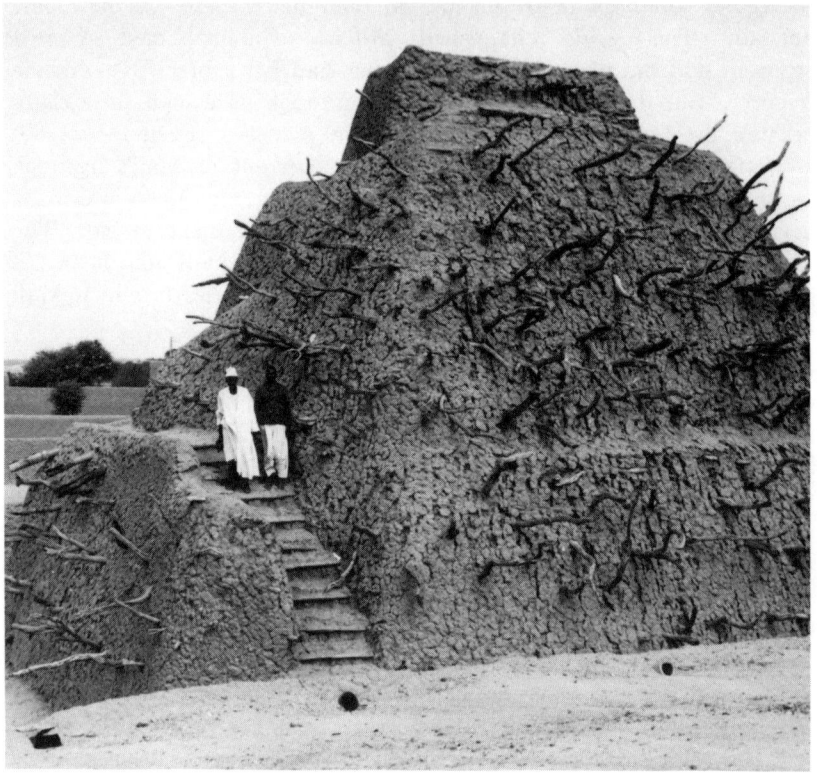

FIGURE 46. The tomb of the Askias at Gao as seen from the roof of the ancient mosque. Local legends recount that a gold canoe and a vast treasure lie buried in the center of the monument.

center of town in a long rambling building across the road from the market place. It had a large courtyard in which his children kept a pet ostrich. His office was a long room which faced the roadway and through the open doorway you could see all of the diverse peoples of the Niger Bend going up and down the street and hear the pleasant rumble of bargaining in the vast market place across the street. Nearby, on the northern periphery of the market was the Hotel Atlantide which was being enlarged and renovated at the time. It had a large gravel covered forecourt which was a delightful place to sit in the evening with a breeze from the river blowing through the high encircling archways which formed a wall.

In the hot dry season, March through June, the temperature in the shade in Gao averages 140 degrees Fahrenheit and at night it rarely falls below 100 degrees. It was impossible to sleep in the hotel rooms or in any room for that matter and so most people slept outdoors. At the Hotel Atlantide, guests slept in beds arranged on a roof terrace where they caught an occasional fresh breeze from the river. Some drenched themselves in the showers with their night clotes on and then went to bed with the fan blowing on them. This worked well when it came to getting to sleep because the exaporation of water from the skin lowers the body temperature. I never slept well at night during the hot season in Gao and always woke up early in the morning completely dehydrated. It would take two liters of water and salt tablets to put me back into fluid and electrolyte balance, a balance which was soon disrupted again as soon as I started moving around. Out in the bush, I always slept near the river where the air was cooler and where there were no masses of buildings radiating heat which had been stored up during the day. But in Gao, no one would hear of this and so I was always provided with a large room either at Dr. Diarra's house or at a government maison de passage.

The majority of Europeans who come to Gao do so in transit and few come specifically to see the place. There are those who take the river streamers from Koulikoro to Gao, a five day trip, and arrive in the afternoon, spend the night on the steamers and then return to Bamako by plane the next morning. Another smaller group is represented by those who cross the Sahara via Tessalit, Bidon V, Reggane and Colomb Bechar. It is 1,137 miles from Gao to Colomb Bechar and from there to the Mediterranean Sea another 439 miles. It takes five days to cross the desert, the best time being between the months of November and January when the temperatures are moderate. Some cross in a single vehicle and others wait for a convoy of trucks to leave Gao. The Malian administration in Gao always advises travelers to go in a convoy because in the past single vehicles have broken down and their occupants have died from thirst and heat stroke. Having traveled so much through the sahel and the southern portion of the Sahara, I never had the urge to cross the desert.

When we arrived in Gao, the town was not so much preoccupied with the threat of cholera as with the story of a Mossi marabout who had poisoned several people. This marabout had come into Gao several months before claiming that he could multiply money. The first of his victims was the engineer at the public works department. He brought the marabout fifty thousand francs and asked that he double it. The marabout agreed and gave the engineer a small bag of powder, instructing him to mix it with water and then to drink it in a latrine at eight in the evening. The marabout then told him that the multiplication would not take place if the powder were not consumed in absolute secrecy. He also told him to throw the glass down into the cesspool below after he had swallowed the magical potion. The engineer did as he was told and promptly died an hour lated. Sudden unexplained deaths are common in Africa, being laid to the will of God, and so no one thought it unusual that a young man in excellent health should suddenly die. The same pattern occurred with three other victims. Finally, the clerk at the local bank came to the marabout late one night and confessed that he had embezzled the equivalent of four thousand dollars. The bank auditors were due to come to Gao from Bamako in a week's time and he wanted to replace the money. The marabout naturally told him that this was a simple problem to solve. All that the clerk had to do was to bring the same amount of money to him and he would double it and then the whole sum could be returned.

The bank clerk did as he was told and after delivering the money went home to drink the so called magical potion in his latrine. He found the taste so bad that he only drank a small portion of it and then began vomiting. He put the glass with the unfinished liquid down on the ground and then went to his room. When Dr. Diarra was called in, he suspected that the man had been poisoned and sent the contents off to Bamako from where they were sent to Paris for analysis. Within two days the telegraphic reply came back — arsenic and strychnine. The bank clerk recovered and managed to recuperate the second sum of money, but was subsequently arrested for having embezzled the original sum. When the marabout was finally arrested, it was discovered that he had poisoned a large number of people in bush villages as well. He was brought to trial in 1972 and condemned to death.

In Gao, Dr. Diarra's decisions were never questioned and invariably he was proven right whenever they were. Many said that he ran the health services of the region in an extremely autocratic fashion, a fashion I always felt well worth adopting in a region where anarchy was the natural individual tendency. He was respected by all and feared by most and his sudden surprise visits to a dispensary or medical post always put everyone in a panic. He got by with very little sleep, perhaps five hours a day at most, between midnight and 5:00 A.M. and was on the go the remainder of the time. This was scarcely to the liking of his staff because in effect they were vulnerable to surprise inspection for nineteen hours a day. And inspect them he did, even at 2:00 A.M. if he happened to wake up. He had two drivers who between them were on duty twenty-four hours a day and who had to be ready on a moment's notice to drive Dr. Diarra either somewhere in the town or else as far away as Goundam. Much to the regret of the medical personnel, the drivers were never given advance notice as to where they were going so they were unable to warn anyone.

I never saw Dr. Diarra remove his hat in anyone's presence, except when we visited Captain Diby Silas Diarra, the former commandant

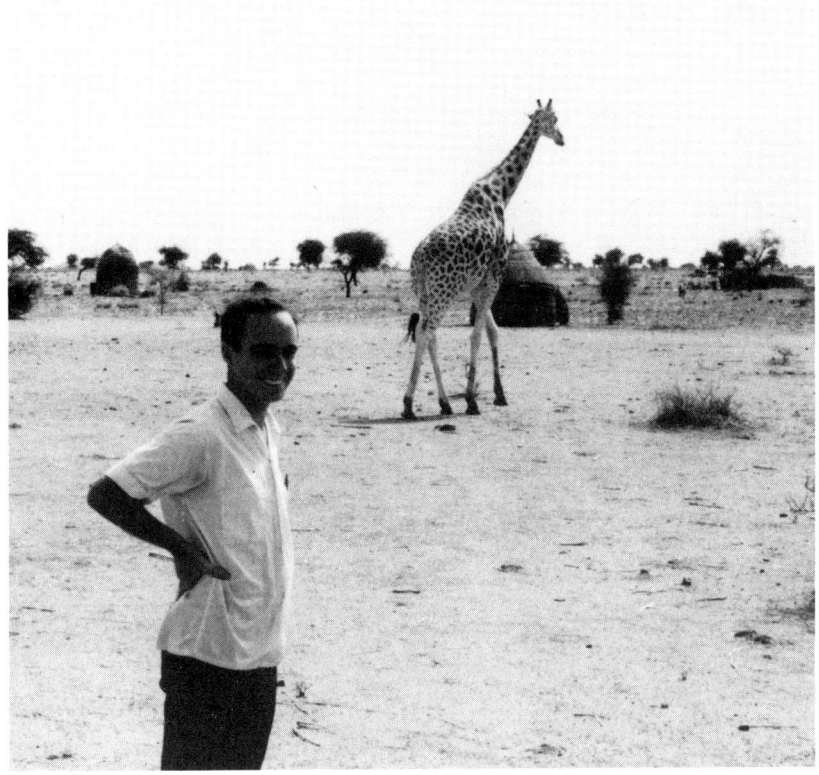

FIGURE 47. Dr. Imperato with a giraffe near Ouatagouna in the southern portion of the cercle of Ansongo. The giraffe in this area are extremely docile and, although wild, graze close to villages. Their lack of fear of man is due in part to their not being hunted by the local population.

of Kidal who was the governor of Gao for a while. But even in the presence of this greatly feared individual, Dr. Diarra was in command of the situation.

After several days in Gao, during which time we vaccinated the town and organized the cholera prevention program for the cercles of Gao, Ansongo and Menaka, Dr. Diarra and I drove down south to Ansongo. It was late in the afternoon when we left Gao and the famous Rose Dune on the other side of the river had already changed its color from yellow to rose under the light of the lowering sun. I had not been to Ansongo in almost two years, since the time we vaccinated the cercle against measles. I had first gone there five years before when smallpox came up the river from Niger, the disease which the Songhoi of Lellehoi said was carried by the wind. Now cholera, another unknown illness to these people, was coming down the river. The past would not be difficult for them to bring to memory, I thought, and the moment they saw me I knew that they would talk about the battle we had waged together against smallpox on this part of the river. It was going to be hard for me to tell them about cholera for they saw in me the solution which had always triumphed over the plagues which had entered their lives in the past. The harmony of our understanding would not suffer from what was bound to be our less than successful mutual effort, but they would be disappointed this time that the jet guns alone would not be able to chase away their common misery. We drove on into the quiet world of sand dunes, thorn trees and the river.

Chapter XXII
Farewell

The cholera epidemic lasted six months in Mali before it moved out of the country into the Niger Republic and Nigeria. The disease remained behind in scattered places, on the Bandiagara Plateau and up near the Mauritanian frontier in Nioro and Niono. In the end, it was estimated that ten thousand cases had occurred in Mali and five thousand deaths, but this is a low estimate and we will never be able to know how many people fell victim to the disease. When this great epidemic was over, the feeling came over me that my work in the country had come to an end and that I should leave. The Malians had demonstrated their ability to meet every manner of health emergency and could now carry on quite alone. Smallpox had been eradicated, measles controlled, hundreds of people trained in valuable new skills and thousands of lives saved and made healthier and happier. I had accomplished what I had come to do and perhaps somewhat more. The rains were ending and the grass and fields of millet stood tall and green across the land. It was the end of the cycle of seasons and it struck me that it was an appropriate time to leave.

I had some time before formulated in my own mind a program for leaving the country in a gradual way. For, after having been there for so many years, it was just not possible to uproot myself abruptly. No one had ever told me that I should leave and indeed all of those around me urged that I stay. All the same, I had been in the country for over five full years and the inner voices of accomplishment and fulfillment were very strong. The Malians around me were in some unexplicable way aware of my state of mind, even though I had never spoken to them about it. They tried their very best to induce me to stay on and constantly pointed out reasons why to their way of thinking

I had to remain. The first they ever spoke to me of this was at the time a strange happening took place while I was in the old village of Kangaba near the Guinean frontier.

The night before I had slept at home in Bamako and was awakened at 5:00 A.M. by a strange nightmare. I dreamed that I was in Kangaba and that a man had been bitten by a snake. I thought nothing more of it, but when my staff arrived at 8:00 A.M. I told them the story and reminded Ahmadou to make sure that he put the anti-venom in the ice chest. There was little need for me to have reminded Ahmadou about this since over the years he had never failed to do it. When we were half way to Kangaba we stopped beneath a kapoc tree for a short while in order to drink some water and it was then that I discovered that Ahmadou had forgotten to put the anti-venom in the ice chest. My staff and I laughed about it ,saying that in all of the years of travel we had never used the serum on anyone and so there was no reason to be concerned now. We spent the morning in Kangaba with the medecin chef and at 11:00 A.M. went to pay our respects to the commandant. While we were in his office a man came rushing in, in a state of panic, and blurted out that a man in his village had been bitten by a viper just before sunrise. "We don't have any anti-venom here," gasped the medecin chef. "But surely you must have some," he said turning to me.

Before that time, I had not believed in extrasensory perception, nor am I entirely convinced of it now. But the Malians with me did and that same day they told me that as I had known that the man in the bush had been bitten by a snake so too did they know that I was planning to leave them. After that, I spoke freely of my leaving, but they did not take it too seriously at first. Gradually, and in the course of the year which followed this event, they came to believe that I would really leave them. I knew that it would mean as much of an upheaval in their lives as in mine. The thread of my life had run between the skyscrapers of a great city and the open plains of Africa, but theirs had always rested in Africa. Where our lives met was all they knew and they could not imagine that my life had its roots in a world far different from theirs. In a sense then, they were never able to fully understand me for they knew nothing of the world from which I came.

The fate of my staff and my servants weighed heavily on my mind, but they themselves made no attempt to arrange their futures. They waited patiently for destiny to come and carry their lives off onto a new path. For many months, Ahmadou and I packed up and inventoried my massive collection of African art and artifacts. I thought that our doing so would impress on him and the other servants the certainty of my going. But to the contrary, it did not, for they viewed the collection as a non-essential part of the household which when gone would not alter our lives. When it had been cleared out of the house and taken to the embassy warehouse, the rooms resounded with those echoes of barrenness which had been there when I first moved in and the servants suggested that I buy pictures to hang on the walls to give some warmth to the house.

Shortly before my departure, I was asked by the Center for Disease Control to visit Mauritania, the Gambia, Guinea and Senegal in order to meet with the ministers of health about continuing the maintenance vaccination phase of the program. During my several weeks away, Ahmadou packed up most of the household effects and sent them off to the embassy warehouse so when I returned the house was empty except for some of the furniture. It wasn't in any sense cold and lonely, but more noble and spartan, the way devout Moslems like Ahmadou preferred it. He was very pleased when I told him that it would have been better had he had it this way all the time. Then he ventured to say what I knew he thought all the time, that there had been too much wood in the house. He was at heart a Moslem iconoclast and did not enjoy being associated with so many masks and statues. Yet he was an extremely courteous person and so he never spoke of these feelings to me.

Ahmadou asked if I would pay a last visit to his home village in Segou to say goodbye to all of the people there. Boussin is a fairly large village of close to a thousand people, all of whom are Marka. It lies on a vast sandy plain in a grove of thorn trees and ancient baobabs. Like several other Marka villages in this part of Mali, Boussin was for centuries an island of Islam in a sea of Bambara animism. The first European to visit Boussin was Captain Briquelot, the French resident of Segou who passed through the village and camped there for several days in February, 1892. Captain Briquelot was enroute for the Minianka country near Bla where a revolt had broken out against recently imposed French rule. Captain Briquelot was the second French resident in Segou, having succeeded Captain Underberg, the man who executed Mari Diarra, the Bambara king whom the French restored to power after having driven the Toucouleur conqueror, Ahmadou, out of Segou in 1890. Once restored to power, Mari Diarra planed to kill Captain Underberg, but the latter, learning of the plan, acted first. Because of his high handedness in this affair, Captain Underberg was replaced by Captain Briquelot who spent most of his time pacifying the country.

Captain Briquelot's visit to Boussin was not preserved in local oral tradition, although at the time it must have been an event of enormous importance. The old men in Boussin knew nothing of his passage nor of the revolt of the Minianka in Bla. But they spoke at great length about the French administrator who lived in Boussin in the 1920's and often showed me the place where his compound had been. All that remained of it were a few shrubs which once formed part of a large enclosure. After I had researched Boussin's recorded history in the archives in Segou, I explained my findings to the old men and the minstrels and much to my surprise many months later I heard the minstrels singing of Captain Briquelot, the first *toubabou-ke* (white man) who had come to Boussin. Modern research had uncovered a fragment of the past and placed it into the mainstream of local oral history.

We left for Segou late one afternoon in the Dodge truck and drove through the cool scent which fills the late hours of the day at that time of year. There is a large forest preserve between Bamako and Fana, called the Faya, and I asked Modibo to stop on top of one of the high rises in the road so that I could look over the tops of the trees and on across to the river. It gave me much peace of mind to rest in such a tranquil setting because the previous months had been full of so much upheaval and turmoil. I climbed on top of the roof rack and sat there alone for a while. It had rained that morning and off on the southern horizon a fine drizzling rain was falling over the green forest, coming down like a misty curtain over the valley through which the Bani River flows. Below me Ahmadou and Modibo talked in muffled tones with the apprentice, Karim, at a low pitch which was in harmony with the whispering of the trees. My staff always had great reverence for my solitude, for it was a quality not outside of their own understanding and one which they themselves valued. It is not a quality generally held up to imitation by many Africans. Segments of their conversation drifted over to me. In Bambara, they lamented my departure in tones which were like a mournful dirge. For them it was a bereavement, the turning of a great page in their book of life.

It was sunset when we arrived in Segou and drove onto the new tarmac road which leads to Markala and the river. A few miles on we left it and went onto the red laterite track which cuts through the thorn bush to Dioro. The evening air had grown cold and was full of drifting mist and drizzle. In the shadowy world of sundown, the foliage opened up reluctantly as we drew closer to the great white sandy plain near the village of Togou. The baobabs which mark the trail to Ahmadou's village looked fantastically big in the fading light and came upon us all of a sudden beyond a great curve in the road. Large puddles of water still lay around the plain, for although this was a dry country it did not take much rain to soak it through to saturation. During the rainy seasons the trails in this area were virtually impassable, covered with two feet of water. But often when we were working in the region I had to cross the terrain in spite of water and then I often felt as if the truck were a large boat for water lay all around us. Beneath the water were large holes and we often fell into them quite suddenly and unexpectedly, giving us a terrible sense of fright.

A full moon came up over the trail and when the clouds parted they left behind a perfect sky full of silver constellations. We lost the trail at one point and fell onto a narrow foot path which cut through a millet field. It was impossible for the truck to get through and so we got out, looking for the main trail, and stood in silence in the tall stalks which were bent heavy with ripened grain. Ahmadou finally found it several hundred yards away and guided the truck over a harvested field until it was back on course.

The people from the villages in the region decided to hold a great festival in my honor because they had heard that I was going away. They all knew me well because the year we had worked in the region of Segou, I had set up my field headquarters in Boussin, in Ahmadou's father's compound. This venerable old man had three wives and many children, of whom Ahmadou was the oldest. He was a man who carried himself with great dignity and commanded much respect in the village. He was grieved at the time of my departure by the death of Ahmadou's brother's wife, a young vivacious girl of eighteen who began hemorrhaging in the seventh month of her pregancy. They had tried their local remedies first and when these failed they placed her on a two wheeled donkey cart and set off for the hospital at Markala where a team of Chinese physicians from the People's Republic of China worked. Somewhere in the bush she delivered a premature baby girl and then hemorrhaged to death in the cart. A few hours later the baby died.

One morning a few days after our arrival in Boussin, the people began to arrive at sunrise with orchestras of drums and xylophones, masks and masquerades. Groups of hunters came in their colorful costumes, playing their guitars and minstrels came with their lutes. From one village young people came with beautiful antelope headdresses,

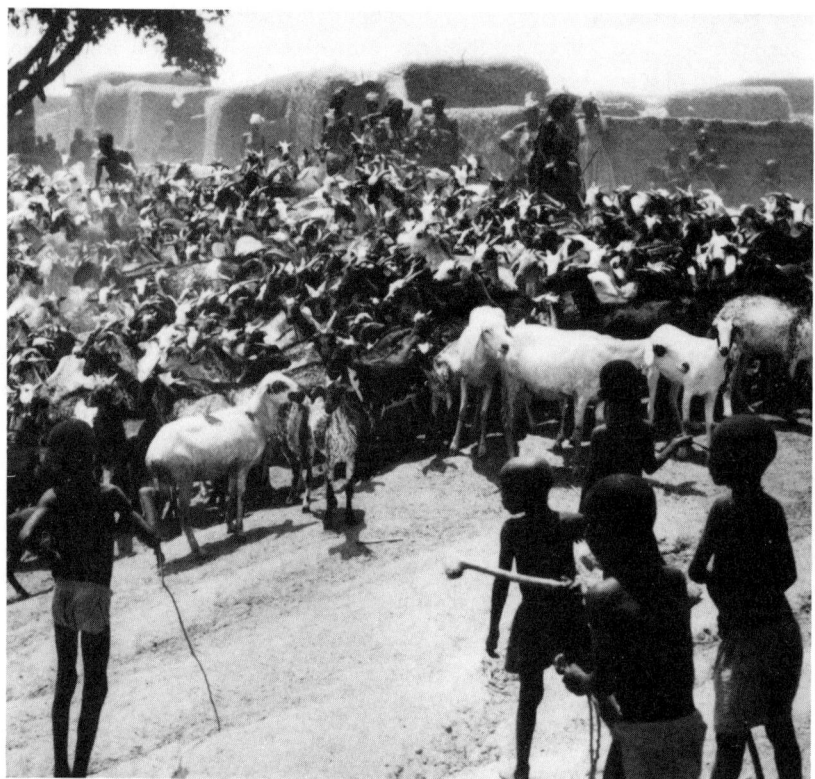

FIGURE 48. The goats and sheep of Boussin, Ahmadou's village, being gathered together at mid-day for a drive out into the bush. During the growing season the animals are taken each day by Peul herdsmen into the bush beyond the village fields. At sundown, they are brought back to the village, each animal returning on its own to its master's compound. During the dry season when crops are not being planted, the animals are allowed to roam freely.

the *tyi wara*, which represent the Bambara spirit of agriculture. All of the people assembled on the great village square which was shaded by several fig trees. The men started the festival off by firing their muskets and the air filled up with puffs of white smoke and the shouts of the crowd. Then the dances began. The Bambara boys from Zambougou performed acrobatic tricks; the Bozo men from Koke danced with their giant puppets mounted atop large camouflaged frames and the Marka age set association from Sanogobougou danced with bronze covered masks called *Djoboli Koun* which represent a beautiful woman.

It was a great gathering of people, over two thousand, and the dancing continued on into the afternoon. The chief of Boussin held a *mechoui* in my honor, a dinner consisting of roasted sheep. There were also large calabashes of rice and *toe,* a pudding made from millet. Then towards sunset, they danced with the tyi wara. The dancers moved slowly across an open field, bent over on wooden canes, carrying on their heads the beautifully sculptured antelopes. They were completely covered with a costume of blackened fibers from the *da* plant, which dangled from their headdresses and fell down over their shoulders to the ground. There is a quiet dignity to the dance of the tyi wara and one senses that it is the expression of a sacred and ancient belief. The dance honors those who farm well and reminds man of the mythical being, also known as tyi wara, who was half man and half animal, who taught man how to farm. By creating this elaborate and meaningful agricultural ritual honoring those who farm well, the Bambara established safeguards for their society as a whole, and in so doing they gave support and prestige to an undertaking which is essential for man's survival and for the preservation of his kind.

During the evening and late into the night, the minstrels and hunters performed, filling the village with the hypnotic din of their lutes. There was one minstrel who came from the arrondissement of Sansanding who played a violin-like instrument which was fashioned in part from an empty can which once held BP number 50 oil. This minstrel came often to Boussin and even the local population considered his music as noise. We nicknamed him *Huile Cinquante* because of the oil can instrument he carried. Huile Cinquante loved to play on into the early hours of the morning and there was no way of stopping him. I once tried to quiet him by giving him a handsome gift of money, but this backfired because he was so happy that he played until dawn. The vaccinators often revenged themselves on Djigui by having Huile Cinquante sit down quietly next to the cot where Djigui was sleeping and of suddenly erupting with his screeching music. Huile Cinquante once turned up at my office in Bamako, and started playing his music, oblivious to the fact that I was in the middle of a meeting with the Director General of Health. He had with him a note from his uncle, in which it was explained in the most eloquent syntax that Huile Cinquante was being presented to me as a permanent gift and that the entire family was sure that I would take good care of him. It took Djigui an entire day to undo this forced adoption and in the end we took

Huile Cinquante back to Boussin from where he returned to Sansanding with my eloquent reply in hand.

My last night in Boussin passed quickly and the excitement of these hours seemed to sweep away all thoughts of my going away.

When the day finally arrived for me to leave Bamako, I felt a soothing calmness of spirit. For I had already sent my heart and life back across the ocean and all that remained now was for the plane to transport the lighest part of me there. I had gotten up very early in the morning before the sun rose so that I could be alone to pack up my last few things. But when I opened the door, I found the garden full of people, standing as a somber congregation and contrary to their usual manner so silent that I only heard the breeze whispering through the trees. They who were never on time were now present before the hour. They had gone out with me on so many occasions to show me the way and now they looked to me for a trail to the future. Modibo and Djigui came forward and entered the house as I went into my room to dress.

Although it was a cool morning I had decided to wear an African shirt, a white cotton emblazoned with whirls of gold colored embroidery. It would please them I thought as I put it on, but when I entered

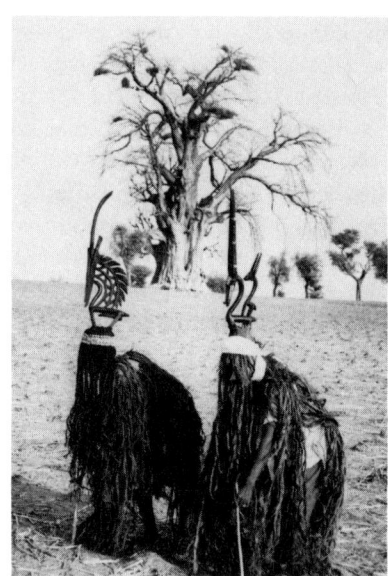

FIGURE 49. The Dance of the *Tyi Wara*.

the living room neither Djigui nor Modibo noticed it. They both blinked and fidgeted a great deal; it was hard for them to weather this ordeal. When Ahmadou came and saw me ready to leave, he gave a deep sigh of resignation. Until the very end he had hoped for a Koranic miracle.

There were no goodbyes to be said at the house for everyone was coming out to the airport. Modibo drove me in my car along with Ahmadou and Djigui and behind us followed Maxine Bradrick, our embassy nurse, with her Peugot station wagon filled with vaccinators. Maxine had been in Mali for four years then and had taken excellent care of all of the personel at the embassy, including myself. Behind the cars came a convoy of trucks full of people. Many of my friends came out to see me off. Monsieur Lastouillas and his wife were there as was Boundiar and Dr. Paul Jean-Joseph and a delegation of Bamako's leading African art merchants. The women and children of many families came, but when they saw so many officials they lost heart and fled away after saying a nervous goodbye. Ambassador Blake and his family were there and the officers from the embassy as well as the officials from the Ministry of Health. I walked out across the tarmac towards the plane and then turned to look at the large crowd waving in front of the large red terminal. It was the end of a great happiness for us all.

TABLE I

Smallpox and Measles Immunizations Given in the Attack Phase of the Smallpox Eradication and Measles Control Program

(Republic of Mali, 1966-1970*)

Time Period	Cercle	Estimated Population	Smallpox Vaccinations	Measles Immunizations
	Bamako	183,000	146,592	47,314
	Dioila	98,560	89,375	26,983
	Koulikoro	66,552	57,017	23,456
	Kangaba	39,600	36,995	4,603
	Banamba	61,153	56,013	15,003
1966-1967	Kolokani	110,000	105,813	34,912
	Nara	93,583	79,785	26,690
	Macina	86,075	96,304	25,688
	Ansongo	60,000	42,034	0
	SUBTOTAL	798,523	709,928	204,649
	Koutiala	201,700	183,566	49,022
	Yorosso	58,000	45,336	8,664
	Tominian	93,400	66,943	14,488
	San	120,000	112,565	24,777
1967-1968	Bandiagara	120,600	120,925	22,204
	Douentza	117,300	106,800	19,073

Time Period	Cercle	Estimated Population	Smallpox Vaccinations	Measles Immunizations
	Koro	118,100	122,952	25,157
	Bankass	103,100	114,992	21,108
	Mopti	139,600	289,923	47,320
	Djenne	89,600	91,852	17,495
	Tenenkou	80,400	69,396	15,100
	Niafounke	162,500	87,558	18,590
	Timbuctoo (City)	11,000	12,752	2,069
	SUBTOTAL	1,415,300	1,425,560	285,067
	Menaka	34,225	35,701	7,198
	Ansongo	**	46,398	10,371
	Kidal	19,917	11,743	2,138
	Bourem	95,345	74,822	14,563
	Gao	87,943	68,261	14,355
	Rharous	60,177	30,561	7,517
	Timbuctoo	45,810	48,582	9,618
	Goundam	86,050	65,250	13,631
1968-1969	Dire	62,129	51,800	12,284
	Kolondieba	80,000	63,529	18,049
	Bougouni	151,000	118,017	29,469
	Kadiolo	70,200	45,242	11,468
	Sikasso	217,800	205,656	60,577
	Koutiala	**	3,723	467
	Yanfoilla	75,700	85,258	16,381
	Niafunke***	25,000	30,192	5,609
	SUBTOTAL	969,741	981,012	233,228
	City of Bamako	300,000	278,337	59,679
	Nioro	172,300	130,562	28,443
	Yelimane	57,000	40,643	10,989
	Kayes	130,000	152,841	34,010
1969-1970	Kenieba	70,000	54,096	12,395
	Bafoulabe	79,000	62,979	13,968
	Kita	120,000	97,159	25,691
	Segou	240,000	195,388	53,411
	Niono	62,000	62,103	16,556
	SUBTOTAL	930,300	1,054,108	255,142
	TOTAL	4,053,864	4,170,608	978,086

*The populations of most cercles are estimates. These estimates are high for cercles such as those vaccinated in 1969-1970 where emigration has occurred in recent years. Estimated populations are less than the population actually vaccinated in some cercles due to the presence of nomads from other areas and low estimates.

**The population of Ansongo is included in the 1966-1967 data.
The population of Koutiala is included in the 1967-1968 data.

***Data presented is for the population in the arrondissements of Koumaira, Ambari and Banikane.

TABLE II
Drivers and Vaccinators of the Smallpox Eradication-Measles Control Program, Republic of Mali, 1966-1972

Drivers

Seydou Camara
Koniba Coulibaly
N'Golo Diarra
Mamadou Diawara
Diadouga Fane
Bassirou Kane

Modibo N'Faly Keita
Seydou Kone
Zamble Kone
Kassim Sangare
Cheick Tawaty
Bakary Traore
Zahn Sabake Traore

Vaccinators

Sekou Bagayoko
Aliou Ballo
Seydou Camara
Bama Cisse
Lassana Cisse
Amady Coulibaly
Cheick Oumar Coulibaly
Konatie Coulibaly
Moussa Coulibaly
Khalifa Dembele
Sandiougou Dembele
Djigui Diakite
Abdoudramane Diallo
Bandiougou Diallo
Mamadou Diallo
Silamakan Diallo
Zantigui Diallo
Abdoulaye Diop
Lassana Doumbia
Saga Demba Doumbia

Dionke Kaladioula
Famory Keita
Idrissa Keita
Issouby Keita
Seydou Keita
Yacouba Koita
Kelicouma Konate
Bakary Kone
Lamine Kone
Mamadou Kone
Yiriba Sako
Dramane Samake
Oua Samake
Sina Samake
Zina Samake
Bekaye Sangare
Issa Sanogo
Karamoko Sanogo
Mamadou Soumare
Mamadou Sissoko
Moulaye Traore

TABLE 3
TRANSHUMANCE IN THE FLOOD PLAINS OF MALI
BY MONTH

Month	Flood Plain	Height of Niger at Bamako 1965	Height of Niger at Mopti 1965	Peul from Nouna and Tougan in Upper Volta (SE Periphery) Seno	Peul from Macina, Nampala and Niafounké (NW Periphery) Farimake	Peul from Douentza, Bandiagara and Koro (NE Periphery) Kounari	Bozo on the Niger	Bozo on the Bani
July	Rain	1.36m	2.28m	Move SE out of flood plain	Move away from shores of Lake Debo	Move east off flood plain. Peul with goats leave Dori in U.V. and move towards Koro and Bandiagara	Move from Lake Debo towards Mopti and from Macina towards Diafarabé	Move towards Mopti from San and towards Segou from San
August	Rain	2.26m	4.57m	Arrive in home villages in Upper Volta	Herdsmen move into Mauritania and northern Nieno. Families and helpers move to home village in Macina, Nampala and Niafounké	Everyone in home village on the plateau	Arrive in home villages	Arrive in home villages
September	Rain Flood Plain Flooded	2.54m	5.78m	In home village. Some Peul cultivate	Families in home villages. Herdsmen in sahael, in Mauritania & northern Nione	Everyone in home village. Some Peul cultivate	In home village	In home village
October	Rains Stop Plains flooded with from 10' and more of water. Borgus grass growing on all plains.	3.23m	6.41m	Peul who don't cultivate move towards the flood plain. Herdsmen move first after last rains with main herds. Women and children & helpers follow 2 weeks later with milking cows and castrated bulls.	Herdsmen leave home villages and start for flood plain.	Peul who don't cultivate begin to move towards flood plain. Peul with goats move down into U.V. to Dori in search of Samori herbs.	Home	Home
November	Water Begins to Recede at Edge of Plains	2.45m	6.84m	Two groups on the move towards the flood plain. Peul who cultivate begin to move.	Herdsmen on way to Diafarabé and six other crossings on the Diaka. Bororo Peul of Nampala not yet on the move.	Those with goats on way to Dori. Five separate Egguirgols 1. To Kona 2. To Nimitogo 3. To Mopti 4. To Sofara, Kabio and Kouna 5. To Korientze	Home	Home

TABLE 3 (Continued)
TRANSHUMANCE IN THE FLOOD PLAINS OF MALI BY MONTH

Month	Flood Plain	Height of Niger at Bamako 1965	Height of Niger at Mopti 1965	MOVEMENTS OF PEUL AND BOZO					
				Peul from Nouna and Tougan in Upper Volta (SE Periphery) Seno	Peul from Macina, Nampala and Niafounké (NW Periphery) Farimake	Peul from Douentza, Bandiagara and Koro (NE Periphery) Kounari	Bozo on the Niger	Bozo on the Bani
December	Water Receding			Herdsmen and families joined in one group in Cercles of San, Koutiala, Tominian and Yorosso. One group passes through Kouia and then enters the flood plain at Tako & goes to Yonga. Second group travels via Tominian & Mansara towards Mounia.	Cross with cattle at Diafarabé and six other traditional points on the Diaka River and move. Bororo Peul move without wives & children to the flood plain. Peul crossing at Diafarabé go to Yonga & south of Mopti. Those crossing lower on Diaka go to Lake Debo.	Move onto the Flood Plain between Sofara and Kona, (traditional route established by Peul Emperor, Cheikou Ahmadou (19th century) Some to Lake Korarou.	Home	Move from Mopti and Segou to San
January	Water Receding			In southern flood plain near Mounia and Yonga.	In flood plain. Some wives & children present.	In the borgu of the plain near Kona, Sofara, Mopti, Kouna, Kabio & Nimitogo	Move up to Debo and Korientze, Markala and Macina	In San Area
February	Water Receding			In southern flood plain near Mounia and Yonga.	Moving towards Debo, Yonga and Mopti.	In borgu	At Debo & Korientze, etc.	In San Area
March	Water Receding			In southern flood plain near Mounia and Yonga.	Moving towards Debo, Yonga and Mopti.	From Kona to L. Debo. From Mopti & Nimitogo to L. Debo. From Kouna to south of Mopti. From Kabio & Sofara to Yonga.	At Debo & Korientze, etc.	In San Area
April	Plain Dry Except Near L. Debo			In southern flood plain near Mounia and Yonga.	Nearing shores of L. Debo at Dintaka & Walado, nearing Mopti & Yonga.	From Kona to L. Debo. From Mopti & Nimitogo to L. Debo. From Kouna to south of Mopti. From Kabio & Sofara to Yonga.	At Debo & Korientze, etc.	In San Area
May	Plain Dry Except Near L. Debo			In southern flood plain near Mounia and Yonga.	All at Lake Debo, Yonga and Mopti.	From Kona to L. Debo. From Mopti & Nimitogo to L. Debo. From Kouna to south of Mopti. From Kabio & Sofara to Yonga.	At Debo & Korientze, etc.	In San Area

Bibliography on Mali by the Author

1. Traditional Beliefs About Smallpox and its Treatment Among the Bambara of Mali, *Journal of Tropical Medicine and Hygiene,* 71:224-228, 1968.
2. The Practice of Variolation Among the Songhoi of Mali, *Transactions of the Royal Society of Tropical Medicine and Hygiene,* 62:868-873, 1968.
3. The Use of Markets as Vaccination Sites in the Republic of Mali, *Journal of Tropical Medicine and Hygiene,* 72:8-13, 1969.
4. Traditional Beliefs About Measles Among the Bambara of Mali, *Tropical and Geographical Medicine,* 18:62-67, 1969.
5. Histoplasmin Skin Sensitivity in Mali, *American Journal of Tropical Medicine and Hygiene,* 18:264-267, 1969.
6. A Comparison of Edmonston-B and Schwartz Measles Vaccine in Malian Children, *Lancet,* 7596:665-667, 1969.
7. Anaphylaxie Fatale à la Suite de la Vaccination Contre la Rougeole Chez un Enfant Malien, *Afrique Médicale,* 69:301-303, 1969.
8. Leishmaniasis in the Republic of Mali, *Transactions of the Royal Society of Tropical Medicine and Hygiene,* 63:236-241, 1969.
9. Leishmanin Skin Sensitivity in Timbuctoo, *Journal of Tropical Medicine and Hygiene,* 72:216-218, 1969.
10. Traditional Attitudes Towards Measles in the Republic of Mali, *Transactions of the Royal Society of Tropical Medicine and Hygiene,* 63:768-780, 1969.
11. *An Outline to the Movements of the Pastoral Peul and the Migratory Bozo Fishermen in the Inland Delta of the Niger,* Atlanta, U.S. Department of Health, Education and Welfare, U.S. Public Health Service, 1969.
12. A Miracle in Africa, *Alumni Today,* Spring/Summer, State University of New York, Downstate Medical Center, pp. 32-37, 1969.

13. Indigenous Medical Beliefs and Practices in Bamako, a Moslem African City, *Tropical and Geographical Medicine,* 22:211-220, 1970.
14. Bokolanfini, Mud Cloth of the Bamana of Mali, *African Arts,* III, 4:32-41, 1970.
15. The Transmission Pattern of Smallpox in a West African School Population, *Journal of Tropical Pediatrics and Child Health,* 16:204-209, 1970.
16. A Doctor in Africa, *Alumni Bulletin,* St. John's University, Summer, pp. 2-11, 1970.
17. Leishmanin Skin Sensitivity in Northwestern Mali, *Acta Tropica,* 27:260-265, 1970.
18. The Dance of the Tyi Wara, *African Arts,* IV, 1:8-13, 71-80, 1970.
19. The Transmission Pattern of Smallpox in Eastern Mali, *Acta Tropica,* 28:175-179, 1971.
20. *Histoplasma duboisii* Infection in the Republic of Mali, *Tropical and Geographical Medicine,* 23:79-83, 1971.
21. Twins Among the Bambara and Malinke of Mali, *Journal of Tropical Medicine and Hygiene,* 74:154-159, 1971.
22. Contemporary Adapted Dances of the Dogon, *African Arts,* V, 128-33, 68-72, 1971.
23. Incidence of and Beliefs About Onchocerciasis in the Senegal River Basin of West Africa, *Tropical and Geographical Medicine,* 23:385-389, 1971.
24. The Epidemiology of Smallpox in the Republic of Mali, *Transactions of the Royal Society of Tropical Medicine and Hygiene,* 66:176-182, 1972.
25. La Variole En République du Mali, *Afrique Médicale,* 105:983-994, 1972.
26. Masks and Masquerades of the Bambara, in *Manding Art and Civilization,* edited by Guy Atkins, London, Studio International, pp. 8-14, 1972.
27. Jet Guns for Africa's Cliff Dwellers, *Sign,* 52, 3:20-26, 1972.
28. Nomads of the Niger, *Natural History,* 81:60-69, 78-79, 1972.
29. Histoplasmin Skin Sensitivity in the Inland Delta of the Niger, *Tropical and Geographical Medicine,* 24:246-248, 1972.
30. Door Locks of the Bamana of Mali, *African Arts,* V, 3:52-56, 1972.
31. Wool Blankets of the Peul of Mali, *African Arts,* VI, 3:40-47, 1973.
32. The Persistence of Smallpox in Remote Unvaccinated Villages During Eradication Program Activities, *Acta Tropica,* 30:261-268, 1973.
33. Positive Leishmanin Skin Sensitivity in the Absence of Clinical Leishmaniasis, *Journal of Tropical Medicine and Hygiene,* 76:132-134, 1973.

34. Mass Campaigns and Their Comparative Operational Costs for Nomadic and Sedentary Populations in Mali, *Tropical and Geographical Medicine,* 25:416-422, 1973.
35. Covers and Blankets of the Bamana and Maninka of Mali, *African Arts,* VII, 3:56-67, 1974.
36. Recent Observations on Variolation Practices in Africa, *Tropical and Geographical Medicine,* 25, 1974, (in press).
37. Intradermo Reaction à la Leishmanine Dans le Cercle de Kita, Mali, *Afrique Médicale,* 13, 120:411-414, 1974.
38. *Health and Nutrition Services of the Sahel Relief and Rehabilitation Program in Mali,* 54 pp., Washington, D.C., The American Public Health Association and The United States Agency for International Development, 1974.
39. Leishmanin Skin Sensitivity in the Inland Delta of the Niger, *Tropical and Geographical Medicine,* 25:303-306, 1974.
40. Cholera in Mali and Popular Reactions to Its First Appearance, *Journal of Tropical Medicine and Hygiene,* 78, 1974, (in press).
41. Nomads of the West African Sahel and the Delivery of Health Services to Them, *Social Science and Medicine,* 8:443-457, 1974.
42. Bambara Masks, *Natural History,* 84, 1975, (in press).
43. Bamana and Maninka Twin Figures, *African Arts,* VIII, 1975, (in press).
44. Strategie et Tactique Pour la Vaccination des Populations du Delta Interieur du Fleuve Niger, *Afrique Médicale,* 14, 1975, (in press).
45. The Delivery of Health Services to Desert Nomadic Populations in West Africa, *Tropical Doctor,* 1975, (in press).
46. The Effect of the Drought on Health Services for the Populations of the Sahel in Mali, *Journal of Tropical Medicine and Hygiene,* 79, 1975, (in press).
47. The Detection of Diabetes Mellitus in Three Population Groups in Mali, *Diabetes,* 1975, (in press).
48. Traditional Medical Practitioners Among the Bambara of Mali and Their Role in the Modern Health Care Delivery System, *Transactions of the Royal Society of Tropical Medicine and Hygiene,* 1975, (in press).
49. Traditional Medical Beliefs and Practices in the City of Timbuctoo, *Bulletin of the New York Academy of Medicine,* 51, 1975, (in press).
50. The Medical Care Program for the Refugee Populations in the Drought Stricken Sahel of Mali, *Lancet,* 1975, (in press).

BAGUILY SY

M'Bodo yétouma na fevii, ha é n'dier bérdame

Index

- A -

Abidjan, 39, 148
Adams, Robert, 313
Adrar des Iforas, 331
African art,
  procurement of, 268-269
African art collection, 343
African art merchants, 234-235, 269, 349
Ahmadou, *See* Sanogo, Ahmadou
Ahmadou Ahmadou, 85
Ahmadou Checkou, 85
Air Mali, 31, 285
Akaramby, iron gates of, 9
Albert, 233-234
Amirou-nai, 106, 114-115
Anderamboukane, 334
Ansongo, 7-9, 328, 340
Antinov-2, 285
Antinov-24, 279
Apollo, 295
L'Aquarium, 316-317
Archinard, General, 184
Ardo, 81-82, 83
Arma, 320
Askia the Great, 310
Askia, tomb of, 310
Atlanta, 14
Awa society, 187
Azalais, 314

- B -

Badalabougou, 39
Badirou Sekou Kouyate, 236
Badjai, 122-124

Bafoulabe, 275, 277, 289
Baguily Sy, 356
Baker, Robert, 86, 150, 229
Baker, Patty, 227, 229, 241
Ba Labo, 85
Bamako, 7, 27, 97, 100, 146, 164, 225-226, 228
  air pollution in, 41-42
  American women in, 35-36
  austerity in, 39-40
  buildings in, 39
  climate of, 50-51
  clothing in, 44
  commerce in, 44-45
  description of, 31-52
  fires in, 41
  flood in, 139-140
  foreigners in, 47-48
  homes in, 33
  meaning of, 31
  meningitis epidemic in, 261-264
  mosquitoes in, 43
  population of, 46
  quarters of, 41
  sporting clubs in, 38
  travel restrictions, 36
  water supply of, 40
Bamako Region, 63
  vaccination campaign in, 65-67
Bamba, 324, 331
Bambara, 23-24, 25, 90, 103, 105, 153-157, 176-177, 181, 241-242, 346-347
Bambara-Maounde, 306
Bambuk, 23
Banantou, 33
Banco, 32

357

Bandiagara Cercle, 188
Bandiagara Cliffs, 220-221
  description of, 128-129
Bandiagara Plateau, 183
Bandiagara, town of, 183, 184, 189
Bani River, 122, 138, 148, 170, 174-175, 207, 212, 344
Bankass, 133-136
Baobabs, 90
Baoule wilderness, 272
Bar du Mali, 122
Barth, Heinrich, 9, 11, 314
Beledougou, 237
Bella, 319, 334
Ber, 323-324
Berabich, 320
Bignat, Monsieur, 207-208
Bignatville, 207
Bilma, 3
Biton Coulibaly, 81
Bla, 150, 343
Blake, Robert O., 147, 349
Bobo, 213
Bobo-Dioulasso, 148
Bobo-Ule, 103
Bolibana, 234
Borgnis des Bordes, General, 42, 52
Borgus grass, 73
Borko, 188
Boundiar, 93, 96-98, 101, 103, 110, 123-125, 126, 127, 130, 132-135, 148, 269, 349
Boure, 23
Bourem, 22, 324, 331-332
Boussin, 228, 292-293, 343-348
Bozo, 75, 162, 165, 179, 204, 215-216, 218, 224
Bozo Fishing Cooperative, 213, 215-216
Bozola, 139, 261
Bradrick, Maxine, 349
Brahima, 22, 232-233, 241
Bramane, 148-159, 171, 188, 196, 201-202, 211, 214, 216, 218, 223-224, 226
Bridge, Niger River, 328
Briquelot, Captain, 343-344
Broussards, 37
Burti, 114

- C -

Cairo, 19
Caillie, Rene, 313-314
Camera, 226, 233, 241

Carola, Monsieur, 326
Center For Disease Control, 14, 15, 16, 263-264, 278, 343
Centre Muraz, 226
Cheikou Ahmadou, 77, 81-84, 161, 312
Chinese, Communist,
  Comportment in Bamako, 47
  embassy of, 48
  meeting with, 127
  motel built by, 124-127
  products of, 49
  technicians, 27
Cholera epidemic, 295-305
Christiano, Dorothea, 223
Christiano, Joseph, 222-223
CIA, 56, 97
Cisse, Astan, 293
Cissoko, Bassaumana, 252
Cissoko, Fily Dabo, 248
Clark, G. Edward, 255, 262, 289
Clark, Stanley, 199-200
Clark, Ted, 219-221
Conakry, 295, 296, 300
Consegula, 150
Coulibaly, Bakary, 283
Coulibaly, Biton, 81
Coup d'etat, 246-256

- D -

Daba, 21
Dabanani, 45
Daga, 319
Dakar, 7, 34, 38, 39, 42, 51, 62, 94, 145, 198, 263, 276, 277
Dama ceremony, 186-187
Daniells, Peter, 35
Dao, 199
Debo, *See* Lake Debo
Degal festival, 161-169
Desplagnes, Lieutenant Louis, 184
Dia-Bozo, 165
Diafarabe, 161-169, 302, 303, 325
Diaka River, 165
Diakite, Djigui, 93, 98-99 ,103, 110, 112, 126, 130, 136, 146, 153, 155-157, 159, 161, 163, 166-168, 195, 217-218, 231, 267, 321, 347, 349
Diallo, Alfarou, 103-112
Diallo, Ibrahima, 263-264
Diallo, Seydou, 302
Diamou, 289
Diarra, Diby Silas, 247-248, 256

INDEX 359

Dolo, Ogobara, 190-194, 202, 219
Dolo, Somine, 201-202
Don Fodio, Ousmane, 81-82
Douentza, 103, 128, 138, 188, 204
Drivers, 91-93
Drought, 332, 334-335
Dyingerey Ber, 310
Dyula merchants, 302, 304

- E -

Ecole William Ponty, 111
Edson, John, 225
El Hadj, 62-70
El Hadj Omar, 85, 118, 158, 279, 281
Elisofon, Eliot, 315-318
Ellert-Beck, Rudolph, 201
Energie du Mali, 65
El Tor Cholera, 298-299
L'Essor, 49-50

- F -

Faladie, 289
Fana, 344
Faraba, 293
Farimake, 83, 218
Faro, 155
Faya Forest, 344
Fignabana, 174
Flood plains, 114-116, 119, 138-139
  vaccination campaign in, 217-218
Fofana, Benintieni, 261, 296, 297, 298
Fouta, Djalon, 42
French Sudan, 20
French West Africa, 20
Friedman, Jay, 59, 93, 95, 144, 145, 146, 161, 164, 198, 200, 203, 217, 226

- G -

Gabibi, 320
Gabon, 150
Gabriel Toure Hospital, 291, 304
Gallieni, General, 94
Gambia, 294
Gangaran, 294
Gao, 7, 123, 213, 242, 335, 337
  Songhoi Empire of, 23-24
Garti, 114
Gatineau, Monsieur, 316-317
General Soumare, 164, 212-213, 223, 246, 249-250

Ghana, 213
Ghana Empire, 23, 25, 310
Gobir, 81
Gossi, 328
Gouina waterfalls, 275
Goundam, 318, 332
Gourma-Rharous, 318, 324-328
Gourmiers, 327
Grandes Endemies Service, 58-59, 62, 146-149
Grand Hotel, 254
Great Mask, 189
Griaule, Marcel, 185-187, 192
Griots, 81
Guandusu, 270
Guardians, 41
Guidado, 81
Guinea, 139, 295-296
Gum arabic, 21

- H -

Hamdallaye, 77, 78, 82-83, 85
Hammalists, 279-281
Handelsman, Milton, 224-225
Handelsman, Sophie, 224
Harmattan, 42
Haute-Senegal Niger, 20
Henderson, D. A., 15-18
Hotel de L'Amitie, 39
Hotel Atlantide, 337
Hotel, Grand, 254
Hombori, 128, 204, 238
Hounkoum, 5-7
Huile Cinquante, 347-348
Hunter, Edward, 236-237

- I -

Ibrahim es Saheli, 310
Ilyushian-18, 31
Imam of Djenne, 77-79
Indigo dyers, 214-215
Inland Delta of the Niger, 73-75, 162
  plan for vaccination of, 138, 141-142
Ippolito, John, 225
Irieli, 219-220
Islam, 25-26
  fatalism of, 76-77
Ivory Coast, 22, 23, 26, 213

- J -

Jaja, Monsieur, 210-211
Jardin, 50

Jean-Joseph, Paul, 261, 349
Jet injectors, 62, 173

- K -

Kaarta, 23
Kabara, 313, 314
Kangaba, 242, 342
Kassambara, Mabo, 188-191
Kassaro, 267, 270
Kassonke, 287
Kati, 141, 249, 289-290
Kayes, 97
Kayes, Region
　description of, 275-276
　vaccination campaign in, 277-294
Kendie, 188
Keita, Lamine, 318, 328
Keita, Madeira ,247, 254
Keita, Mamadou, 94
Keita, Modibo N'Faly, 93-96, 101, 103, 126, 130 ,135, 144, 148, 153, 155-156, 159, 218, 223, 286, 292, 293, 344, 349
Keita, N'Faly, 94
Keita, President Modibo, 49, 99, 119, 257-259, 269
　coup d'etat against, 29
　fall of, 245-256
　leadership of, 28
　personality cult of, 29
Keita, Sundiata, 42, 52
Keita, Togunta, 94
Kenieba, 277, 289, 293, 294
Khasa, 107
Kidal, 248, 256, 331, 340
Kimparana, 157-158
Kinkeleba, 294
Kirane, 284
Kita, 94, 277
Kita, Badinka, 294
Kita, cercle of, 265-267
Kita Kourou, 294
Koblenale, 270
Koke, 346
Kommugel, 205
Komo, 99, 155-157
Komo de, 155
Komo Tigui, 155-156
Kona, 218
Konare, Dr., 212
Kone, Zamble, 304
Kora, 236

Koran, 44, 130, 142
Koro, 130-132
Koroti, 179
Korporokenie-na, 133
Koulikoro, 139, 164-165
Koulouba, 35, 42, 68
　water reservoir on, 40
Kouniana, 149, 150
Koutiala, 100-101, 103, 109-112, 138, 141, 144-160

- L -

Laing, Majar Gordon, 313-
Lakamane, 286-288
Lake Agagoungou, 218
Lake Debo, 75, 116, 118, 138, 213, 216, 217-218, 223-224
Lake Do, 218, 306, 328
Lake Faguibine, 321
Lake Korientze, 218
Lake Niangaye, 218, 306
LaPointe, Mark, 226, 233, 246-247, 251-252, 264, 278-279, 289-290, 292, 293, 326
Lastouillas, Jean Paul, 58-59, 140-141, 145, 146, 158, 164-165, 195, 349
Lazaret, 261-262
Lellehoi, 4-13, 340
Lenz, Oscar, 314
Leonard, Thomas, 247
Leydi, 115
Liberia, 300-301

- M -

McKinney, Francis J., 185, 202-203, 222
McKinney, Laura, 185
Macina, 81-82, 164
Maga Diallo, 81
Mali, 1, 2, 13, 16-18
　arrival of author in, 32
　coup d'etat in, 246-256
　crops in, 21-22
　cultural revolution in, 28
　currency of, 26
　departure of author from, 342-349
　economic problems, 23
　expatriates in, 36-37
　French influence, 38-39
　Frenchmen in, 37-38
　geographic location, 20

gross national product, 22-23
housing, 18
population of, 22
Post Report on, 18
preparations for trip to, 19-20
size of, 21
socialism in, 26-29
socialist option, 26
state owned enterprises, 26
tribalism in, 25
Mali Empire, 22-23, 42
Mali Federation, 21
Malian Tourist Office, 190-192
Malians, difficulties in working with, 57, 71
Malinke, 23-24
Manding Hills, 31, 89, 262, 267
Mandinka, 23
Mansa Moussa, 23, 310
Mao buttons, 44, 47, 48, 50, 125, 129, 160
Mao, pictures of, 49
Marabout, 4, 5, 13 ,123, 337-338
chants of, 52
in Hamadallaye, 82-83
Marena, 267, 270-274
Marka, 105
Markala, 127, 164, 246, 344
Markala Dam, 139
Markets, 150-151
Marshall, David, 307
Marshall, Eleanor, 307
Marshall, Frank, 307-308
Masks, production of, 268
Mather, Cotton, 8
Maure, 46, 284
Mauritania, 150, 200, 343
Measles, 35, 71, 75
epidemic of, 174-181
indigenous treatment of, 178
in West Africa, 15-16
Medina-Coura market, 232, 239
Menaka, 334, 340
Meningitis belt, 260
Meningitis epidemic, 261-264
Military Committee, 255
Militia, 151, 174, 255, 258
surveillance activities of, 56-57
See Popular militia
Minianka, 103, 104, 109-112, 148-149
Missionaries, 26
Molobala, 150
Molinari, Jean, 192

Montague, Lady Mary Wortley, 8
Moore, C. Robert, 140, 199
Mopti, 75, 100, 165, 201, 218
City of, 117-119, 122, 126
campement in, 122-124
cholera in, 301-302
commerce, 206
description of, 204-206
dried fish commerce, 22
Europeans in ,207-212
market, 213-214
mosque, 205
motel, 125-127
Moroccan, 10
Moroccan invasion, 81
Moslems, 25-26
Mossi, 310
M'Pessoba, 150

- N -

National Committee, 28
Negala, 272
N'Gouma, 306
Niafunke, 213, 223
Niamey, 2, 3
Niarela, 139
Niger Bend, 328
Niger Republic, 1, 2, 83, 260, 332
Niger River, 1, 2, 9, 73, 103, 120, 138, 161-162
at Bamako, 31
fish resources, 22
flood of, 139-140
genies in, 6
Niger River Bridge, 89
Niono, 291-292
Niono, Ahmadou, 269
Nioro, 273, 278, 279, 282-283, 288
Noukouma, 82
Nyamina, 250

- O -

OCCGE, 147
Office du Niger, 39, 292
Ogobara, *See* Dolo
Onchocerciasis, 146-147
Oua, 198
Ouloguem, Yambo, 186

- P -

Park, Mungo, 42, 52, 158, 312-313
Parthenay, Madame, 54

INDEX

Pate, Lewis, 235-236
Pate, Sonja, 236
Pegue, 221
Peul, 3, 22, 23, 75, 129, 181
    camps, 103-105
    cattle of, 108-109
    cattle crossing, 163-169
    conversion to Islam, 83
    disputes among, 116-119
    history of, 81-85
    nomadic movements, 83-84, 114-120
    oral tradition, 79
    personality of, 105-106
    physical characteristics, 107
    refusal of vaccination, 153
    sedentarization of, 83
Point G. 42
Point G Hospital ,36, 333
Popular militia, 28-30
Postage stamp, 150
Poule Verte, 150, 159

- Q -

Quartier Fleuve, 32-33
Quimby, Lucy, 281

- R -

Radio Mali, 29, 252
Ramadan, 62, 283
Ras el Ma, 321
Richet, General, 147
River blindness, 146-147
Roads, 90-91
Rockefeller, Michael, 315
Rogers, Sadie, 34-35
Roque, Monsieur, 208
Rose Dune, 340
Route des Poissons, 22
Russians, comportment in Bamako, 47

- S -

Sahara, 1, 2
    caravan routes, 23
    Harmattan from, 42
Sahel, 21
Saint Louis, 208
Samake, Bekaye, 286
Samake, Dramane, 67-69
Samake, Faran, 333
San, 157, 159, 171, 172, 246
Sandare, 286

Sanga, 185, 189-190, 192-194, 202, 218-222
Sangare, Kassim, 220-221
Sanogo, Ahmadou, 43, 86, 87, 179, 226-234, 241-242 ,251-252, 292-293, 316, 342-345 ,349
Sanogo, Amineta, 229-230
Sanogo, Djeneba, 230
Sanogo, Karamoko, 158-159
Sanogo, Lassana, 229-230
Sansanding, 313, 348
Sarafere, 302, 303
Sarakole, 45
    description of, 25
    emigration of, 276, 282
    expulsion from Zaire, 282
    villages of, 284
Sarro, 268
Sebekoro, 290
Secret societies, 99
Secteur Numero Trois, 62, 64
Segou, 81, 150, 159, 166, 228, 246-247, 291, 344
    description of, 100
    kingdom of, 23
    road to, 93
Segy, Helena, 219-221
Segy, Ladislas, 219-221
Sencer, David, 202
Senegal, 21, 90, 107, 111, 150, 208, 210, 313, 343
Senegal River, 275
Seno, 103, 106
Service d'Hygiene, 56, 57, 59, 67, 69, 97, 150, 232
    Sevare, 124-125
Shamir, Marli, 237-238
Shamir, Meir, 237
Shanks, Colonel, 198, 200
Sidibe, Karim, 220-221
Sierra Leone, 300
Sigui festival, 189-194
Sikasso, 150, 330
Simone, Henri ,208-209
Simulium fly, 146-147
Sinjan, 42
Sinyare, 106
Sleeping sickness, 146-147, 154
Smallpox, 55, 71
    epidemics, 5-13, 73
    eradication, 14
    distribution in Mali, 73
    plan to eradicate, 73

Smith, Grandma, 17
Smith, Harold, 17
Smith, Marianne, 17
Snow, John, 297-298
SOMIEX, 27, 173, 209
Songhoi, 1
Songhoi Empire, 23-24
Sonni Ali Ber, 310
Sorko fishermen, 324
Sosso, King of, 42
Sossobe, 164, 174-181
Soufroulaye, 164
Soukoba, 45
Soumare, Mohamed, 283, 286, 288
Sow, Ousmane, 277, 289, 326
Stewart, William, 198-202
Sundiata Epic, 258
Sy, Baguily, 356
Szabo, Andre, 100-101, 210-212, 216, 222-223
Szabo, Rosey, 210-212, 222-223

- T -

Tambacara, 286
Tambaoura Escarpment, 275
Tangara, Mama, 216, 224
Taoudeni, 3
  salt from, 27, 314
Tata, 85
Tawaty, Cheick, 327-328
Tellem, 186
Tenenkou, 164, 213
Thoughts of Mao, 125, 129-130
Tiebassa, 267
Tilemsi Valley, 331
Tillaberi, 2, 3, 4, 5
Timbuctoo, 20, 50, 51, 96, 97, 126, 206, 213
  Campement, 320
  explorers' visits, 312-314
  history of, 309-312
  population of, 319
  tourists in, 320
  trade center, 23
  visits by Americans, 25
Tin Essako, 248
Toggue, 83
Togola, Teninko, 277-278, 286, 292
Togou, 345
Tominian, 247
Tondibi, battle of, 311
Toucouleurs, 85
Toukoto, 289

Traore, President Moussa, 255, 257
Trois Caimans, 50
Trypano, 64
Trypanosomiasis ,146-147, 154
Tsetse flies, 50, 146, 153-154
Tuareg nomads, 1, 22, 323
  description of, 3
  revolt of, 247-248
  salt commerce of, 27
  variolation among, 7-8
Tulane University, 14
Tyi Wara, 345-347

- U -

Uganda, 15
Underberg, Captain, 343-344
UNICEF, 127
Union Soudanaise, 26, 154, 250
Upper Volta, 26, 26, 130, 138, 148, 226, 247, 260
USAID, 14
  compound of, 48

- V -

Vaccination campaign, 145-146
  in flood plains, 217-218
Vaccinators, 58-62
  characteristics of, 142-144
Variolation, 8
Vastine, David, 247

- W -

Walado, 233
Wind Illness, 174
Wolklani, 226
World Health Organization, 15, 296, 298
Wunderman, Lester, 316

- Y -

Yame River, 183-184
Yelimane, 268, 275, 278, 282-283, 288-289
Yellow fever epidemic, 289-290
Youga, 192-193
Yougou yougou, 48-49
Youvarou, 219

- Z -

Zaire, 282
Zambougou, 346

INDEX

Smith, Grandma, 17
Smith, Harold, 17
Smith, Marianne, 17
Snow, John, 297-298
SOMIEX, 27, 173, 209
Songhoi, 1
Songhoi Empire, 23-24
Sonni Ali Ber, 310
Sorko fishermen, 324
Sosso, King of, 42
Sossobe, 164, 174-181
Soufroulaye, 164
Soukoba, 45
Soumare, Mohamed, 283, 286, 288
Sow, Ousmane, 277, 289, 326
Stewart, William, 198-202
Sundiata Epic, 258
Sy, Baguily, 356
Szabo, Andre, 100-101, 210-212, 216, 222-223
Szabo, Rosey, 210-212, 222-223

- T -

Tambacara, 286
Tambaoura Escarpment, 275
Tangara, Mama, 216, 224
Taoudeni, 3
  salt from, 27, 314
Tata, 85
Tawaty, Cheick, 327-328
Tellem, 186
Tenenkou, 164, 213
Thoughts of Mao, 125, 129-130
Tiebassa, 267
Tilemsi Valley, 331
Tillaberi, 2, 3, 4, 5
Timbuctoo, 20, 50, 51, 96, 97, 126, 206, 213
  Campement, 320
  explorers' visits, 312-314
  history of, 309-312
  population of, 319
  tourists in, 320
  trade center, 23
  visits by Americans, 25
Tin Essako, 248
Toggue, 83
Togola, Teninko, 277-278, 286, 292
Togou, 345
Tominian, 247
Tondibi, battle of, 311
Toucouleurs, 85
Toukoto, 289

Traore, President Moussa, 255, 257
Trois Caimans, 50
Trypano, 64
Trypanosomiasis, 146-147, 154
Tsetse flies, 50, 146, 153-154
Tuareg nomads, 1, 22, 323
  description of, 3
  revolt of, 247-248
  salt commerce of, 27
  variolation among, 7-8
Tulane University, 14
Tyi Wara, 345-347

- U -

Uganda, 15
Underberg, Captain, 343-344
UNICEF, 127
Union Soudanaise, 26, 154, 250
Upper Volta, 26, 26, 130, 138, 148, 226, 247, 260
USAID, 14
  compound of, 48

- V -

Vaccination campaign, 145-146
  in flood plains, 217-218
Vaccinators, 58-62
  characteristics of, 142-144
Variolation, 8
Vastine, David, 247

- W -

Walado, 233
Wind Illness, 174
Wolklani, 226
World Health Organization, 15, 296, 298
Wunderman, Lester, 316

- Y -

Yame River, 183-184
Yelimane, 268, 275, 278, 282-283, 288-289
Yellow fever epidemic, 289-290
Youga, 192-193
Yougou yougou, 48-49
Youvarou, 219

- Z -

Zaire, 282
Zambougou, 346